CARDIOLOGY RESEARCH AND CLINICAL DEVELOPMENTS

THROMBOSIS: CAUSES, TREATMENT AND PREVENTION

CARDIOLOGY RESEARCH AND CLINICAL DEVELOPMENTS

Additional books in this series can be found on Nova's website at:

https://www.novapublishers.com/catalog/index.php?cPath=23_29&seriesp=Cardiology%20Research%20and%20Clinical%20Developments&sort=2a&page=1

Additional e-books in this series can be found on Nova's website at:

https://www.novapublishers.com/catalog/index.php?cPath=23_29&seriespe=Cardiology+Research+and+Clinical+Developments

CARDIOLOGY RESEARCH AND CLINICAL DEVELOPMENTS

THROMBOSIS: CAUSES, TREATMENT AND PREVENTION

DIMITRI G. MACRI
AND
LAMAR D. PROCACCINI
EDITORS

Nova Biomedical Books
New York

For permission to use material from this book please contact us:
Telephone 631-231-7269; Fax 631-231-8175
Web Site: http://www.novapublishers.com

Library of Congress Cataloging-in-Publication Data

Thrombosis : causes, treatment, and prevention / editors, Dimitri G. Macri and Lamar D. Procaccini.
p. ; cm.
Includes bibliographical references and index.
ISBN 978-1-61668-696-3 (hardcover)
1. Thrombosis--Etiology. 2. Thrombosis--Treatment. 3. Thrombosis--Prevention. I. Macri, Dimitri G. II. Procaccini, Lamar D.
[DNLM: 1. Thrombosis. QZ 170 T5319 2010]
RC694.3.T466 2010
616.1'35--dc22
2010014100

Published by Nova Science Publishers, Inc. ✢ New York

CONTENTS

PREFACE

Thrombosis is the formation of a blood clot inside a blood vessel, obstructing the flow of blood through the circulatory system. When a blood vessel is injured, the body uses platelets and fibrin to form a blood clot, because the first step in repairing it is to prevent the loss of blood. If that mechanism causes too much clotting, and the clot breaks free, an embolus is formed. This book presents and discusses recent research on the causes, treatment and prevention of thrombosis such as thromboembolic complications in childhood nephropathies, renal vein and artery thrombosis in children and the management of portal vein thrombosis.

Chapter I- Conversion of a soluble fibrinogen into insoluble fibrin with thrombin leads to the formation of a hemostatic plug that under physiological conditions is degraded by plasmin. Thrombosis is considered to be a result of an imbalance between procoagulant and anticoagulant activities of blood and the persistent presence of fibrin clots in the coronary, pulmonary or cerebral circulations. The main component of a thrombus is fibrin formed from fibrinogen by the action of thrombin. Human plasma fibrinogen is one of the largest plasma proteins composed of three pairs of polypeptide chains linked together by means of disulfide bonds. It had been observed over a century ago that fibrin-like deposits present in atherosclerotic plaques were morphologically different from those in thrombi formed in the blood circulation system. In experimental models, it has been documented that atherosclerotic fibrin deposits are not readily preventable by anticoagulation and are resistant to fibrinolytic degradation. Therefore, the mechanism of atherogenesis cannot be completely explained in terms of activation of classic blood coagulation cascade. More recent studies indicated, however, a link between atherosclerosis and inflammation that is known to be associated with the excessive production of free radicals. Reactive oxygen species are generally recognized to cause oxidative stress resulting in an undesirable oxidation of carbohydrates, fatty acids, nucleic acids and particularly proteins. However, as recently shown by this author, treatment of fibrinogen with non-oxidizing hydroxyl radicals resulted in a limited reduction of its disulfides. As a consequence, fibrinogen polypeptide chains become unfolded with the exposure of buried hydrophobic epitopes and the formation of insoluble intermolecularly bonded aggregates. In human plasma hydroxyl radicals cause the formation of insoluble aggregates composed of fibrinogen and albumin that cannot be degraded either by plasmin or by other active proteolytic enzymes. *In vitro* prepared fibrinogen-albumin complex, when converted with thrombin to a clot is also refractory to proteolytic degradation.

In vivo fibrinogen-albumin complexes are present in patients with congenital abnormalities associated with thromboses, in which an extra cystein is present in the fibrinogen molecule. A characteristic feature of such a complex is its resistance to fibrinolytic degradation of a fibrin clot induced with thrombin. Apparently, this extra cystein causes reductive unfolding of polypeptide chains similar to that induced with hydroxyl radicals making fibrin clots resistant to fibrinolysis. In this Chapter, it is argued that the hypoxia-induced reductive conditions associated with coronary and/or cerebral thrombosis generate hydroxyl radicals causing, in turn, the formation of fibrin(ogen)-albumin complex refractory to proteolysis. This phenomenon may explain why thrombolytic therapy is ineffective when installed 3–4 hours after the onset of thombosis. It has been recently found that such insoluble complexes can be dissolved by the action of singlet oxygen. The non-radical species oxidizes side chains of certain amino acids involved in the hydrophobic interactions between fibrinogen and albumin resulting in the solubilization of insoluble aggregates. In conclusion, the Chapter will present new ideas on the importance of maintaining proper redox balance in the circulation to prevent and reverse the undesirable effects of hydroxyl radicals generated under the reducing conditions of hypoxia observed in atherosclerosis, cancer, neurological and other chronic diseases.

Chapter II- Several well-recognized glomerulopathies in children may result in nephrotic range proteinuria. A possible complication of nephrotic syndrome and its treatment is thromboembolic complications (TEC). Patients with membranous glomerulopathy with heavy proteinuria and lupus nephritis/antiphospholipid syndrome run the highest risk of thromboembolic complications. A lower incidence of TEC has been found in children with nephrotic syndrome as compared with adults with NS, although children had severe morbidity. Clinically silent thromboembolic complications may be much more common than previously reported in studies designed to collect data only from symptomatic events. Thus, this chapter covers the pathogenesis of thromboembolic complications in children with heavy proteinurias, either with acquired thrombophilia or associated with congenital hemostasis disorders. Moreover, the clinical features of patients experiencing venous and arterial thromboemolic complications in different areas of the body, such as the lungs, kidneys, brain and heart, will be described. The prevention of thromboembolism in patients at high risk, either through drugs or through appropriate management of the main condition, will be emphasized. In addition, treatment options after a thromboembolism has begun will be discussed. Patients with lupus nephritis/antiphospholipid syndrome run the highest risk of thromboembolic complications. Venous thrombosis is more frequent than arterial thrombosis. Systemic lupus eritematosus patients with nephritis are more prone to arterial thromboembolic complications than those without renal involvement. The chapter also covers the pathogenesis of TEC in lupus nephritis patients, with particular emphasis on antiphospholipid antibodies. However, we present the clinical features of patients with either thrombotic microangiopathy or vasal thrombosis and their treatment options. Finally, a concise overview of physiological hemostasis is given.

Chapter III- In newborns, renal thromboembolism has been associated most frequently with umbilical artery catheters. In children, the most common renal disorder associated with hemostatic complications is renal vein thrombosis. The main causes are severe dehydration secondary to sepsis, nephrotic syndrome and related glomerulonephropathy and congenital disorders of hemostasis. Clinical features of the condition in newborns and young children include enlarged kidneys, gross hematuria, thrombocytopenia, hypertension and kidney failure. The severity of the condition depends on whether one or both kidneys are involved. Clinical evaluation is feasible with ultrasound and scintigraphy as well as with other imaging tecniques. The treatment, either pharmacological or surgical, presents both benefits and risks. The prognosis, which is generally poor, champions the need for prevention of thromboembolism and a prompt diagnosis is essential in order to begin appropriate therapy and relative follow-up. Late sequelae include impairment of renal function, shrunken hypoplastic kidney, arterial hypertension and tubular defects. In this chapter, conditions concerning venous or arterial thrombosis associated with terminal renal failure, renal transplantation or tumors are not covered.

Chapter IV- Thrombosis in women is subject to many hormonal influences. Menstruation and pregnancy can be associated with accelerated presentation of either coagulopathies or inherited thrombophilia. There is also a rise in the incidence of arterial thrombosis at the onset of menopause, which had been thought to represent a loss of the protective effects of oestrogen. Not only are there alterations in native hormone levels as women age, but women may also opt to use exogenous hormones, in the form of the oral contraceptive pill, or in later years, hormone replacement therapy.

Thus at certain times in a woman's life, the interplay between the various hormone systems may result in an increased risk of thrombosis due to either physiological factors, or exogenous hormone intake. Underlying conditions such as diabetes, renal failure and smoking may also alter thrombotic tendencies. Thus, it may be advisable to tailor both preventative and treatment options in terms of diet, lifestyle and antiplatelet or anticoagulant therapies in order to incorporate these hormonal variations. Female patients may require somewhat different strategies than their male counterparts. We present a discussion of the mechanisms underlying these processes, and review recent evidence in order to optimize clinicians' awareness of these risks.

Chapter V- Portal vein thrombosis (PVT) is considered a rare event in general population, more common in patients with an advanced liver disease and hepatocellular carcinoma. Local and systemic factors - or a combination of them - may contribute to PVT development, making often difficult to identify certainly its original cause. However, thanks to innovations in non-invasive imaging, the diagnosis of PVT is now possible in the most part of suggestive cases. Clinical experience has also a pivotal role in PVT early diagnosis, even if, sometimes, patients may be completely asymptomatic or may present only few symptoms. In particular, it depends on the modality of PVT onset (acute or chronic) and on the extension of the thrombosis since, sometimes, PVT may progress to intestinal ischemia or cause a massive gastrointestinal bleeding. These extreme consequences are the manifestation of a complex alteration in liver and splanchnic hemodynamic, resulting in portal hypertension, hyperdinamic circulation and impairment in liver function. Thus, a prompt therapeutic management is essential to avoid complications, preserving patients' health and, sometimes, life.

Chapter VI- The investigation of the risk factors, development and treatment of venous thrombembolism (VTE) is probably one of the fields in medicine that possesses one of the most evidence-based labors of knowledge. The complexity of finding and understanding the main causes and pathological mechanism of thrombosis process extended the time of the study. Therefore, there are still several controversial issues in the understanding of thrombosis development. Many factors have played a role in venous thrombosis development. The acquired risk factors such as trauma, surgery, prolonged immobilization, etc. affect many persons, but frequently a combination of some risk factors in one person, is necessary for thrombus formation. Indeed, multiple risk factors are a prerequisite for thrombosis development. In our days, the importance of inherited risk factors in the development of venous thromboembolism, has been increasingly recognized. The knowledge for relatively rare conditions take part in VTE development, such as protein C, protein S and antitrombin III deficiency [1], have been expanded with the discovery of the impact of mutation in coagulation factors. Recently, the most frequent prothrombotic genetic defects in patients with VTE have been considered to be Factor V Leiden mutation [2] (FVL) and Factor II 20210 G>A mutation (FII 20210 G>A) [3]. Along with mutation in natural anticoagulants and factors from cascade of coagulation, an inherited changes in platelet membrane receptors was discussed as a possible cause for abnormal thrombosis development. The surface glycoproteins (integrins), such as the GP Ib/IX/V complex, GP IIb/III, GP Ia/IIa and GPVI , play major roles in platelet activity, and so inherited changes in glycoproteins' structure could be associated with pathologic disorders without change in platelet count. Some of the heritable differences in glycoproteins' structure influence the expression and avidity of these receptors, which lead to enhanced platelet activity and increase risk for thrombus development.

This review discusses the role of inherited changes in cell surface glycoproteins, in increased risk for development of deep venous thrombosis (DVT), venous thrombembolism, as well as thrombotic events in intervillous space of placenta of the pregnant women, which could leaded to pregnancy loss. The establishment of clinically significant inherited changes in cell integrins could help to identify high-risk patients with a genetic predisposition, who have had a permanently risk for venous thrombosis development. An important impact of the genetic profile is into those individuals, who have risk of recurrent venous thrombotic events, as the identification of the polymorphisms in cell surface integrins could have influence in further antithrombotic therapy. This chapter manly focused on carrier status for polymorphism A1/A2 (PL A1/A2) in beta3 subunits of integrins alphaIIb/beta3 (GP IIb/IIIa), because of a common spread of this polymorphism in Caucasian and the important role of GP IIb/IIIa in platelet aggregation, and the risk of thrombus development. The significance of PL A1/A2 in integrin alphaV/beta3 is not connected precisely with thrombosis development, but it could be referred as possible factor in implantation failure of the concepsus in the early part of gestation. The contribution of platelet glycoprotein polymorphisms as genetic risk factors for the disease is a relatively new area of human genomics, that is still evolving. The role of PL A1/A2 in the development of venous thrombosis, as well as the impact in early and late pregnancy loss, needs conformation in more and larger studies.

Chapter VII- An effective, accurate and reliable method for the simultaneous separation and determination of four active components (3,4-dihydroxyphenyllactic acid, protocatechuic aldehyde, puerarin and ferulaic acid) in Chinese medicine 'TONGMAI' oral liquid was developed using reverse phase high-performance liquid chromatography (RP-HPLC) coupled with diode array detection. The chromatographic separation was performed on a Lichrospher C_{18} column (250 mm × 4.6 mm i.d. with 5.0 μm particle size) with a simple linear gradient elution programme. Due to the different UV characteristic of these components, three detection wavelengths were utilized for the quantitative analysis (UV wavelength 250 nm for puerarin, 281 nm for 3,4-dihydroxyphenyllactic acid and protocatechuic aldehyde, and 323 nm for ferulaic acid, respectively). Excellent linear behaviors over the investigated concentration ranges were observed with the value of R^2 higher than 0.99 for all the analytes. The recoveries, measured at three concentration levels, varied from 98.6% to 102.0%. The validated method was successfully applied to the simultaneously determination of these active components in 'TONGMAI' oral liquid from different production batches.

Chapter VIII- Drug eluting stents are associated with significantly lower restenosis rates than bare metal stents. However, recent reports of an increased risk of thrombosis with these devices have cast some doubt on the clinical effectiveness of this new technology. In this review, the most recent studies in this field are evaluated, showing that drug eluting stents are a safe and effective technology when adequately used in its approved indications.

Chapter IX- The integral role of pathologic platelet activation for progression of atherosclerosis and acute clinical events such as myocardial infarction and stroke has been recognized in the last decades. Consequently, treatment with oral antiplatelet agents — particularly acetylsalicylic acid (ASA) and the thienopyridines clopidogrel and ticlopidine— constitutes a cornerstone in the therapy of vascular diseases. Coronary angioplasty and stent implantation furthermore dramatically improved the therapy of coronary artery disease and especially the treatment of acute myocardial infarction. Sustained success with regard to prevention of reocclusion was achieved when dual antiplatelet therapy had been introduced. This combination of ASA and clopidogrel reduced the risk of stent thrombosis to ~1% following elective stenting in stable coronary artery disease. However, targeting more complex lesions or performing the intervention in states of increased platelet reactivity such as in acute coronary syndromes or in diabetic patients is still associated with an increased risk of stent thrombosis. Additionally, incomplete ADP-receptor inhibition by thienopyridine treatment is associated with increased cardiovascular events and mortality after coronary intervention.

This review displays the underlying pathophysiology of stent thrombosis and its pharmacological prevention by dual antiplatelet therapy. Furthermore, it discusses the assessment of antiplatelet therapy by different analytical methods and the phenomenon of clopidogrel non-responsiveness. The last part highlights current strategies in improving the efficacy of clopidogrel treatment as well as the next generation anti-platelet substances such as novel thienopyridines and non-thienopyridine $P2Y_{12}$-receptor blocking agents.

In: Thrombosis: Causes, Treatment and Prevention
Editor: D. G. Macri and L. D. Procaccini, pp. 1-53
ISBN 978-1-61668-696-3

Chapter I

SIGNIFICANCE OF FREE RADICAL-MODIFIED FIBRINOGEN IN THROMBOSIS AND RELATED DISEASES

Boguslaw Lipinski*
Joslin Diabetes Center, Harvard Medical School, Boston, MA 02215, U.S.A.

ABSTRACT

Conversion of a soluble fibrinogen into insoluble fibrin with thrombin leads to the formation of a hemostatic plug that under physiological conditions is degraded by plasmin. Thrombosis is considered to be a result of an imbalance between procoagulant and anticoagulant activities of blood and the persistent presence of fibrin clots in the coronary, pulmonary or cerebral circulations. The main component of a thrombus is fibrin formed from fibrinogen by the action of thrombin. Human plasma fibrinogen is one of the largest plasma proteins composed of three pairs of polypeptide chains linked together by means of disulfide bonds. It had been observed over a century ago that fibrin-like deposits present in atherosclerotic plaques were morphologically different from those in thrombi formed in the blood circulation system. In experimental models, it has been documented that atherosclerotic fibrin deposits are not readily preventable by anticoagulation and are resistant to fibrinolytic degradation. Therefore, the mechanism of atherogenesis cannot be completely explained in terms of activation of classic blood coagulation cascade. More recent studies indicated, however, a link between atherosclerosis and inflammation that is known to be associated with the excessive production of free radicals. Reactive oxygen species are generally recognized to cause oxidative stress resulting in an undesirable oxidation of carbohydrates, fatty acids, nucleic acids and particularly proteins. However, as recently shown by this author, treatment of fibrinogen with non-oxidizing hydroxyl radicals resulted in a limited reduction of its disulfides. As a consequence, fibrinogen polypeptide chains become unfolded with the exposure of buried hydrophobic epitopes and the formation of insoluble intermolecularly bonded aggregates. In human plasma hydroxyl radicals cause the formation of insoluble aggregates composed of fibrinogen and albumin that cannot be degraded either by plasmin or by other active proteolytic enzymes. *In vitro* prepared

* Correspondence concerning this article should be addressed to: Boguslaw Lipinski, Joslin Diabetes Center, Harvard Medical School, One Joslin Place, Boston, MA 02215. Tel.: 617-732-2693; Fax: 617-732-2667; E-mail: boguslaw_lipinski@joslin.harvard.edu.

fibrinogen-albumin complex, when converted with thrombin to a clot is also refractory to proteolytic degradation.

In vivo fibrinogen-albumin complexes are present in patients with congenital abnormalities associated with thromboses, in which an extra cystein is present in the fibrinogen molecule. A characteristic feature of such a complex is its resistance to fibrinolytic degradation of a fibrin clot induced with thrombin. Apparently, this extra cystein causes reductive unfolding of polypeptide chains similar to that induced with hydroxyl radicals making fibrin clots resistant to fibrinolysis. In this Chapter, it is argued that the hypoxia-induced reductive conditions associated with coronary and/or cerebral thrombosis generate hydroxyl radicals causing, in turn, the formation of fibrin(ogen)-albumin complex refractory to proteolysis. This phenomenon may explain why thrombolytic therapy is ineffective when installed 3–4 hours after the onset of thombosis. It has been recently found that such insoluble complexes can be dissolved by the action of singlet oxygen. The non-radical species oxidizes side chains of certain amino acids involved in the hydrophobic interactions between fibrinogen and albumin resulting in the solubilization of insoluble aggregates. In conclusion, the Chapter will present new ideas on the importance of maintaining proper redox balance in the circulation to prevent and reverse the undesirable effects of hydroxyl radicals generated under the reducing conditions of hypoxia observed in atherosclerosis, cancer, neurological and other chronic diseases.

1. Introduction

Thrombosis is a result of activation of intravascular activation of blood coagulation, the physiological function of which is to maintain hemostatic balance within the circulation. The main component of a thrombus is fibrin formed from fibrinogen by the action of enzyme thrombin generated as a result of the coagulation cascade activation. A characteristic feature of a fibrin clot is that one mg of it can hold in place 1 000 mg (one milliliter) of blood thus forming an effective hemostatic plug. However, the same property of fibrin is responsible for thrombosis when the clot is formed inside the blood vessel lumen. Consequently, the most therapeutically useful approach to thrombosis is the inhibition of intravascular blood coagulation with proper anticoagulants and/or thrombin inhibitors. One should, however, bear in mind that thrombosis is not just a quantitative phenomenon, meaning that the greater amount of fibrin will bring about more extensive thrombosis. The reasons are that under physiological conditions intravascular formation of fibrin elicits rapid fibrinolytic response in the form of the plasminogen activator-induced generation of plasmin that, in turn, efficiently degrades the fibrin clot. The best example is a therapeutic defibrination by means of a viper coagulant enzyme—ancrod—that not only does not lead to thrombosis but also in fact prevents it.

In addition to plasmatic components, the size and stability of a thrombus depends on blood cellular elements such as platelets, leukocytes and red blood cells (reviewed by Wohner, 2008). Blood platelets set the stage for the thrombus formation and growth, and also prevent premature fibrin degradation. On the other hand, neutrophil leukocytes promote fibrin clot dissolution by secreting elastase, cathepsin G and metalloproteinases. Red blood cells may also play a role in clot formation, particularly under the conditions of hypoxia and acidosis (Weisel&Litvinov, 2008). Another important factor is blood flow, the proper maintenance of which is secured by regular exercise thus reducing the risk of both arterial and venous thrombosis (Lowe, 2003). Therefore, effective treatment of thrombosis should involve not only anticoagulation but also application of measures aimed at the removal of persistent fibrin clots from the coronary and/or cerebral circulations. In recent years, a number of various plasminogen activators have been available to cardiologists, the best known being tissue plasminogen activator (tPA). Yet even the most specific ones, fail to cause thrombolysis when administered 3–4 hours after the onset of a thrombotic episode. Thus, it is obvious that the persistent presence of thrombi within the circulation must be caused by factors different than the inefficiency of fibrinolytic enzyme alone. Based on recent observations of thrombophilia associated with certain congenital fibrinogen abnormalities, it has been postulated that the inhibition of fibrin clot lysis is caused not by the insufficiency of fibrinolysis, but by a specific modification of fibrin(ogen) structure. In case of abnormal fibrinogens, the best known being fibrinogen Dusart, a substitution A alpha554Arg-->Cys results in the formation of the disulfide linked fibrinogen-albumin complex (Koopman et al. 1993). A characteristic feature of such complex is the resistance to degradation of fibrin clots formed by the action of thrombin. This unusual property of such clots was later confirmed with the *in vitro* prepared fibrinogen-albumin complex (Lipinski, 1995).

These findings coincided with the observation that certain reactive oxygen species (specifically the hydroxyl radicals) convert soluble human fibrinogen into an insoluble fibrin-like aggregate. Such an aggregate when prepared from purified human fibrinogen is refractory to plasmid-induced dissolution. Similarly, exposure of human plasma to hydroxyl radicals (ascorbic acid/ferric ions) caused the formation of an insoluble complex of fibrinogen and albumin that is not digestible even with trypsin. It is not currently understood what kind of structural modification is being introduced by the action of hydroxyl radical. However, the most plausible explanation is that this radical causes unfolding of fibrinogen polypeptide chain(s) with the exposure of buried hydrophobic epitomes that form extremely strong bonds with the hydrophobic side chains of albumin amino acids. Hydrophobic interactions in proteins are known to have dramatic effects on their properties making them refractory to proteolysis degradation. Thus, it can be concluded that the commonly observed thrombolytic resistance in older thrombi might be caused by the fibrin(ogen) modification resulted from the action of hydroxyl radicals generated under reducing condition of chronic hypoxia (Lipinski, 2009).

It was then serendipitously found that the treatment of insoluble fibrinogen-albumin aggregate with a singlet oxygen (non-radical but strongly oxidizing oxygen species) caused its gradual dissolution. In this particular case, singlet oxygen was generated by a mixture of hydrogen peroxide and sodium molybdate. As reported by Stief (1991), chloramine T, another singlet oxygen generating agent, is an effective thrombolytic agent when used in the animal model. A compelling picture emerges from these studies namely that hypoxic conditions lead to undesirable changes in a thrombus, whereas the oxygenation and/or certain oxidizing agents can be beneficial. These arguments are supported by the current therapeutic approaches critically evaluated in this Chapter. Review of these new findings may help solve a number of previously unexplained phenomena such as the mechanism of aggregation of red blood cells, clumping of certain bacteria, pathogenesis of atherosclerosis and certain neurological diseases (e.g., Alzheimer's disease), and last but not least the resistance of cancer cells to immune recognition and killing.

2. Properties and Functions of Fibrinogen

Fibrinogen is a plasma protein of a molecular weight 340 kDa composed of three pairs of polypeptide chains termed A alpha, B beta and gamma joined by 32 disulfide bridges. Molecular weights of these chains are 68 kDa, 56 kDa and 48 kDa respectively. This protein is an elongated dimeric molecule (about 45 nm in length) in which two outer D domains are linked by alpha-helical coils to a central domain E (Hall&Slater, 1959). A fourth nodule (alpha C domain) can be seen in electron microscope pictures as an extension of the A alpha chain attached by a thin filament with the D domain. Two small fibrinopeptides, FP-A (1900 Da) and fibrinopeptide B (FP-B, 2400 Da) is located at the amino-termini of A alpha and B beta chains respectively.

A characteristic feature of fibrinogen is its loss of solubility on a brief heating (3 min.) at 55-56°C that causes a conversion of intramolecular to intermolecular disulfide bonds with the formation of insoluble aggregates. Fibrinogen can also form fibrin-like aggregates by lowering ionic strength of its solutions below 0.05 with the appearance of aperiodic (polar) striation pattern (Gollwitzer et al. 1983). Relevant to this is Alfred Copley's concept according to which thrombogenesis is due to the aggregation of fibrinogen molecules, forming so-called "fibrinogenin" without the participation of thrombin (Copley, 1981). It was later on discovered that heparin, a known thrombin inhibitor, also prevents fibrinogenin formation by interfering with the gelation process that might involve hydrophobic/hydrophilic interactions (Copley&King, 1984).

It has been estimated that in human blood there is over one million of different fibrinogen molecules (Henschen, 1993) modified due to amino acid sulfation, phosphorylation, glycosylation, hydroxylation and limited proteolysis. The heterogeneity of fibrinogen is manifested by differences in solubility (Hartley&Waugh, 1960), electrophoretic mobility, molecular weight, and by differences in chromatographic elution patterns (Finlayson&Mosesson, 1963; Gaffney, 1971). In addition to microheterogeneity of fibrinogen, normal human plasma contains two major components, high molecular weight (HMW-Fbg) and a lower molecular weight (LMW-Fbg, 280-290 kDa) that is lacking a substantial portion of A alpha chain including FP-A. A third minor form of fibrinogen, LMW', was demonstrated by electrophoretic separation of plasma proteins at low concentration (3.5 percent) of a polyacrylamide gel (Lipinska et al. 1974). By contrast to fibrinogen fragments generated by digestion with plasmin, all these major fractions of fibrinogen are clottable with thrombin albeit at a different rate. The slowest was LMW' and fastest clotting time was observed with HMW-Fbg that represents about 70 percent of total fibrinogen. The proportions of these three molecular weight fractions of fibrinogen differed substantially in plasma of patients with various diseases. For example, in patients with liver disease the proportions of both LMW and LMW' components of fibrinogen were shown to be significantly increased (Lipinski et al. 1977). Both LMW-Fbg and total fibrinogen concentrations were recently demonstrated to be increased in diabetic patients (Doronina et al. 2007).

It was originally thought that the lower molecular weight forms of fibrinogen are products of limited degradation by plasmin of the native molecule. More detailed studies have revealed, however, that plasmin degrades fibrinogen in a much more extensive manner. The initial attack of this enzyme involves the carboxy-terminal portion of the A alpha chain and the amino-terminal part of B beta chain. As a result, fragment X is formed which is further degraded asymmetrically into fragment D and Y. It should be noted, however, that despite increased fibrinolytic activity in cirrhotic patients, this type of fibrinogen heterogeneity is not related to blood fibrinolysis, as documented *in vivo* utilizing radioalabeled fibrinogen (Lipinski et al. 1974). We have also demonstrated significant increases in LMW and LMW' components in patients with vascular disease and those after surgery, whereas HMW fraction was drastically elevated in cancer patients (Lipinski et al. 1976). These and other post-translational modifications of fibrinogen affect fibrin clot structure and functions. For example, any modification that has an effect on the rate of fibrin monomer polymerization and subsequent clot fiber thickness, dramatically determines clot susceptibility to fibrinolysis (Gabriel et al. 1999; Weisel&Litvinov, 2007). The effect of calcium and ionic strength on the structure of fibrin has been known for a long time (Shulman&Ferry, 1950). Extensive acetylation of fibrinogen results in the loss of its clottability (Kloczewiak et al. 1974).

Fibrinogen plays an important role not only in hemostasis but also in cellular and matrix interactions, inflammation, wound healing and in cancer. One of the major hemostatic functions of this protein is its ability to support ADP-induced platelet aggregation, which is lost upon digestion with plasmin (Niewiarowski et al. 1977). Kowalski et al. (1959) found that plasmic digestion products of fibrinogen (FDP) when infused into dogs caused bleeding without affecting platelet count. This effect was suggested to be due to a combined inhibitory action of FDP on both platelet function and blood coagulation (Latallo et, 1964). Further studies showed unequivocally that FDP, particularly the early digestion products with plasmin, delay blood coagulation by forming soluble fibrin monomer complexes (SFMC) (Lipinski, 1968).

It was then discovered in the course of determination of plasma fibrinogen concentrations by the method of Clauss (Clauss, 1957), that plasma samples obtained from blood collected on EDTA gave consistently lower values that the citrated ones. Since EDTA but not citrate chelates magnesium (Mg), it was logical to test the effect of this ion on the clottability of fibrinogen with thrombin. Using SDS-polyacrylamide gel electrophoresis we have showed that in the absence of Mg LMW-Fbg was not converted into fibrin, whereas its high molecular form was (Lipinski&Lipinska, 2000). Consequently, determinations of fibrinogen in EDTA plasma by the method of thrombin clotting time with and without magnesium turned out to be a convenient and quick method for quantization HMW and LMW fibrinogens in human plasma. It should be mentioned, however, that very little is known about the role of magnesium in blood coagulation as reviewed by Serebruany et al.(1998).

3. Fibrin and Fibrinolysis

The most important function of fibrinogen is in hemostasis by its conversion into an insoluble fibrin clot. In the first step thrombin splits off FP-A converting fibrinogen into des-A-fibrin, which is further acted upon with this enzyme that splits off FP-B causing lateral aggregation of fibrin fibrils. At the final stage of blood coagulation cascade fibrin becomes stabilized by means of gamma glutamyl-epsilon-lysil crosslinks initiated by the action of Factor XIII (Lorand et al. 1966). Such a clot is mechanically stronger than the non-crosslinked one and is also less vulnerable to premature fibrinolytic degradation. Fibrinolysis is brought about by enzymatic activation of plasminogen by various plasmatic and/or tissue activators, e.g. single chain urokinase-type activator (scu-PA) and tPA. A sequence of events leading to fibrin formation and its degradation is shown in Figure 1.

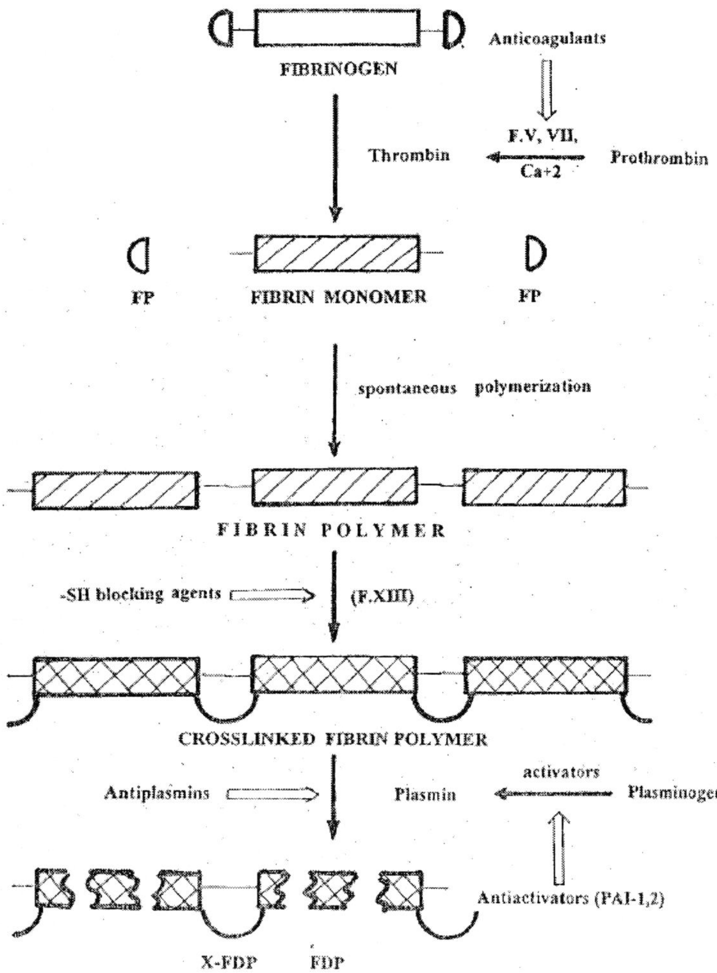

Figure 1. Enzymatic conversion of fibrinogen to fibrin and to its degradation products. FP - fibrinopeptides; X-FDP - crosslinked fibrin degradation products.

One should remember, however, that under physiological conditions plasminogen activators are bound by the plasminogen activator inhibitor(s) (PAI-I and -II) and thus are not available for the conversion into plasmin. Such reaction occurs only in the presence of a solid phase of fibrin that causes *in situ* dissociation of PAI-activator complex (Lipinski et al. 1974). Plasma fibrinogen can only be degraded when the level of activators exceeds that of its inhibitors and/or plasmin inhibitors (eg.alpha-2-antiplasmin). Yet specific products of fibrin degradation (for example D-dimer) have been shown to be increased in numerous pathological states associated with thrombosis and with inhibition of fibrinolysis as measured by functional methods e.g. euglobulin clot lysis (Kowalski et al. 1959). This paradoxical phenomenon is explained later on in this review. Structure of fibrin network and its susceptibility to proteolytic degradation is known to be influenced by physical, biochemical and genetic factors that operate under various pathological conditions. Thus, the clot architecture determines the size of pores which, in turn, determines the rate of blood perfusion making thick fibrin fibrils more susceptible to fibrinolysis that the thin ones.

It has been well documented that, under normal conditions, intravascular fibrin deposition induces a powerful fibrinolytic response by tPA released from the vascular wall that catalyses the conversion of plasminogen to a proteolytic enzyme plasmin. A thrombin-like enzyme ancrod produces fibrin clots that are particularly susceptible to plasmin degradation; consequently this enzyme has been used for the therapeutic defibrination. The purpose of this type of therapy is two-fold, first to remove all fibrinogen from the circulating blood thus preventing further intravascular fibrin formation. Second, to generate massive amounts of tPA that can attack any existing intravascular and/or extravascular thrombi. Such an idea was behind recently performed clinical trial with intravenous ancrod started within 6 hours after onset of ischemic stroke that, however, did not improve the outcome (Levy et al. 2009). This disappointing result might be explained in terms of fibrin structure modifications recently described in a series of elegant papers by Undas et al. They have found that idiopathic thromboembolism was associated with the formation of significantly less permeable and lysable fibrin clots as compared to healthy subjects (Undas et al. 2009). These authors have also confirmed that these effects were related to the thickness of fibrin fibers, namely the thinner ones being more resistant to proteolytic degradation, and have concluded that these abnormalities may result from free radical stress (Undas et al.2008). In another paper Undas et al. (2008a) described similar altered fibrin clot properties in patients on haemodialysis.

3.1. Fibrin Monomer Complexes

Fibrinogen properties and functions are dramatically altered by its conversion to fibrin monomers and their complexes. Thus, soluble fibrin monomer complexes (SFMC) are very unstable in aqueous solutions and are readily precipitable by a positively charged protein, protamine sulfate in the so-called paracoagulation reaction (Lipinski, 1968). These complexes, rather than undigested molecule, were later on documented to be responsible for staphylococcal cells clumping (Lipinski et al. 1967) that can be explained in terms of their greater hydrophobicity. It is therefore possible that biofilms frequently observed in human

Staphylococcal aureus infections are also formed by their interaction with SFMC molecules that are resistant to proteolytic degradation (Katsuyama et al. 2006). A characteristic feature of SFMC is their ability to form insoluble precipitate upon addition of positively charged protamine sulfate (PS). Based on this property of PS a number of diagnostic tests were elaborated to measure SFMC level in human blood. One such test was utilized to measure soluble fibrin in patients with myocardial infarction (Nowak et al. 1972). This test was based on a previous observation that when protamine is added to oxalate anticoagulated whole blood, a white precipitate is formed that remains on top of packed red cells after brief centrifugation. This precipitate can be quntitated by measuring its height in a hematocrit tube and represent SFMC present in a given blood sample.

It was originally thought that protamine sulfate reacts specially in a dose dependent manner with soluble fibrin complexes by decreasing their net negative charge. However, fibrinogen itself is also precipitable with protamine but at much higher concentrations which is due to the protective action of negatively charged fibrinopeptides. The concept that protamine selectively interacts with fibrin monomers was later on challenged by the following experiment. Oxalated whole blood samples obtained obtained from healthy subjects was incubated at 37°C for 18 hours and the amount of protamine sulfate precipitable protein (PSPP) was determined before and after the incubation. Consistently, in each case there was a highly significant increase in the PSPP as well as in the total fibrinogen level as measured by the fibrin clot functional method (Lipinski&Gurewich, 1972). A high molecular weight protein was subsequently isolated from normal serum that when added to whole blood increased the amount of protamine precipitable protein as well as the size and weight of fibrin clots. It should be emphasized that the experimental conditions for the generation of PSPP were unintentionally set up exactly as those known years later to produce hydroxyl radicals that involves the presence of iron leaking from RBC and the sustained hypoxia. The later condition was abrogated by bubbling air through the incubated samples thus eliminating the reducing milieu of the whole blood samples and preventing PSPP formation (Lipinski&Gurewich, 1972). Therefore, all the reactions described previously for the use of protamine sulfate are applicable to the current concept of hydroxyl radical-modified fibrinogen complexes. This is due to the fact that positive charges enhance hydrophobic interactions (Andrews et al. 2005) leading eventually to the loss of protein solubility.

It was discovered years later that plasma obtained from diabetic patients contained a macromolecular protein complex (MPC) the properties of which are similar to those of PSPS. Although unclottable with thrombin, MCP significantly increased the amount of fibrin when mixed with purified fibrinogen (Lipinski et al. 1995). Similar type of a plasma complex, termed *Advanced Oxidation Protein Products* (AOPP) was found to be significantly increased in uremic patients (Witko-Sarsat et al. 1996). Although AOPP has been considered by these authors to be formed as a result of oxidative stress, it is most likely a product of the hydroxyl radical modification of plasma proteins (Lipinski, 2001). A link between leukocyte activation, hydroxyl radical generation and MCP formation is schematically presented in Figure 2.

A major modification of fibrinogen structure and function is also introduced by forming a complex with human serum albumin (HSA) by virtue of a disulfide exchange reaction (Lipinski, 1995b). The fibrinogen-albumin complex still clots with thrombin, albeit much slower as compared to native fibrinogen, yielding a fibrin network that is resistant to fibrinolytic degradation. It is of interest to note that this type of fibrinogen modification occur in congenital dysfibrinogenemias, in which one of the amino acids is substituted by cysteine (Soria et al. 1983; Koopman et al. 1993; Tarumi et al. 2000). Patients with this type of dysfibrinogenemia have history of thrombotic events that is caused by the resistance of modified fibrin to fibrinolysis. Apparently an extra cysteine introduced to the fibrinogen molecule is sufficient to reduce some of the intramolecular disulfide bonds followed by the exposition of hydrophobic epitopes that form a stable complex with albumin with properties similar to that formed *in vitro*. Similar fibrinogen modification leading to altered fibrin structure has also been observed in patients with homocysteinemias (Sauls et al. 2006).

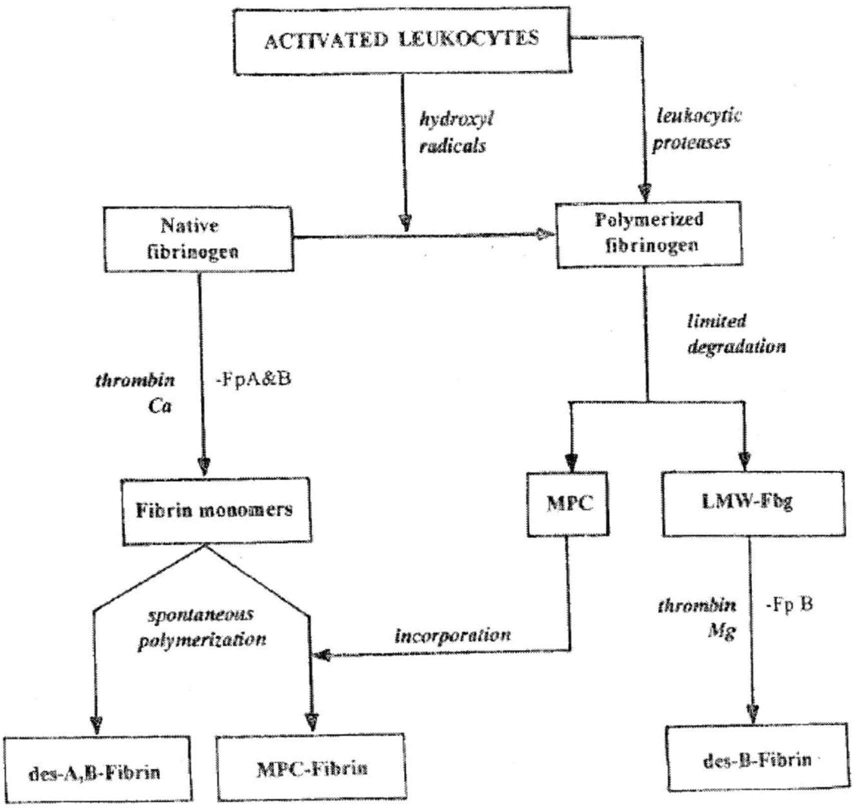

Figure 2. Sequence of events leading to the formation of lower molecular weight fibrinogen (LMW-Fbg), macromolecular protein complex (MPC) and their interactions with fibrin. Fp - fibrinopeptide; Mg - magnesium.

4. Oxidative Stress versus Free Radical Stress

In order to better understand the consequences of free radical modification of fibrinogen, it is essential to review current concepts of their *in vivo* generation. It is commonly believed that the conversion of biomolecules into corresponding oxy-derivatives is induced by reactive oxygen species (ROS). However, oxidation reaction in biological systems may also occur by a non-radical pathway, for example by hypochlorous acid and/or hydrogen peroxide. In both cases, the products of their action are molecules that are enriched in one or more oxygen atoms that are generally considered to be markers of oxidative stress. Yet the mere presence of extra oxygen does not tell us whether a given product is generated by a single (free radical) or two-electron oxidation reaction. The situation is further complicated by a well known, albeit usually neglected fact, that oxidation can occur without the addition of oxygen atom(s) to the affected molecule. According to the principles of electrochemistry, oxidation is defined as a transfer of an electron from a donor (oxidized substrate) to an acceptor (an oxidant). A classical example of such a redox couple is oxidation of Fe+2 to Fe+3, which occurs without participation of oxygen.

In living organisms there are two major reactive oxygen species, superoxide radical and hydroxyl radical that are being continuously formed in a process of reduction of oxygen to water. Both radicals are considered to be active oxidants, however, under reducing condition and in the presence of transition, metals (copper and iron) the predominant species formed is a non-oxidizing hydroxyl radical (Halliwell&Gutteridge, 1984). Hydroxyl radical (HO*) is known to be the most biologically active species that are formed *in vivo* under hypoxic conditions (Michiels, 2004). This type of radical is commonly measured by so-called aromatic hydroxylation method in which salicylic acid is converted to 2,3-dihydroxybenzoic acid (Liu et al. 2002). Another method is based on the reaction of the hydroxyl radical with coumarin-3-carboxylic acid, which is then determined by measuring fluorescence of its hydroxylation product (Manevich et al. 1997).

In addition to the essential role of hypoxic/reducing conditions in the *in vivo* generation of hydroxyl radicals, there is another important, although not generally recognized factor, namely free iron circulating in so called labile iron pool (Kruszewski, 2004). Protein-bound iron, in addition to hemoglobin and myoglobin is stored in ferritin, and the excess of this element is incorporated into hemosiderin and may also be sequestered by the reticuloendothelial system. It has been shown that under hypoxic conditions of inadequate oxygen supply, ferric ion is reduced to ferrous state that, in turn, participates in the Fenton reaction to generate hydroxyl radical. It was suggested some years ago that iron therapy might promote the formation of hydroxyl radicals thus contributing to atherosclerosis (Sengoelge et al, 2005; Reis et al. 2005). In connection with this, it is of importance to note that excessive accumulation of stored iron is observed in atherosclerotic lesions (Ramakrishna&Cooper, 2003). In a recent paper GJ Brewer (2007) reviewed the roles of both iron and copper in aging-related diseases. He discusses pros and cons for the question whether or not relative availability of iron and copper contribute to aging-related diseases. With 136 references the Brewer's review is highly recommended to any researcher seriously interested in this important aspect of aging.

It should be emphasized that according to the concept of oxidative stress, peroxidation and degradation of vulnerable biological molecules is caused by oxygen-centered radicals generated, in turn, by excessive blood oxygenation. However, this conclusion is based on studies of ischemia/reperfusion cases in which periods of prolonged hypoxia are followed by a sudden supply of oxygen. In patients with extracorporeal circulation the appearance of lipid and/or nucleic acids oxidation products is accepted as signs of oxidative stress. In order to solve this so important problem of what causes oxidative stress, researchers have initiated investigation of an intriguing phenomenon of the lack of signs of peroxidation in ringed arctic seals. These marine mammals hunt for fish by diving for periods of time up to 30 minutes. Yet when their blood and organs are analyzed after they emerge from water and start breathing, no signs of oxidative stress are found (Vasquez-Medina et al. 2006). It is generally accepted that the high content of unsaturated fats in seals serve only a purpose of insulation against cold, which may well be the case. But there is another explanation for this phenomenon, namely that the numerous double bonds of this type of fatty acids serve as effective scavengers of hydroxyl radicals generated during extensive periods of hypoxia.

4.1. Antioxidants, Oxidants and Free Radical Scavengers

The uncritical acceptance of the fact that the presence of additional oxygen atom(s) in biomolecules is a sign of oxidation, led to a misleading definition of an antioxidant. An antioxidant must be, according to the principles of electrochemistry, endowed with a reductive property, but except ascorbic acid (vitamin C) and glutathione very few natural substances have reducing properties. Therefore, it is not surprising that these types of substances not only failed to prevent consequences of oxidative stress, but on the contrary exhibited deleterious effects particularly in the presence of transition metals (Sharma et al. 2004; Fang et al. 2002). These facts present a paradox exemplified by a failure to demonstrate a significant effect of antioxidant therapies in diseases believed to be associated with oxidative stress such as atherosclerosis (Patterson et al. 2000) and hypertension (Ward&Croft, 2006). Several attempts were made to explain this problem in a series of publications (Sies, 1997; Davies, 1995; Davies, 2000). Another example of antioxidant paradox are successful trials to combat oxidative stress with the use of substances such as polyphenols, carotenoids and unsaturated fatty acids that not only are non-reducing substances but act as *oxidants*.

This paradox can, however, be explained in terms of a strong affinity of hydroxyl radicals to double bonds that become reduced to single bonds (Czapski, 1984). Despite the fact that hydroxyl radicals *in vivo* have very short half-life, they readily reacts with lipids, proteins and nucleic acids leading to stable products the presence of which can be assessed by various chemical and/or immunochemical methods. In the case of unsaturated fatty acid (PUFA) the product formed is a hydroxy-fatty acid that in the presence of molecular oxygen can form peroxides further decomposing to aldehydes and ketones. This very important fact is an ultimate source of confusion, since these specific peroxidation products are accepted as markers of oxidative stress. Yet by contrast to expectations and according to epidemiological studies, PUFAs exert beneficial effects in those diseases that are known to be associated with free radical generation (Schmidt, 1997) e.g. complications of diabetes mellitus (Mori et al. 2003). Both omega-3 fatty acids and polyphenolic natural substances were shown to have protective effect in Alzheimer's disease in preclinical trials (Cole et al. 2005), as well as in cancer (Cognaut et al. 2000) that is known to be linked to the persistent free radical stress (Toyokuni et al. 1995). Similarly to PUFAs, beta-carotene scavenges hydroxyl radicals by virtue of the addition of hydroxyl groups to its multiple double bonds (Plyakov et al. 2001).

Biological activity and health beneficial effects of natural carotenoids have been extensively reviewed by Stahl and Sies (2005).

In addition to the aforementioned substances, certain biologically active substances containing phenolic rings in their structure have the capacity to scavenge hydroxyl radicals by virtue of aromatic hydroxylation. One of such recently discovered scavengers is resveratrol that was shown to have a protective effect on ischemia-induced cerebral neuron damage (Lu et al. 2006). The most widely used benzene ring class of drugs, salicylates have been shown to protect against free radical injury *in vitro* (Podhaisky et al. 1997) and *in vivo* (Kim et al. 2001). The beneficial effect of salicylic acid in diabetes mellitus (DM) was first observed almost 100 years ago (Williamson&Lond, 1901). Significant reduction of a risk of myocardial infarctions in diabetic patients has been attributed to the hydroxyl radicals scavenging activity of salicylates (Ghiselli et al.1992). Cardiovascular consequences of excessive hydroxyl radical production in diabetes may be explained in terms of their modification of fibrinogen molecule that becomes deposited in kidneys in the form of a fibrin-like aggregates (Lipinski, 2001). Protective effect against hydroxyl radical-induced damage in biological systems has been documented by the use of natural polyene and polyphenol class of substances, such as flavonoids, present mostly in fruits and vegetables (Areias, 2001; Benedek et al. 2006). The addition of hydroxyl group to double bonds may explain beneficial effects of quercetin on modification of LDL molecule (Moon et. al. 2001), and of phenolic compounds in virgin olive oil that may also be due to their capacity to scavenge hydroxyl radicals (Tuck et al. 2001). Moreover, genistein, a naturally occurring isoflavone present in soybeans, was recently documented to be an effective hydroxyl radical scavenger by virtue of the addition of a hydroxyl group to double bonds of its aromatic rings (Zielonka et al, 2003).

There are a number of publications concerning the importance of fruit and vegetable diet in the prevention of cardiovascular disease dealt with by Hu et al. (2003) and Calabrese et al. (2006) and most recently reviewed by Dauchet at al. (2009). It is well known that plant products contain also vitamins such as A, B, C and E, the beneficial effects of which have been attributed to their antioxidant properties. However, as mentioned before only very few of them are reducing agents and thus they cannot be classified as antioxidants and the remaining ones are either neutral or mild oxidants. Nevertheless, these natural phytochemicals, particularly polyphenols, have been shown to provide protection against many chronic diseases by virtue of their free radical scavenging properties (Stocklet et. al. 2004). The best known and already used in clinical practice is resveratrol, which neutralize hydroxyl radicals by means of the aromatic hydroxylation reaction. Similar action against hydroxyl radicals exerts ferulic acid that belongs to the family of hydroxycinnamic acid with the chemical structure similar to curcumin (Srinivasan et al. 2007). Ferulic acid is found in leaves and seeds of many plants, especially in brown rice, whole wheat and oats, apples, artichokes, oranges and pineapples. Curcumin (turmeric yellow) exerts anti-inflammatory activity, prevents atherosclerosis and have protective action on brain. This compound also binds cadmium and lead thus having additional benefits for human health. Likewise, extracts of *Sesamus indicum* seeds were shown to scavenge hydroxyl radicals and chelate metals (Visavadiya et al. 2009). Last but not least is the cardiovascular protective effect of fish oil that enhances fibrinolysis *in vivo* (Sorensen, 1994). Unsaturated fatty acid present in this type of oil act also as scavengers of hydroxyl radicals converting them to hydroxy-fatty acids (Czapski, 1984). These facts support observations that people who consume fruits, vegetables and fish supplemented with red wine (so called Mediterranean diet) experience less cardiovascular mortality and morbidity than the other populations. In addition to these natural substances, a synthetic hydroxyl radical scavenger similar to ferulic acid was recently synthesized and shown to protect against stroke and cardiovascular diseases. Edaravone (*3-methyl-1-phenyl-pyrazolin-5-one*) when administered within 72 hours after onset of ischemic stroke produced sustained benefits in functional outcome during 12 months follow-up period (The Edaravone, 2003).

4.1.1. Oxygen and other Oxidants

Comparing oxidative stress to rusting of metals by oxygen led some researchers to an improbable conclusion that oxygen is deleterious to our health. It is being forgotten, however, that modern man lives in conditions under which we breathe less and less oxygen due to the industrial pollution and indoor living style. The latter has been shown to be associated with a depletion of air of its negative charge so important for the proper oxygen utilization (Lipinski, 1977). It was demonstrated by the largest epidemiological study conducted in Italy in the second half of this century that life expectancy was best correlated with high levels of respiratory indices, specifically vital capacity (Menotti et al, 1983). Moreover, oxygen therapy has also been shown to have beneficial effect in various diseases. For example, tumor radiosensitivity is enhanced by increasing tumor oxygenation (Crokart et al, 2005) that, in turn, may be explained by the effect of oxygen on the radiation-induced degradation of aggregated proteins (Davies & Delsignore, 1987). The positive effect of hyperbaric oxygen in tumor radiation therapy was reviewed in two recent papers (Bennett et al, 2005; Suzuki et al, 2006).

In connection with this it is noteworthy that powerful oxidizing agent ozone was shown to selectively inhibit growth of human cancer cells (Sweet et al, 1980) and to enhance the therapeutic effectiveness of 5-fluorouracil (Zanker et al, 1990). Contrary to adverse effects of ozone in the polluted air on human respiratory tracts, this agent was shown to be beneficial when properly administered into the circulation with ozone treated blood (Bocci, 2009). Diabetic complications are also believed to be associated with oxidative stress; nevertheless diabetic ulcers were successfully healed with nothing else but a hyperbaric oxygen therapy (Boykin, 2000). Last but not least is the health beneficial influence of moderate exercise, particularly in the prevention of cardiovascular disease and consequences of aging (Larson et al, 2006) possibly by activating fibrinolytic activity (Jahangard et al. 2009). This effect is mediated by increased blood oxygenation, thus counterbalancing the damaging effect of hypoxia-induced generation of hydroxyl radicals. It is therefore obvious that the adequate supply of oxygen is protective against free radical-induced tissue and organ damage, and thus oxygen can paradoxically be viewed as the most efficient "antioxidant". It was recently reported that in a population of healthy individuals maximal oxygen consumption was negatively correlated with plasma viscosity and fibrinogen concentration (El-Sayed, 2009) that can be explained in terms of reduced plasma content of hydroxyl radicals. Physical immobility and lack of adequate oxygen supply may also increase the risk of venous thrombosis associated with airplane flights (Bendz et al. 2000).

Another class of oxidants is the substances with disulfide groups in their structure that become reduced to thiols (Bader et al. 1999). One of such substances is lipoic acid (LPA) incorrectly classified as an antioxidant (Packer, 1994). Reactivity of LPA is a classical example of oxidation without the addition of an oxygen atom but just a transfer of an electron from an oxidized substrate to a disulfide bond. The non-oxygen assisted oxidation reaction is also exhibited by human serum albumin (HSA). This most abundant plasma protein contains sixteen intramolecular disulfide bonds that in the process of scavenging of hydroxyl radicals become reduced, unfolded and aggregated (Lipinski, 2002). Relevant to this is a finding that aggregation of proteins is a result of their protective action in hypoxia/ischemic injury (Gifford et al. 2004).

4.1.2. Selenium

Selenium has a special place amongst substances believed to be antioxidants because of its presence in the active centers of ROS decomposing peroxidases and superoxide dismutases (Berry et al. 1991). There is a wide spectrum of selenium concentrations in soil (from 0.1 mcg to 1000 mcg per kg), thus its content in food products depends very much on a geographical area they are grown. On an average in the US the daily intake of selenium is from 60 to 300 mcg/day, but only about 80 percent is being absorbed in human alimentary track. Amongst organic forms of selenium the most abundant is selenocysteine that is now recognized as the 21st amino acid being present in about fourteen mammalian selenoproteins (Gladyshev, 2001). Selenium in inorganic compounds exists in two forms: sodium selenite (Se+4) and sodium selenate (Se+6). Despite a relatively minor difference in their structure, these two types of compounds differ dramatically in their chemical reactivity. Thus selenite, but not selenate, reacts rapidly with sulfhydryl groups of proteins and enzymes oxidizing them to disulfides (Frenkel et al. 1991) according to the following reaction:

$$P\text{-}[SH]_2 + Na_2SeO_3 \text{ ----> } P\text{-}S\text{-}S\text{-}P + NaOH + SeO$$

in which four-valent selenium is reduced to two-valent reddish-colored oxide.

Similarly, oxidative properties of selenite can be demonstrated by the reaction with ascorbic acid that becomes oxidized to dehydroascorbic acid. Thus, it is obvious that sodium selenite is an oxidant and not antioxidant as it proclaimed in medical literature. Oxidative properties of selenite have been demonstrated by researchers in various biological systems (Kramer&Ames, 1988; Terrada et al. 1999). This particular property may explain the augmentation of the function of natural killer cells so important for cancer prevention and therapy (Kiremidjian-Schunmacher et al. 1996).

Among the medical community there is an exaggerated concern about toxicity of selenium, with little or no attention being paid to their chemical nature (Daniels, 2004). Yet data on selenium toxicity and cancerostatic activity was already available since 1994 (Spallholz, 1994). In this study LD50 dose for selenite in rats was established to be 4.1 mg/kg body weight which is a thousand-fold greater than a maximum safe dose for humans (Whanger, 2004). In his review the author stated that such a dose is about 600 mcg/day, and the toxic symptoms in the form of reversible hair loss and nails brittleness occur with a dose of 1000 mcg/day in a span of year or so. Metabolism of selenium *in vivo* has been extensively studied showing a complex pathway of a conversion of inorganic into organic forms, as well as into some volatile derivatives. Importance of selenium in biological systems and its crucial role in health maintenance was extensively reviewed by Rayman (2002) and more recently in two other papers (Schrauzer&Surai, 2009; Vincent&Forceville, 2008). Selenium in relation to oxidative stress and health status was also dealt with in a paper by Sies and colleagues (Brenneisen et al. 2005). Recent work has demonstrated that deficiencies in selenium result in increased viral pathogenecity and altered immune responses changing benign viruses into virulent ones (Beck, 2007). Although this aspect of selenium is of extreme importance for the prevention and possible therapy of swine and other influenza viruses, little attention is being paid by health officials to this potential beneficial property of selenium. Last but not least is the beneficial effect of high dose administration of sodium selenite in septic shock patients (Forceville X, 2007).

5. Hydroxyl Radical-induced Modification of Human Fibrinogen

Fibrinogen is the most hydrophobic plasma protein and thus it is very unstable in aqueous solutions and is readily adsorbed on various surfaces (Jung et al. 2003). In fact, the conversion of fibrinogen to fibrin by the action of thrombin renders fibrin monomers even more hydrophobic thus facilitating their spontaneous polymerization (van Oss, 1990). In addition to the enzyme-induced modification of fibrinogen molecules, certain chemical agents and free radicals can also alter its properties that may or may not affect prothrombotic readiness of blood (Vadseth et al. 2004). Exposure of purified fibrinogen to the ascorbic acid/cupric ion system results in the formation of an insoluble fibrin-like precipitate (neofibe) (Marx&Chevion, 1985). It was later on documented that the precipitation of fibrinogen in the iron (III)/ascorbic acid system is caused by hydroxyl radicals (Lipinski, unpublished observation). As can be seen from Figure 3, the amount of precipitated protein is proportional to the number hydroxyl radicals consumed in the process of fibrinogen modification in this system.

Formation of insoluble aggregates under the influence of hydroxyl radicals is due to a limited reduction of intramolecular disulfide bridges followed by exposure of buried hydrophobic epitopes that form non-covalent intermolecular bonds resistant to the action of plasmin. Interestingly enough, acetylation of fibrinogen prior to the reaction with hydroxyl radicals rendered it susceptible to fibrinolysis (Upchurch, 1998). It is very likely that this effect of salicylates is due to the introduction of a negative charge to the protein, thus diminishing hydrophobic interactions. An example of the effect of negative charge in the form of sulfate groups is sulfitolysis of proteins that completely unfolds their polypeptide chains and yet maintains their complete solubility. A well-known effect of exogenous negative charge of dodecyl sulfate is utilized in polyacrylamide gel electrophoresis of proteins after their reduction that normally renders them insoluble.

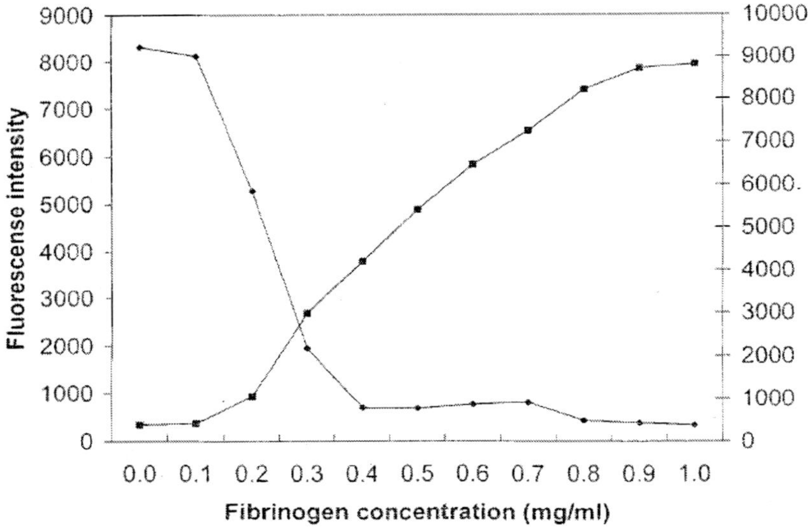

Figure 3. Fluorescence intensity of hydroxy-coumarin-3-carboxylic acid, as a measure of hydroxyl radicals, and the formation of insoluble fibrinogen polymer registered as optical density at 450 nm. Decreasing concentration of hydroxyl radicals with increasing concentration of soluble fibrinogen is a result of their consumption in the process of molecular modification of fibrinogen.

It is of interest to note that when normal human plasma is exposed to hydroxyl radicals produced by ferric ions in the presence of ascorbic acid, an insoluble fibrin-like precipitate is also formed that has, however, different properties than that obtained from purified fibrinogen. Such a precipitate when allowed to react with hydroxyl radicals for longer that 3 hours, is resistant not only to degradation induced with plasmin but also with an active proteolytic enzyme, chymotrypsin (Lipinski&Lipinska, 2002). It is important to note that the insoluble precipitate when exposed to a system generating singlet oxygen yields a solution containing various molecular weight complexes of fibrinogen with albumin (Lipinski, preliminary observation). Singlet oxygen ($^1O_2$) can be generated by a variety of chemicobiological reactions (e.g. chloramine and hypochlorate) as well as by physical factors such as ultrasound and ultraviolet light. In this particular case singlet oxygen was produced in a molybdate ions catalyzed disproportionation of hydrogen peroxide (Aubury et al. 1989) according to the following reaction:

$$2H_2O_2 + MoO_4^{-2} = 2H_2O + MoO_6^{-2} \dashrightarrow MoO_4^{-2} + {}^1O_2$$

Singlet oxygen is known to oxidize histidine, methionine, tyrosine and tryptophan side chains thus reducing their hydrophobicity and consequently increasing solubility of aggregated proteins. Hence, this method might be very useful for the detection and identification of insoluble protein aggregates bound by means of hydrophobic forces. It is known that hydrophobic groups attract each other forming protein bonds that are even strongest than the covalent ones (Lins&Brauser, 1995). Such bonds, by contrast to the disulfide linkage, cannot be broken by the reduction in the presence of chaotropic solvents and boiling in alkali, as exemplified by a recent study of fungal hydrophobins (Kwan, 2006).

Because of this important, although not generally known fact, protein aggregates formed as a result of hydrophobic interactions are frequently mistaken for covalently bonded protein complexes. The hydrophobic phenomenon can thus explain a failure to identify individual components of many fibrillar deposits that are formed under numerous pathologic conditions. For example, because of its resistance to proteolytic degradation, it is not known what are the protein components of the fibrillar islet amyloid (Badman et al. 1998). Another non-reducible and non-extractable deposit containing fibrinogen and HSA was recently detected by immunohistochemical methods in silica dust-induced lung nodules (Kim et al. 2005). An example of a special function of a protease resistant fibrinoid is placenta of pregnant women (Kaufman et al. 1996). It is important to note that that the placental villi accumulate fibrinogen/albumin complexes that are particularly resistant to fibrinolytic degradation and thus serve as an effective feto-maternal barrier (Wasiutynski et al. 2002).

In addition to the modification of fibrinogen by hydroxyl radicals, similar effects occur after exposure of this protein to certain sulfhydryl compounds. This phenomenon can be explained in terms of the reduction of intramolecular disulfide bonds followed by their intermolecular exchange with the exposition of buried hydrophobic regions of the plasma proteins. For example, incubation of human plasma with dithiothreitol resulted in a gradual formation of protein aggregates until all plasma components formed a huge copolymer (Lipinski&Egyud, 1992). It is, therefore, possible that *in vivo* formed similar aggregates known as fibrinoids or amyloids are also composed of hydrophobically bound plasma proteins. Fibrinogen has already one free cysteine residue per molecule and the introduction of a second one has a very profound effect on its structure. Thus, preincubation of plasma and/or purified fibrinogen with homocysteine produced fibrin gels in a dose depended manner that was significantly less permeable and more resistant to fibrinolysis than the control ones (Quintana, 2009). This may be explained in terms of a reaction of homocysteine thiolactone with amine groups of lysines (Jakubowski, 1999). As a result a homocysteamide-protein adduct is formed that introduces an extra free sulfhydryl group to the molecule of fibrinogen. This event may be just a sufficient trigger for a limited reduction of its disulfide bonds with all its structural consequences. This reaction may also offer an explanation why even a mild elevation of plasma homocysteine represents and independent risk for atherosclerosis, myocardial infarction and/or stroke (Hankey&Eikelboom, 1999), that are known to be associated with the inhibition of fibrinolysis (Undas et al.2008a) and prothrombotic state (Hoffman et al. 2008).

6. Hydroxyl Radical-modified Fibrinogen in Various Pathologic Conditions

6.1. Cardiovascular Disease

Accumulating evidence within last several decades points out to the important role of hemostatic abnormalities in the pathogenesis of atherosclerosis and cardiovascular disease (CVD). Most recently Becker and his colleagues published a review on the significance of hypercoagulable states in CVD (Chan et, 2008). In addition to acquired factors leading to hypercoagulable states the authors have emphasized the role of inherited ones in pathophysiology of CVD (Figure 4).

Numerous epidemiological and large prospective studies have documented that one of the most important risk factors for heart diseases and strokes is increased blood level of fibrinogen (Levenson et al. 1995; Kannel et al. 1987). Cigarette smoking is also known to contribute to atherosclerosis by altering fibrin clot dynamics and architecture which may also be caused by hydroxyl radicals generated under hypoxic conditions (Barua et al. 2009). A consensus exists that the higher fibrinogen concentration the greater chance of thrombus formation, therefore everything should be done to lower its blood concentration. Although it is a desirable goal, it should be remembered that the critical event in thrombosis does not depend on the amount of clottable protein, but how long does the thrombus persist in the circulation. Perhaps the example is the use of a viper venom (ancrod) for the therapeutic defibrination (Marsh&Williams, 2005) to prevent thrombosis. The reason for this paradoxical phenomenon is that desA-fibrin formed in the circulation immediately activates fibrinolytic system that effectively degrades fibrin clots. As soon, however, as this system is inhibited, for example with Aprotinin, widespread deposition of fibrin is observed (Muller-Berghaus&Mann, 1973). Inhibition of fibrin degradation in atherosclerotic lesions may be caused by the presence of insoluble albumin (Zhang et al. 1993) that when hydrophobically bound to fibrin makes it resistant to fibrinolysis. Undas and her colleagues have also demonstrated reduced fibrin clot permeability and its resistance to fibrinolytic degradation that were associated with inflammation and free radical generation (Undas et al. 2008).

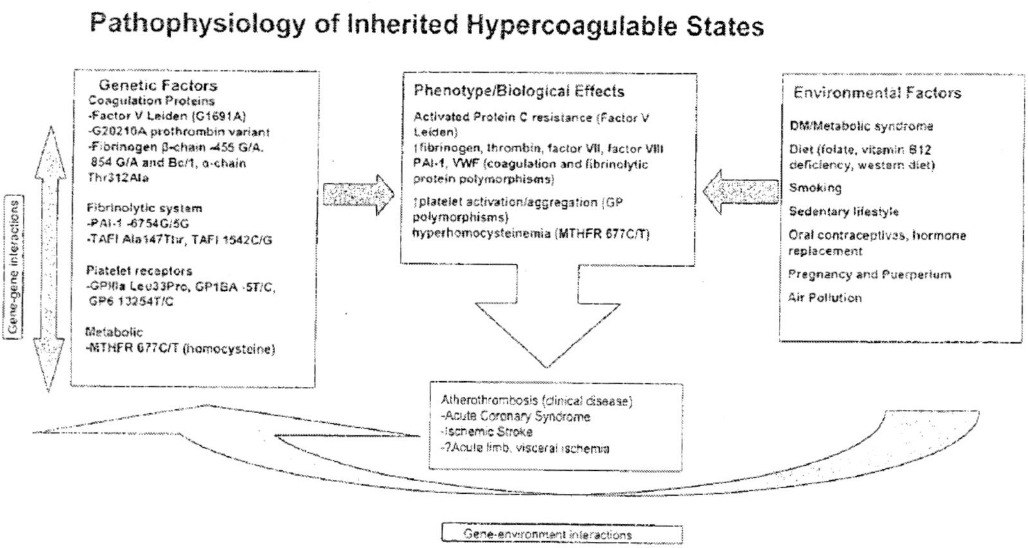

Figure 4. Pathophysiology of inherited hypercoagulable states. (Reproduced from *Circulation, vol. 118*, p. 2287, 2008).

As explained beforehand, the mere activation of blood coagulation does not offer a satisfactory explanation in view of the powerful fibrinolytic potential of human blood (Astrup, 1956). The presence of fibrin-like material in atherosclerotic plaques was first observed by Rokitansky over 150 years ago (quoted in 1952) and a century later confirmed by Duguid (1946) and later on by others (More et al. 1957; Woolf, 1961; Haust et al. 1964; Shainoff&Page, 1972). Elspeth Smith in a series of elegant papers had documented the existence of soluble fibrin(ogen)-related antigens (FRA) in both soluble and insoluble fractions of atherosclerotic intima (Smith et al.1976; Smith, 1994). According to this author fibrin is detectable at the surface as well as deep inside of the plaque thus providing scaffolding for migration and proliferation of smooth muscle cells (SMC). Moreover, fibrin degradation products, specifically fragment E, are endowed with mutagenic activity further contributing to atherogenesis. It is well known that intravascular thrombi are usually formed at sites of narrowing and/or plaque rupture of atherosclerotic vessels. However, this fact obscures identification of fibrin deposits in the vessel walls prior to thrombosis onset that may explain why the role of fibrin in atherogenesis has been so difficult to be generally accepted. Of course, the other more obvious reason is that the attention of investigators has been directed mainly to the role of cholesterol and lipoproteins.

The presence of fibrin-like material in atherosclerotic plaques can also be explained in terms of the loss of a negative charge of the arterial vessel wall (Lipinski et al. 1972). It was demonstrated that the amount of saline-extractable acid mucopolysaccharides (AMPS) in the arterial intima was significantly reduced as compared to healthy subjects. According to this concept AMPS would form soluble complexes with cationic proteins thus preventing fibrin monomers from their anchoring and deposition on the endothelial cells. An alternative and more plausible explanation for this phenomenon is now being offered by the interaction of hydroxyl radical-modified fibrin(ogen) with hydrophobic epitopes on endothelial cells which is preventable by acidic polymers. Cardiovascular health effects of aspirin can also be explained in terms of increasing negative charges of the modified fibrinogen molecules through acetylation of lysine epsilon-NH_3^+ groups. Evidence for role of hydroxyl radicals in the pathogenesis of atherosclerosis and CVD is indirectly obtained in an experimental study in which a potent scavenger, edaravone, was shown to significantly reduce myocardial infarct size in rabbits (Onogi et al. 2006). In addition, a higher prevalence of plaque iron may contribute to the increased incidence of atherosclerosis by virtue of participating in the hydroxyl radical production (Moreno et al. 2008). Moreover, hydroxyl radical-induced damaged proteins were detected in atherosclerotic plaques (Fu et al. 1998). Therefore, it becomes clear that the best strategy for the prevention of atherosclerosis is by the administration of direct hydroxyl radical scavengers in combination with those substances that can increase the net negative charge of fibrinogen. So far the only drug that can do both is aspirin, thus its beneficial effects in variety of chronic disorders associated with fibrin deposition should not be surprising. Cardioprotective effect docosahexanoic acid (McLennan et al. 1996) can also be explained by its hydroxyl radical scavenging properties (Green et al. 2001).

6.2. Cancer

Another pathologic condition in which fibrin(ogen) has been implicated, is neoplasia and uncontrolled cell growth. An increased tendency to thrombosis in cancer was observed over one hundred years ago (Trousseau, 1895) and confirmed more recently (Goodnight, 1974).

Yet considerable literature on this subject does not completely explain association of neoplasia with thrombosis. Thus, anticoagulation with warfarin has been shown to be practically ineffective in patients with breast cancer (Thomes, 1974). Even more important was the observation of deposition in cancer tissue of fibrin-like material without thrombin generation (Constantini et al. 1991). Therefore, this obvious paradox can only be explained in terms of mechanisms of fibrin(ogen) deposition other than classical thrombosis. Most recently new concepts have been presented according to which chronic inflammation plays an important role in age-related disease including cancer, diabetes and cardiovascular diseases (Allavena et al. 2008; Khansari et al. 2009). Chronic inflammation is, in turn, associated with the excessive production of free radicals (Hold&El-Omar, 2008) that facilitate cellular malignancy and proliferation (Cook et al. 2004; Schafer&Werner, 2008). According to Ames (1995), chronic infection and inflammation contributes to approximately one-quarter of all cancer cases worldwide. Another factor that has been suggested to contribute carcinogenesis is iron overload through its known role in hydroxyl radical production (Reizenstein, 1991; Sahu, 1992; Huang, 2003).

Whatever the mechanism, the most important fact is that fibrin(ogen) deposits persist in the cancer tissue due to their resistance to fibrinolytic degradation (Egyud&Lipinski, 1991). Some researchers suggested that this resistance is a result of increased content of argentine-rich peptides in fibrin clots obtained formed in cancer patients (Farbiszewski et al. 1973). Still another piece of this puzzle is the well known fact of increased production of tissue plasminogen activator by neoplastic cells specifically those in prostate cancer giving rise to elevated concentration of fibrin(ogen) degradation products (FDP). This, in turn, was incorrectly interpreted as a sign of activation of fibrinolysis being associated with cancer. It is now understood that FDP are product of a secondary degradation of fibrin(ogen) deposited at the perimeter of the cancer tissue. Importance of inhibition of fibrinolysis in cancer is further supported by the finding that aprotinin and EACA treatments of mice have significantly increased lung B16F10 melanoma metastasis (Kirstein et al. 2009).

It is of interest to note that, in addition to fibrin(ogen) deposits, cancer tissue especially lung carcinoma and breast cancer, contain insoluble forms of human serum albumin (HSA) (Soreide, 1991). In view of the fact that polymerized insoluble HSA was shown to be associated with fibrinolysis inhibition (Rockwell&Ehrlich, 1990), it is possible that a similar phenomenon occurs in cancer. Based on these observations a hypothesis was presented according to which insoluble fibrin(ogen)-albumin complexes coat tumor cells thus presenting them as 'self ' to natural killer cells (Lipinski&Egyud, 2000). This hypothesis emphasizes a defect in the immune surveillance rather than the failure of immune system being responsible for the uncontrolled growth of malignant cells. Over 100 years ago, William Coley, a New York surgeon, reported tumor regression in patients injected with pyogenic bacterial extracts (Wieman&Starnes, 1994). Due to lack of understanding, Coley's therapy has been ignored for many years. However, in the 60th new data has emerged indicating that certain viruses and bacteria can induce the destruction of tumors in cancer patients (Csatary, 1971; Kirshner, 1995). Moreover, it was also demonstrated that exotoxins of group A streptococci can function as 'superantigens' capable of activating T cells followed by their massive infiltration of the tumor (Dohlsten et al. 1995). These findings indicate that a superantigen therapy is directed not so much at stimulating the host's immune system, but at improving the surveillance capability of the cellular defense system. The proposed mechanism of this type of therapy is based on a strong interaction between the hydrophobic regions of fibrin-albumin coat on tumor cells and the apolar side chains of a superantigen. As a consequence such a sandwiched cell becomes 'non-self' and is subsequently recognized and attacked by NK cells (Figure 5).

There has been plethora of publications on the preventive and therapeutic role of selenium in cancer (Spallholz, 1994; Combs&Gray 1998; Whanger, 2004; Thompson, 1984). Apparently due to their different chemical reactivity, not all forms of selenium are equally effective. In view of the fact that selenite specifically oxidizes sulfhydryl groups, this compound was suggested to play an important role in the treatment of cancer (Lipinski&Egyud, 1992). It was then hypothesized that selenite prevents the formation of a fibrinogen-albumin coat on the surface of cancer cells thus unmasking specific tumor antigens which allow for immune recognition and subsequent elimination by natural killer cells (Lipinski, 2005). Selenite is also known to directly activate NK cells (Kiremidjian-Schumacher et al. 1996) and inhibit angiogenesis as well (Jiang et al. 1999). In addition to solid tumors, selenite was also shown to have an anti-leukemic effect (Jiang et al.1992) and can be a potential drug for the treatment of multi drug resistant acute myeloid leukemia (Olm et al. 2009). Hydroxyl radical scavenging properties of double bonds may also explain anticancer effect of unsaturated fatty acids (Pariza&Ha, 1990).

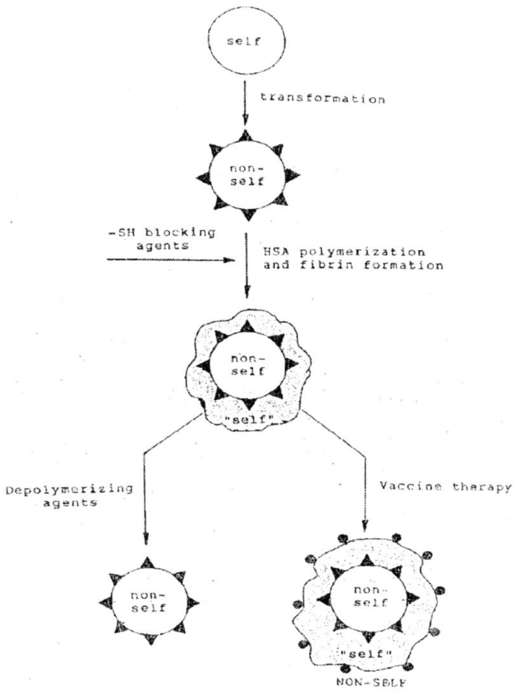

Figure 5. Hypothetical role of fibrinogen-human serum albumin (HSA) complex in the transformation of "non-self" cancer cells to those not recognized by natural killer (NK) cells. Attachment of vaccine antigens to a protective coat by means of hydrophobic interactions makes such a cell a target for immune recognition and killing. Alternatively, the same effect can be achieved by prevention of the coat formation and/or by its enzymatic or chemical depolymerization.

It has also been argued that diet plays an important role in the development and prevention of cancer. Specifically, red meat and its processed products were shown to be positively associated with advanced prostate cancer (Sinha et al. 2009). In view of the fact that red meat contains free iron, its overload in human body may accelerate hydroxyl radical generation and thus contribute to breast cancer (Bae et al. 2009; Kabat&Rohan, 2007). Intake of meat iron was also shown to contribute not only to cancer of prostate but also to lung, colorectal and ovarian cancers (Ferrucci et al. 2009). On the other hand, consumption of fruit and vegetable products rich in polyphenolic substances, iron chelating agents (e.g. citric acid) and epigallocatechin-3-gallate (a major component of green tea) may prevent cancer by virtue of free radical scavenging (Mandel et al. 2006). Consumption of cruciferous vegetables was emphasized at a conference on this subject (Kim&Park, 2009) and was also shown to increase cell protection against DNA damage (Riso et al. 2009). Isothiocyanates present in cabbage and broccoli are suggested to be of therapeutic value not only in cancer but also in liver cirrhosis, chronic renal and lung diseases, diabetes and Alzheimer's disease (Bengmark et al. 2009).

There is still another class of dietary agents that are considered to play an important role in the prevention and treatment of cancer. These are polyunsaturated fatty acids present in fish and certain plants oils, specifically omega n-3 fatty acids (Calviello et al. 2009), as well as conjugated linoleic acid that was demonstrated to inhibit tumor cell proliferation (De la Torre et a. 2005). Over a quarter of century ago a German scientist, Johanna Budwig suggested that flaxseed oil may prevent cancer growth by means of the interaction of the double bonds of unsaturated fatty acids of this oil with sulfhydryl groups on the tumor cell membrane (Budwig, 1971). Only very recently her ideas seem to find support by other researchers who are showing that flaxseed oil have a chemoprotective effect on colon cancer (Bommareddy, 2006). Even more important is a comprehensive review by Radin in which this author emphasizes the role of unsaturated allylic bonds in the interaction with sulfhydryl groups of tumor cells (Radin, 2007). Allylic moieties are present not only in ubiquitous sphingolipids but in many anticancer drugs (e.g. doxorubicin, tamoxifen) and antibiotics such as tetracycline and rapamycin, as well as in vitamin D3. Therefore, an inescapable conclusion can be drawn from these studies that dietary factors are of great importance for the prevention of cancers by virtue of their neutralizing effect on protein sulfhydryls with all its consequences (see Figure 5).

6.3. Lung Diseases

Pulmonary embolism accounts for over 300,000 deaths annually in the US. Acute and chronic lung diseases are characterized by excessive and persistent interstitial fibrin deposition (Wygrecka et al. 2008). The presence of alveolar fibrin, enhanced by inhibition of fibrinolysis, promotes lung dysfunction and acute inflammatory response (Idell, 2003). Extravascular pulmonary fibrin accumulation has also been observed in sarcoidosis (Hasday et al. 1988) and in idiopathic pulmonary fibrosis (Kotani et al. 1995; Kubo et al. 2005). It is known that fibrin and fibrin degradation products are potent chemotactic agents that enhance neutrophil recruitment in the lung, increase vascular permeability and activate inflammation

(Wygrecka et al. 2008). Inhibition of fibrin dissolution in the alveolar compartment of experimental animals and in patients with acute and chronic lung disease is well documented and is very likely caused by hydroxyl radical modification of fibrinogen. A possible relationship between pulmonary fibrin formation and hydroxyl radicals was demonstrated in dogs in which administration of edaravone protected the animals against lungs ischemia-reperfusion injury (Akao et al. 2006). Current understanding of the role of coagulation and fibrinolytic abnormalities in the development of lung infectious injury was recently reviewed (Bastarache et al, 2006). It is of interest to note that the thrombolytic therapy with alteplase can be enhanced by concomitant heparin administration (Konstantinides, 2004) suggesting that negative charges of this substance may destabilize hydrophobic bonds of thrombi. There is an increasing evidence of activation of the extrinsic blood coagulation pathways in the airways of asthmatic patients (Brims et al.2009). Treatment of severe asthma with inhaled corticosteroids resulted in the inhibition of fibrinolysis in the airways that may explain side effects of long-term therapy. Therefore, prevention of fibrin deposition might have a therapeutic potential in severe asthma. In connection with this it is of interest to note that the protective effect of the dietary intake of selenium was reported for the large London population (Shaheen et al. 2001). These findings were supported by another study of supplementation with sodium selenite at 100 mcg/day that showed significant improvement in patients with asthma (Hasselmark et al. 1993).

6.4. Kidney Diseases and Diabetes

It is well established that patients with chronic kidney disease exhibit a higher burden of cardiovascular risk factors including inflammation, hypertension, dyslipidemia, hypercoagulability and inhibition of fibrinolysis (Adams&Bird, 2009; Ceriello, 1993). Metabolic syndrome, defined by abdominal obesity, elevated blood pressure, fasting glucose and triglycerides was reported to be associated with increased risk venous thromboembolism (Ay et al. 2007). In addition, diabetic patients were shown to have significantly higher levels of fibrinogen, plasma viscosity and red cell aggregation as compared to non-diabetic patients (Jax et al. 2009). Role of blood coagulation and the persistent presence of fibrin in glomerular sclerosis were recently emphasized (Hertig&Rondeau, 2004). In type 2 diabetic patients with silent myocardial ischemia fibrinogen cut off value was shown to be 400 mg/dl (Guardado-Mendoza et al. 2009). It is of interest to note that RBC aggregation is closely, albeit not perfectly, correlated with the plasma fibrinogen concentration (Khodabadenhlou&Le Devehat, 2004). It is possible that the aggregability of red cells is influenced mostly by those fibrinogen molecules, which had been modified by hydroxyl radicals, thus increasing the chance of hydrophobic interactions with corresponding epitopes on cell membranes. Similarly to atherosclerotic plaque, fibrin-like material present in diseased glomeruli often referred to as "fibrinoid" has been identified by specific histochemical and/or immunological analysis (Takemura et al. 1987). Fibrinogen A alpha chains have frequently been detected in renal amyloidosis (von Hutten et al. 2009).

It was also shown that fibrinogen which appears in Bowman's space in proteinuric conditions have the capacity to activate podocyte cytokines and thereby accelerate their injury (Motojima et al. 2009). Moreover, increased plasma levels of D-dimer, a product of cross-linked fibrin degradation, observed in renal patients is believed to be an evidence for the intraglomerular fibrin deposition and its gradual, albeit incomplete dissolution, very likely due to hypofibrinolysis (Collet et al. 1999). Marked alterations in fibrin clot properties found in patients on chronic peritoneal dialysis (Sjoland et al. 2007) might be caused by hydroxyl modification of is structure. Concomitant with the presence of fibrin in renal failure is the occurrence of reactive oxygen species in diabetic patients thought to be a result of auto-oxidation of glucose (Miyata et al. 1999). Evidence was also provided for the accumulation of oxidatively modified products prior to the development of diabetes (Matteucci & Giampietro, 2000), that might be augmented by disturbances in the transition metal redox balance (Monnier, 2001). In addition, increased level of ROS in type 2 diabetic patients was implicated to contribute to thrombolytic resistance (Collier et al. 1992) by inhibition of fibrinolysis (Skrha et al. 1996). Also excessive production of free radicals and protein oxidation was associated with the accelerated loss of residual renal function in hemodialysis patients (Loughrey et al. 1993). It was suggested that combination of fibrinolysis inhibition with alteration of fibrin structure creates a prothrombotic condition in diabetes mellitus (Grant, 2007). As documented by others, fibrinolysis defect may contribute to chronic renal failure, chronic dysfunction of the renal transplants and to catheter obstruction in patients in patients on peritoneal dialysis (Opatrny et al. 2007).

I was suggested many years ago that kidney failure in diabetes is due to the loss of tubular negative charges. This important concept has been supported in many experimental studies showing the beneficial effect of heparin and other highly negatively charged biopolymers (Ishikawa et al. 1988; Groggel et al. 1990). Long-term high dose heparin therapy was also shown to ameliorate the course of chronic glomerulonephritis (Cade et al. 1971). However, the use of heparin in kidney diseases is hampered not only by its powerful anticlotting effect but also by inducing thombocytopenia (Warketin et al. 1995). Although heparin may exert its beneficial effect in renal diseases by inhibiting thrombin formation, it may have another very important non-anticoagulant influence on fibrin formation and dissolution (Diamond&Karnovsky, 1989). Relevant to this is a report that negatively charged biopolymers prevent albumin binding to the glomerular capillary wall (Adal et al. 1995). These findings can be explained in terms of counteracting effect of negative charges on hydrophobic interactions thus making hydroxyl radical modified fibrin(ogen) vulnerable to proteolytic degradation.

One of the most extensively studied animal models of renal cortical necrosis is so called generalized Shwartzman reaction (GSR) induced with bacterial lipopolysaccharide endotoxins (Thomas&Good, 1952). When rabbits are treated with two 24-hour spaced sublethal doses of *E.Coli* endotoxin, massive fibrinoid deposits are formed in the kidney cortex. Despite the fact that such deposits were morhologically very different from classical thrombi, a prevailing opinion was that GSR is caused by intravascular blood cogulation initiated by the endotoxin-induced platelet activation (Margaretten&McKay, 1969). It was later on documented that not blood platelets but leukocytes are involved in this reaction to endotoxin (Horn, 1973). The presence of protamine sulfate precipitable protein was originally believed to be related to thrombin elaboration and the formation of soluble fibrin complexes in plasma of endotoxin treated animals (Lipinski&Jeljaszewicz, 1969). However, it became only very recently known that this material has all the characteristic of hydroxyl radical-modified fibrin(ogen) formed as a result of hypoxic conditions caused by endotoxins.

The involvement of oxygen-centered free radicals in renal diseases has recently been supported by the findings of the beneficial effects of free radical scavengers (Ho &Bray, 1999; Keaney et al. 1999; O'Brien et al. 2000; Devaraj & Jialal, 2000). From the point of view of the effects of hydroxyl radicals, it is important to note that a variety of substances which are not antioxidants have been shown to be of benefit in diabetes, specifically dietary flavonoid quercetin and phenolic compounds contained in food products (Struck et al. 1994; Doi et al. 2004). A synthetic free radical scavenger, edaravone, was also shown to counteract the development of streptozotocin-induced diabetes, indicating that hydroxyl radicals may be a causative factor in diabetes (Fukudome et al. 2008). One of the most powerful free radical scavengers is alpha-lipoic acid (6-thioctic acid), a coenzyme of hydrogen transfer and acyl group transfer reaction (Deneke, 2000). Treatment with alpha-lipoic acid was shown to have beneficial effects in diabetic patients with poor glycemic control and albuminuria (Borcea et al. 1999).

Modification of insulin by hydroxyl radicals resulting in its increased hydrophobicity may also explain the phenomenon of hyperinsulinemia in type 2 diabetes (Inoue&Hirobe, 1986). The hydrophobic effect in protein folding and unfolding was well theoretically and experimentally explained by Lins&Brasseur (1995). Under physiological conditions insulin circulates in blood in a monomeric form, but its hydrophobically bonded dimers exhibit impaired hormone-receptor interactions (Pocker&Biswas, 1981) and have markedly reduced potency to stimulate glucose uptake (Nanjo et al. 1987). *In vitro* exposure of insulin to hydroxyl radicals generated in the Fenton reaction resulted in its polymerization without affecting its immunological characteristics (Lipinski, preliminary observation). This phenomenon may explain why in hyperinsulinemic patients there is an increased concentration of this blood hormone that is, however, biologically inactive due to the free radical-induced modification of its molecular structure.

6.5. Arthritis

It was observed many years ago that plasma obtained from patients with rheumatoid arthritis (RA) contained soluble fibrin complexes (Szpilman et al. 1972). Although fibrin(ogen) deposition within joints of RA patients has recently been confirmed (Flick et al. 2007), its contribution to the debilitating joint damage remains largely unexplored. However, it has been suggested that intracavitary fibrin clots may initiate pannus formation and the immunopathology of RA (Sanchez-Pernaute et al. 2003). As in other pathological cases, it is not a mere fact of fibrin formation but its persistent presence in the joint cavity that results in an arthritic condition (So et al. 2003). Rice bodies composed of fibrin and fragments of collagen present in chronic synovial fluid inflammation (Busso, 2002) may thus be responsible for the defective fibrinolysis. Yet there is data indicating that both blood coagulation and fibrinolysis are activated in RA joints (Weinberg et al.1991; Wallberg-Jonsson et al. 2000). In experimental arthritis active fibrinolytic system is essential for prevention and amelioration of joint inflammation (Yang et al. 2001) and so is inhibition of fibrin formation (Marty et al. 2001). So et al (2003) have documented elevated plasma D-dimers in RA patients that is usually interpreted as a sign of enhanced fibrinolysis. This paradox can be now explained in terms of the plasmin attack on those fibrin fibers that had not yet been modified and thus remain susceptible to proteolytic degradation.

Significance of effective fibrinolysis for the protection of tissues against persistent deposition of fibrin is exemplified by normal wound healing. It is well recognized that the wound will not heal properly until all fibrin is completely, albeit gradually, removed to give place to a connective tissue for a regrowth (Clark, 1985). Arthritic lesions may therefore be considered as wounds that do not heal. There is increasing evidence that hydroxyl radicals play important role in osteaoarthritis of temporomandibular joint (TMJ) (Dijkgraaf et al. 2003). These free radicals were suggested to be formed from the catalytic action of iron released from the extravasated hemoglobin. In arthritic joints a five-fold increase in iron concentration has been detected in the synovial linings. According to Dijkgraaf and coworkers, intracapsular adhesions are initiated by free radical modification of proteins leading to the formation of stable biopolymers resistant to proteolytic degradation. Using spectrophotometric turbidity measurements and light-scattering methods, these researchers have documented that fibrinogen and fibronectin formed insoluble aggregates under the influence of free radicals generated in the Fenton reaction. The aggregates, of molecular weight up to 400 kDa were shown by PAGE under reducing conditions to be covalently bonded. These authors have also emphasized that under normal conditions the fibrous adhesions can be dissolved by plasmin within a few days. By contrast, matured TMJ adhesions are resistant to fibrinolytic degradation, despite the fact that the fibrinolytic capacity is increased (Holmdahl, 1997). It can be therefore concluded that adhesions and fibrosis in arthritis may be formed as a result of free radical-induced crosslinking in fibrinogen and fibronectin molecules that are resistant to fibrinolytic degradation. Relevant to this is a recent paper in which it was demonstrated that heat-aggregated fibrinogen enhanced the extracellular release of reactive oxygen species from activated macrophages (Jozefowski&Marcinkiewicz, 2009) that, in turn, cause tissue injury.

6.6. Neurological Diseases

There is an increasing evidence for the role of hemostatic factors in neurological diseases and in Alzheimer's disease (AD) especially (Gupta et al. 2005; Kalaria, 2003). In one study, isoforms of fibrinogen gamma chain were identified among insoluble proteins in AD brains (Choi et al. 2003), and in another one it was shown that fibrin interacted with beta-amyloid protein (Merkle et al. 1996). Other researchers have demonstrated, by immunocytochemical methods, the perivascular leakage of fibrinogen around brain microvessels in AD and HIV-related neurological disorders (Fiala et al. 2002) and the presence of fibrin in CNS (Inoue et al. 1997). The existence of a protease-resistant complex of fibrinogen and albumin, indicative of their hydroxyl radical modification, was demonstrated in AD brains (Lipinski&Sajdel-Sulkowska, 2006). Moreover, Paul and Strickland (2007) document that fibrin accelerates neurovascular damage in AD. In acute cerebral lesions of multiple sclerosis tissue plasminogen activator was colocalized with fibrin(ogen) on large diameter axons that was interpreted as an attempt to remove fibrin deposits and restore normal axon function (Gverie et al. 2001). Brain injury accompanied by cerebrovascular fibrin deposition was revealed in a hypertensive stroke model (Ninomia et al. 2000). Regulation of fibrin clearance and/or deposition was suggested to be a key regulatory mechanism for Schwann differentiation and nerve cell damage (Akassoglou et al. 2002). It is also of interest to note that high blood fibrinogen is associated with an increased risk of AD (Van Oijen et al. 2005), and that antibodies to beta-amyloid peptide react with individual chains of fibrinogen (Stern et al. 1990). Moreover, amyloid fibrils were shown to contain fibrinogen A alpha chain among other diverse proteins and peptides (Kourie&Henry, 2001). A concept that any protein with exposed hydrophobic sites has the potential to aggregate and fuse with cellular membranes seems to be supported by the theoretical considerations of this subject by Klonowski&Klonowska (1986).

Yet despite intensive research we still do not understand well how fibrin is being formed in cerebral microcirculation, especially following episodes of hypoxia/ischemia. By contrast to coronary tissue, very few blood components are present in extravascular brain space due to a selective permeability of blood-brain-barrier (BBB). Perhaps it is not surprising that one of such component is tissue plasminogen activator (tPA), which might serve as the first line of defense against fibrin formed from plasma leaked after damage to BBB (Grevie, 2001). On the other hand, it has been suggested that this activator in conjunction with plasmid may aid the clearance of Abeta peptide as shown in the brains of patients with Alzheimer's disease (Melcher, 2003). On the other hand, plasmin formed in the cerebral extravascular space can be neurotoxic, by activating metaloproteinases that are known to degrade basement membrane matrix (Kaur et al. 2004). Utilizing immunochemical methods it was shown that tPA is abundant in amyloid-rich areas of AD brains, but not in control subjects (Medina&Moreno-Otero, 2005). Interestingly enough, no plasmin was found to be associated with increased levels of tPA (Ledesma et al. 2000) that may be explained in terms of either absence of plasminogen or inactivity of tPA as shown by zymography in the brains of mouse model of AD (Melcher, 2003).

The involvement of free radicals in pathogenesis of neurological diseases has been documented by numerous recent investigations, particularly in the disease of aging (Szweda et al. 2002). Free radical-induced protein aggregates resistant to proteases were suggested to be responsible for the amyloid formation (Squier, 2001). As recently emphasized by Roher et al. (2006) there is in AD a significant degree of brain hypoxia/ischemia that results from impaired total cerebral blood flow and is associated with increased levels of risk factors for atherosclerotic disease. It is worth noting that one of the risk factors for AD is diabetes mellitus, in which excessive generation of free radicals was indicated to play a major pathogenic role (Lipinski, 2001). There is another factor suggested to be involved in pathogenesis of AD, namely copper and iron known to generate hydroxyl radicals in hypoxia. These transition metals are present in normal brain tissue, but are significantly increased in cerebrospinal fluid of AD patients (Multhaup et al. 1995) and in AD brains (Markesbery&Carney, 1999; Altamura&Muckenthaler, 2009). Moreover, transition metals have been implicated in the generation of oxygen-centered free radical and the aggregation of amyloid protein in the brains of Alzheimer's patients (Adlard&Bush, 2006). Role of iron in neurotoxicity was recently reviewed by Stankiewicz&Brass (2009), and the iron load in the early stages of life was suggested to induce cognitive impairment by causing oxidative damage in the brain (de Lima et al. 2005). It is possible that under reducing conditions of hypoxia, these metal ions generate hydroxyl radical with all its pathological consequences (Rotilio et al. 2000; Dajas-Bailader et al. 1998). Reduced levels of ceruloplasmin, a copper binding glycoprotein expressed in nervous system, may also potentiate the free radical-generating effect of copper ions (Maltais et al. 2003). It was suggested that extravasation of albumin into ischemic brain may provide neuroprotection due to binding of transition metals by this protein (Gum et al. 2004). An imbalance between free radical generation and scavenging was suggested to be one of the earliest pathological events in AD (Moreira et al. 2005).

Additional evidence for the involvement of hydroxyl radicals in pathogenesis of Alzheimer's disease comes from the experimental investigations showing the protective effect of a free radical scavenger ferulic acid, in mice brain against Abeta 1-41 peptide toxicity (Yan et al. 2001). Also inhibition of hydroxyl radical production *in vivo* was shown to delay neuronal death in a transient cerebral ischemia (Yamamoto et al. 1997). Evidence for the involvement of free radicals in neurological disease comes from experimental studies with the use of edaravone a potent scavenger of hydroxyl radicals generated by a Fenton reaction (Abe et al. 2004). On the basis of its scavenging properties, this compound was approved in Japan for the treatment of acute cerebral infarcts within 24 h after onset (Wanatabe et al. 1997). It was shown that edaravone exerts an early neuroprotective effect and thus may act as an important extension of the therapeutic time window in stroke patients (Zhang et al. 2006). As reviewed by Yoshida et al. (2006) this phenolic compound significantly reduced brain infarct volume and produced sustained benefits in functional outcome during 12 months follow-up period (The Endaravone, 2003). During the early stage of ischemic insult edaravone suppressed the accumulation of 4-hydroxy-2-nonenal-modified proteins and of 8-hydroxy-deoxyguanosine in the penumbra area (Zhang et al. 2005). Also early treatment with this free radical scavenger decreased mortality during the acute stage in stroke patients (Toyoda et al. 2004). It was reported that edaravone protected against endoplasmic reticulum dysfunction caused by the accumulation of unfolded proteins induced by cerebral ischemia (Qi et al. 2004). Experiments conducted in an animal model showed that a combination therapy of edaravone and tissue plasminogen activator significantly increased the survival rates of rats with transient occlusion of middle cerebral artery (Zhang et al. 2004). At the same time post-reperfusion brain edema and hemorrhagic events induced by thrombolytic therapy were reduced by pretreatment with edaravone (Yoshida et al.2006). Three-day therapy with this substance was demonstrated to offer protection against white matter lesions in rats subjected to chronic hypoperfusion (Ueno et al. 2009). Diabetic neuropathy was also shown to be prevented by edaravone in an animal experimental study (Saini et al. 2007). Perhaps, the best evidence for the connection between hypoxia and hydroxyl radical production was provided by showing the protective effect of edaravone in fetal lamb brain after umbilical cord occlusion (Nakajima et al. 2006).

Brain is known to contain high concentration of polyunsaturated fatty acids (PUFAs) that paradoxically do not become oxidized by oxygen present in the brain at such a high concentration. By contrast, PUFAs have been shown to have a neuroprotective effect that can be explained in terms of their double bonds acting as scavengers of hydroxyl radicals by converting them to corresponding hydroxy-fatty acids (Song&Horrobin, 2004; Yavin et al. 2001). A highly unsaturated eicosapentanoic acid was also shown to offer neuroprotection in hippocampus of gamma-irradiated rats (Lonergan et al. 2002). Concentrations of essential fatty acids in plasma and red blood cell phospholipids were found to be lower in patients with Alzheimer's disease, and supplementation with fish oil of AD patients substantially improved their memory (Corrigan et al. 1991). It is of interest to note that the adequate blood oxygenation in combination with edaravone therapy was shown to prevent neuronal damage after focal cerebral ischemia (Nonaka et al. 2008). Resveratrol, another scavenger of hydroxyl radicals, was also reported to have a protective effect in cerebral ischemia-induced neuron loss (Lu et al. 2006). Chiuch et al. (2000) suggested that natural and man-made free radical scavengers could be employed as part of preventative and neuroprotective treatments in Parkinson's disease. In view of the importance of oxidation reactions in neutralizing hydroxyl radicals, it is not surprising that hyperbaric oxygen therapy had a neuroprotective effect as well (Yang et al. 2009).

6.7. Erythrocyte Sedimentation Rate

Elevated erythrocyte sedimentation rate (ESR) is a phenomenon observed practically in all degenerative, acute and/or chronic diseases. It was initially thought that the variations in ESR observed in pathological states were ascribed to the disturbances in the albumin/globulin ratio. However, the essential role of fibrinogen in the erythrocyte sedimentation was documented over a hundred years ago by Edmund Biernacki, (Biernacki, 1897). He had shown that washed red blood cells (RBC) obtained from patients with elevated ESR rate did not sediment at all in sera obtained from the same blood samples. The clinical significance of RBC sedimentation was later on emphasized and elaborated as practical clinical tests (Westegren, 1924; Wintrobe&Landsberg, 1935). It was then found out that the velocity of red cell sedimentation is influenced not so much by fibrinogen itself but its complexes with fibrin monomers, thus linking this phenomenon to thrombosis. Soluble fibrin monomer complexes (SFMC) represent a great variety of high-molecular weight fibrinogen derivatives (Lipinski, 1968), characteristic feature of which is their instability in aqueous solutions and adsorption on hydrophobic surfaces and cell membranes. It was later on observed that the addition of protamine sulphate (PS) to whole blood obtained from patients with high ESR reduced it to zero (Lipinski et al. 1969). The most important fact was that after PS treatment washed red cells resuspended in normal plasma did not sedimentate at all. These experiments clearly demonstrated that SFMC form bridges between individual RBCs dramatically increasing their size thus resulting in their accelerated sedimentation.

On the basis of these findings it was concluded that the elevated sedimentation rate is a manifestation of intravascular thrombin generation leading to thrombosis. There have been, however, data that did not fit to this concept, specifically lack of the association between ESR and the blood coagulation activation. One of such paradoxes was the experimental demonstration of increased ESR in rabbits treated with mercuric chloride which does not activates blood coagulation but does increase PS precipitable protein (Worowski&Farbiszewski, 1970). One should also bear in mind that erythrocytes can spontaneously aggregate just by removing plasma proteins from their surfaces. A simple method was elaborated in which red cells were washed with 0.3 M sucrose and their spontaneous aggregation recorded by optical density measurements (Lipinski et al., unpublished report). Alternative exposure of washed RBC to positively charged protamine and negatively charged heparin resulted in their aggregation and disaggregation. In view of the fact that hydroxyl radical-induced modification renders fibrinogen very hydrophobic, it becomes obvious that such modification might be responsible for the enhanced interaction with hydrophobic epitopes on red blood cells. Therefore, association of increased ESR with soluble fibrin should be considered not so much as evidence of intravascular coagulation (Bokarev et al. 2006), but of the generation of hydroxyl radicals occurring in numerous pathologies associated with hypoxic states and deficiencies of free radical scavengers. In a recent study it was shown than ESR was inversely correlated with nocturnal oxygen saturation in patients with sleep apnea (Min et al. 2009). It can therefore be argued that the presence of erythrocyte aggregates may impair blood oxygenation and in this way initiate a vicious cycle of hypoxia and excessive hydroxyl radical generation with all its pathological consequences.

6.8. Thrombolysis

It is well recognized that thrombolytic therapy in acute thrombotic episodes is effective only when installed not later than 3-4 hours after the onset (Leya&Deplanque, 2006). Even the discovery of more fibrin-specific plasminogen activators (Husain et al. 1981) had not helped to solve this clinically so important problem (Gurewich&Liu, 1998; Hill&Buchan, 2005). It is being argued that the ineffectiveness of current thrombolytic therapies results from the excessive blood content of activator inhibitor (PAI). Yet it has been known for a long time that in the presence of a solid phase of fibrin clot, PAI-activator complex becomes dissociated allowing for the effective fibrinolysis (Lipinski et al. 1974). Thus it is clear that the thrombolytic resistance must be caused by factors other than ineffective fibrinolytic agents. It was recently suggested that this phenomenon could be explained in terms of hydroxyl radical-induced modification of fibrin(ogen) in a thrombus that makes it resistant to proteolytic degradation (Lipinski, 2010). Similar mechanism might also be responsible for the thrombolytic episodes in patients whose circulation is assisted with mechanical devices (Nielsen e al. 2008).

On the other hand, *in vivo* studies with intravenous administration of submillimolar blood concentration of chloramine-T resulted in thrombolysis after about 30 min as compared to 90 min after injection of urokinase alone (Stief, 1991). This was the first report of thrombolysis achieved by physical rather than enzymatic method. In addition, experimental investigations in animals have demonstrated that thrombolysis with tPA was significantly accelerated by the application of ultrasound (Differtshofer&Hennenci, 2006; Tsivgoulis et al. 2008). In human subjects sonothrombolysis with microspheres and tPA was shown to enhance recanalization and clinical recovery rates as compared to tPA alone (Meairs&Culp, 2009). Moreover, application of transcranial ultrasound for thrombolysis was recently reviewed by Molina (2009). The findings described above indicate that successful thrombolysis after 3-4 hours windows of opportunity can be achieved by the methods, which counterbalance the hydrophobic modification of fibrin, thus making thrombi vulnerable to fibrinolytic degradation. It is, however, possible that such an effect can be obtained with certain proteolytic enzymes (e.g. nattokinase) that may split fibrin(ogen)-albumin aggregates in the vicinity of hydrophobic bonds (Hsu et al. 2009; Hsia et al. 2009). Last but not least is a beneficial effect of hydroxyl radical scavengers and iron chelating agents administered together or prior to the installment of thrombolytic therapy.

7. Conclusion

It is generally believed that thrombosis occurs as a result of a breakdown in the safety checkpoints at any of the stages of the coagulation cascade. Therefore, widespread occurrence of thrombosis in modern times may be considered an evolutionary failure. However, it is difficult to imagine that such a finely tuned balance between pro- and anticoagulants would so easily be shifted into deadly thrombosis thus acting against evolutionary purposes. Moreover, evolution has elaborated an ultimate defense mechanism in the form of a powerful fibrinolytic enzyme system based on the plasmin generation activated at a solid phase of the fibrin network. Under physiological conditions, the blood fibrinolytic system is in a constant state of readiness with all of its components circulating in inactive forms, and becomes activated only in the presence of the fibrin network. Yet with the dawn of a modern civilization, persistent fibrin deposits that are resistant to thrombolytic therapy are being observed in numerous diseases such as atherosclerosis, infections, cancer, arthritis, lung, kidney and neurological diseases.

Naturally, one may explain this thrombotic trend in terms of relatively recent changes in human life style to which evolution had no time to adapt. There are two main factors believed to contribute to so-called civilization diseases—one is diet and the other is a sedentary life style. Atherosclerosis, being a special case of chronic thrombosis, is attributable to a cholesterol and saturated fatty acid-rich diet and lack of certain essential nutrients, e.g., vitamins and minerals. In addition, the importance of exercise in the prevention of cardiovascular diseases and cancer should not be overlooked. There are numerous metabolic advantages of physical exercise that may contribute to its preventive power, yet one obvious albeit not generally recognized factor is outstanding, namely blood oxygenation. It was demonstrated over a quarter of a century ago that amongst all risk factors contributing to overall mortality, the most important one was the volume of air inhaled with breathing. According to this study people with low vital capacity had a shorter life span than those with normal or higher capacity. This may be explained in terms of a beneficial effect of oxygen circulating in their blood. In addition, low oxygen concentration in air observed in recent times, particularly in the industrialized countries, and sedentary life style may also contribute to a decreased content of oxygen in human blood.

The question arises what is so special about having sufficient level of oxygen in blood? In addition to obvious reasons, one aspect is not so obvious and in fact is rather controversial. Widespread acceptance of deleterious effects of so-called oxidative stress led some researchers to proclaim that oxygen is bad for us. An incredible comparison was even made between the human body and a piece of iron that rusts when exposed to air! Scientists have arrived at this erroneous conclusion on the basis of their findings of oxidation products of biological molecules in numerous human pathologies, particularly in the ischemia/reperfusion cases. As indicated in a previous section of this chapter, this conclusion arose from the lack of understanding of the principles of electrochemistry. Oxidation does not have to be accompanied by the addition of oxygen to a bimolecular, and vice versa the presence of extra oxygen atom in not necessarily a result of oxidation reaction. Moreover and more importantly, oxygen atoms are effectively introduced to lipids and proteins by reducing hydroxyl radicals formed under the condition of ischemia and hypoxia in the presence of transition metals (iron and copper). Therefore, it is proposed here that the oxidation and peroxidation products of biomolecules found in numerous chronic diseases are initiated during the stage of hypoxia/ischemia by hydroxyl radicals and fully formed only after reoxygenation.

Fibrinogen is a unique protein that in a single enzymatic event is converted into insoluble fibrin, a characteristic feature of which is its susceptibility to fibrinolytic degradation and dissolution. Although it is generally believed that thrombosis is a result of activated blood coagulation, no explanation is being offered for the persistent presence of fibrin deposits in the thrombotically affected organs. A classical example is stroke in which thrombolytic therapy is effective only during the first 3–4 hours after the onset of thrombosis. This phenomenon can now be explained in terms of the modification of fibrin(ogen) structure induced by hydroxyl radicals generated during the period of ischemia caused, in turn, by blocking of blood flow within obstructed vessels. The aforementioned modification involves intra-to inter-molecular disulfide rearrangement induced by a reductive power of hydroxyl radicals that result in the exposition of buried hydrophobic epitopes. Such epitopes react readily with hydrophobic regions of other proteins forming linkages stronger than the peptide covalent bonds rendering them resistant to proteolytic degradation. However, the formation of hydrophobic complexes can be prevented by the negatively charged substances, e.g., heparin-like and polycarboxylic molecules contained in certain food products, especially in onions.

In circulating blood, free radical-induced alteration of fibrinogen molecules involves human serum albumin that forms a mixed copolymer with fibrinogen that cannot be degraded not only with plasmin but with other active proteolytic enzymes as well. In view of this fact, in *vivo* and/or *ex-vivo* detection of such insoluble copolymers is extremely difficult to achieve with conventional analytical methods. Yet the use of direct immunochemical procedures have allowed us to demonstrate the existence of insoluble deposits of fibrin and human serum albumin in chronic diseases such as cancer, rheumatoid arthritis, renal, lung and Alzheimer's diseases, as well as in a normal human placenta. In the latter case such a copolymer serves as barrier against recognition and elimination of fetus by the maternal immune system. The ability of albumin to form a complex with fibrinogen does not mean that this ubiquitous protein is harmful—on the contrary, its role is to scavenge hydroxyl radicals and thus protect other biomolecules from undesirable free radical modifications. However, the excessive generation of hydroxyl radicals, being a consequence of chronic hypoxia due to the lack of exercise and sedentary life style, give rise to the formation of a complex of fibrinogen with albumin. When clotted with thrombin such a complex becomes resistant to fibrinolytic degradation by conventional proteases. However, as documented in recent trials, insoluble fibrin(ogen)-albumin copolymer can be broken down by singlet oxygen generated by (bio)-chemical reactions or physical forces (ultrasound).

Obviously, the best way to prevent the formation of hydroxyl radicals is to eliminate chronic hypoxia/ischemia through sufficient saturation of blood with oxygen by regular physical exercise and/or proper breathing. Since redox balance of blood is also controlled by the dietary factors, it is essential to supplement it with natural pro-oxidants such as n-3 polyunsaturated fatty acids and with substances containing aromatic rings that directly scavenge hydroxyl radicals. As indicated in previous sections of this chapter, the formation of hydroxyl radicals is catalyzed by free iron and copper ions. In connection with this it is very important for the prevention of thrombosis to regularly consume fruits and vegetables that contain transition metals chelating substances. Finally, it should be emphasized that life styles and food habits of so-called primitive societies contained all the necessary God-given ingredients that for centuries protected humanity from chronic diseases. Only after we had embraced modern life styles, we started to experience epidemics of such killer diseases as cancer, heart attacks and strokes, not to mention neurological and other debilitating conditions.

References

Abe S, Kirima K, Tsuchiya K, Okamoto M, Hasegawa T, Houchi H, Yoshizumi M, Tamaki T. The reaction rate of edaravone (3-methyl-1-phenyl-2-pyrazolin-5-one-MCI-186) with hydroxyl radicals. *Chem Pharm Bull (Tokyo),* 2004,52:186-91.

Adal Y, Smitt MF, Osicka TM, Comper WD. Albumin interaction with glomerular capillary wall in vitro. *Kidney Int.* 1995,47:1031-1038.

Adams RL, Bird RJ. Review article: Coagulation cascade and therapeutics advance: relevance to nephrology. *Nephrology (Carlton),* 2009,14:462-470.

Adlard PA, Bush AI. Metals and Alzheimer's disease. *J Alzheimer's Disease,* 2006,10:145-163.

Akao T, Takeyoshi I, Totsuka O, Arakawa K, Muraoka M, Kobayashi K, Konno K, Matsumoto K, Morishita Y. Effect of the free radical scavenger MCI-186 on pulmonary ischemia-reperfusion injury in dogs. *J Heart Lung Transplant.* 2006,25:965-971.

Akassoglou, K., Komrinck, K.W., Degen, JL. Strickland, S. Tissue plasminogen activator-mediated fibrinolysis protects against axonal degeneration and demyelination after sciatic nerve injury. *J Cell Biol.*2000,149:1157-1166.

Akiyama H, Ueda M, Kanzaki H, Tada J, Arata J. Biofilm formation of Staphylococcal aureus strains isolated from impetigo and furuncle: role of fibrinogen an fibrin. *J Dermatol Sci.* 1997,16:2-10.

Allavena P, Sica A, Solinas G, Porta C, Mantovanii A. The inflammatory micro environment in tumor progression: the role of tumor-associated macrophages. *Crit Rev Oncol Hematol.* 2008,66:1-9.

Altamura S, Muckenthaler MU. Iron toxicity in diseases of aging: Alzheimer's disease, Parkinson's disease and atherosclerosis. *J Alzheimers Dis.* 2009,16:879-895.

Ames BN, Gold LS, Willet WC. The cause and prevention of cancer. *Proc Natl Acad Sci. USA,* 1995,92:5258-5265.

Andrews BA, Schmidt AS, Asenjo JA. Correlation for the partition behavior of proteins in aqueous two-phase systems: effects of surface hydrophobicity and charge. *Biotechnol Bioeng.* 2005,90:380-390.

Areias FM, Rego AC, Oliveira CR, Seabra RM. Antioxidant effect of flavonoids after ascorbate/Fe2+-induced oxidative stress in cultured retinal stress. *Biochem Pharmacol.* 2001,62: 111-118.

Astrup T. Biological significance of fibrinolysis. *Lancet,* 1956,2:565-568.

Aubry JM, Cazin B, Duprat F. Chemical sources of singlet oxygen. 3. Peroxidation of water-soluble singlet oxygen carriers with hydrogen peroxide-molybdate system. *J Org Chem.* 1989,54:726-728.

Ay C, Tengler T, Vormittag R, Simanek R, Dorda W, Vukovich T, Pabinger I. Venous thromboembolism - a mnifestation of the metabolic syndrome. *Haematologica,* 2007,92:374-380.

Bader M, Muse W, Ballou DP, Gassner C, J.C.A. Bardwell JCR. Oxidative protein folding is driven by the electron transport system. *Cell,* 1999, 98: 217-227.

Badman MK, Pryce RA, Charge SBP, Morris JF, Clark A. Fibrillar islet amyloid polypeptide (amylin) is internalised by macrophages but resists proteolytic degradation. *Cell Tissue Res.* 1998,291:285-294.

Bae YJ, Yeon JY, Sung CJ, Kim HS, Sung MK. Dietary intake and serum levels of iron in relation to oxidative stress in breast cancer patients. *J Clin Biochem Nutr.* 2009,45:355-360.

Barua RS, Sy F, Srikanth S, Huang G, Javed U, Buhari C, Margosan D, Ambrose JA. Effects of cigarette smoke exposure on clot dynamics and fibrin structure. An ex vivo investigation. *Arterioscler Thromb Vasc Biol.* 2009 (in press).

Bastarache JA, Ware LB, Bernard GR. The role of the coagulation cascade in the continuum of sepsis and acute lung injury and acute respiratory distress syndrome. *Semin Respir Crit Care Med.* 2006,27:365-376.

Beck MA. Selenium and vitamin E status: impact on viral pathogenecity. *J Nutr.* 2007,137:1330-1340.

Benedek B, Weniger B, Parejo I, Bastida J, Arango GJ, Lobstein A, Codina C, Antioxidant activity of isoflavones and biflavones isolated from Godoya antioquiensis. *Arzneimittelforschung.* 2006,56:661-664.

Bengmark S, Mesa MD, Gil A. Plant-derived health: the effects of turmeric and curcuminoids. *Nutr Hosp.* 2009,24:273-281.

Bennett M, Feldmeier J, Smee R, Milross RC. Hyperbaric oxygenation for tumour sensitization to radiotherapy. *Cochrane Database Syst Rev.* 2005,19:50-57.

Benz B, Rostrup M, Sevre K, Andersen TO, Sandset PM. Association between acute hypobaric hypoxia and activation of coagulation in human beings. *Lancet,* 2000,356:1657-1658.

Berry MJ, Banu l, Larsen PR. Type I iodothyronine deiodinase is a selenocysteine-containing enzyme. *Nature,* 1991,349:438-440.

Bocci V, Borrelli E, Travagli V, Zanardi I. The ozone paradox: ozone is a strong oxidant as well as a medical drug. *Medic Res Rev.* 2009, 29:646-682.

Bokarev IN, Nemchinov EN, Ermolaeva OA. Thrombus precursor protein (soluble monomeric protein) in patients with acute coronary syndrome. *Klin Med (Mosk).* 2006,84:27-30.

Bommareddy A, Arasada BL, Mthees DP, Dwivedi C. Chemopreventive effects of dietary flaxseed on colon tumor development. *Nutr Cancer,* 2006,54:216-222.

Borcea V et al. Alpha-lipoic acid decreases oxidative stress even in diabetic patients with poor glycemic control and albuminuria. *Free Radic Biol Med.* 1999,26:1495-1500.

Boykin JV. The nitric oxide connection: hyperbaric oxygen therapy and diabetic ulcer management, *Adv Skin Wound Care,* 2000,13:169-174.

Brenneisen P, Steinbrenner H, Sies H. Selenium, oxidative stress, and health aspects. *Mol Aspects Med.* 2005,26:256-267.

Brewer GJ. Iron and copper toxicity in diseases of aging, particularly atherosclerosis and Alzheimer's disease. *Exp Biol Med. (Maywood),* 2007,232:323-325.

Brims FJ, Chauchan AJ, Higgins BR, Shute JK. Coagulation factors in the airways in moderate and severe asthma and the effect of inhaled steroids. *Thorax,* 2009, 64:1037-1043..

Budwig J. Photo-elements of life as an anti-carcinoma factor, successful as a preventive and in progressive state of the illness. *Minerva Ginecol.* 1971,23:115-117.

Busso N, Hamilton JA. Extravascular coagulation and the plasminogen actiator/plasmin system in rheumatoid arthritis. *Arthritis Rheum.* 2002,46:2268-79.

Cade et al. The effect of long-term high dose heparin treatment on the course of chronic proliferatve glomerulonephritis. *Nephron,* 1971,8:67-80.

Calabrese V, Guagliano E, Sapienza M, Mancuso C, Butterfield DA, Stella AM. Redox regulation of cellular stress response in neurodegenerative disorders. *Ital J Biochem.* 2006,55:263-282.

Calviello G, Serini S, Piccioni E, Pessina G. Antineoplastic effects of n-3 polyunsaturated fatty acids in combination with drugs and radiotherapy: preventive and therapeutic strategies. *Nutr Cancer,* 2009,61:287-301.

Ceriello A. Coagulation activation in diabetes mellitus. *Diabeteologia,* 1993,36:1119-1125.

Chan MY, Andreotti F, Becker RC. Hypercoagulable states in cardiovascular disease. *Circulation,* 2008,118:2286-2297.

Choi J, Malakowsky CA, Talent JM, Conrad CC, Gracy RW. Identification of oxidized plasma proteins in Alzheimer's disease. *Biochem Biophys Res Commun.* 2002,293:1566-70.

Clark RAF. Cutaneous tissue rapair: basic biological considerations. *J Am Acad Dermatol.* 1985,13:701-724.

Clauss A. Gerinnungsphysiologische Schnellmethode zur Bestimung des Fibrinogens. *Acta Haematol.* 1957,30:84-85.

Cognaut, M. Jourdan ML, Germain E, Pitavy R, Morel E, Durand G, Bougnaux P, Lhuillery, C. Effect of an alpha-linolenic acid-rich diet on rat mammary tumor growth depends on the dietary oxidative status. *Nutrit Cancer,* 2000,36:33-41.

Colafranceschi M, Gliuliani A, Colosimo A. Primary structure of proteins as space-dependent signals. *Biophys Bioeng Letters,* 2009,1(2):1-19.
Cole GM, Lim GP, Yang F, Teter B, Begum A, Ma Q, Harris-White ME, Frautschy SA. Prevention of Alzheimer's disease: Omega-3 fatty acids and phenolic anti-oxidant interventions. *Neurobiol Aging,* 2005, 265:S133-S136.
Collier A, Rumley AG, Peterson JR, Leach JP, Lowe GDO, Small M. Free radical activity and hemostatic factors in NIDDM patients with and without microalbuminuria. *Diabetes,*1992,41:909-913.
Collet J-P, Mishal Z, Lesty C. et al. Abnormal fibrin clot architecture in nephrotic patients is related to hypofibrinolysis: influence of plasma biochemical modifications. *Thromb Haemost.* 1999,82:1482-1489.
Constantini V, Zacharski LR, Memoli VA, Kisiel W, Kudryk BJ, Rousseau S. Fibrinogen deposition without thrombin generation in primary human breast cancer tissue. *Cancer Res.* 1991,51:349-351.
Cook JA, Gius D, Wink DA, Krishna MC, Russo A, Mitchell JB. Oxidative stress, redox, and the tumor microenvironment. *Semin Radiat Oncol.* 2004,14:259-266.
Copley AL. Hemorheological aspects of the endothelial fibrin lining and fibrinogen gel clotting. Their importance in physiology and pathological conditions. *Clin Hemorh.* 1981,1:9-72.
Copley AL, King RG. A survey of surface hemorheological experiments of the inhibition of fibrinogenin formation employing surface layers of fibrinogen system with heparins and other substances. *Thromb Res.* 1984,35:237-256.
Corrigan FM, Van Rhijn A, Horrobin DF. Essential fatty acids in Alzheimer's disease. *Ann NY Acad Sci.* 1991,640:250-252.
Crokart N, Radermacher K, Jordan BF, Baudelet C, Cron GO, Gregoire V, Beghein N, Bouzin C, Feron O, Gallez B. Tumor radiosensitization by anti-inflammatory drugs: evidence for a new mechanism involving the oxygen effect. *Cancer Res.* 2005,65:7911-7916.
Csatary LI. Viruses in the treatment of cancer. *Lancet,* 1971,2:825.
Czapski G. Reactions of OH radical. *Meth Enzymol.* 1984,105:209-215.
Daffertshofer M, Hennerici M. Sonothrombolysis: experimenatal evidence. *Front Neurol Neurosci.* 2006,21:140-149.
Dajas-Bailador FA, Martinez-Borges A, Costa G, Abin JA, Martignoni NG, Dajas F. Hydroxyl radical production in the substantia nigra after 6-hydoxydopamine and hypoxia-reoxygenation. *Brain Res.* 1998,813:18-25.
Daniels LA. Selenium: does selenium status have health outcome beyond over deficiency? *Med J Australia,* 2004,180:373-374.
Dauchet L, Amouyel P, Dallongeville J. Fruits, vegetables and coronary heart disease. *Nature Rev Cardiol.* 2009,6:599-608.
Davies MJ. Oxidative stress: the paradox of aerobic life. *Biochem Soc Symp.* 1995,61:1-31.
Davies KJA. An overview of oxidative stress. *IUMB Life,* 2000,50:2441-2444.
Davies KJA, Delsignore MA. Protein damage and degradation by oxygen radicals. III. Modification of secondary and tertiary structure. *J Biol Chem.* 1987,262:9908-9913.

De la Torre A, Debiton E, Durand D, Chardigny JM, Berdeaux O, Loreau O, Barthomeuf C, Bauchart D, Gruffat D. Conjugated linoleic acid isomers and their conjugated derivatives inhibit growth of human cancer cell lines. *Anticancer Res.* 2005,25:3943-3949.

Dempfle CE, Pfitzner SA, Schott D, Niessen RH, Heene DL. Fibrinogen heterogeneity in homozygous plasminogen deficiency type 1: further evidence that plasmin is not involved in formation of LMW and LMW'-fibrinogen. *Thromb Haemost.* 1997,77:279-283.

Deneke SM. Thiol-based antioxidants. *Curr Topics Cell Regul.* 2000,36:151-180.

Devaraj S, Jialal I. Oxidative stress and antioxidants in Type 2 diabetes. In: Bendich A. & Deckelbaum RJ. (Eds.) Primary and secondary preventive nutrition (pp.117-125), Humana Press, 2000.

Di Paolo N, Gaggiotti E, Galli F. Extracorporeal blood oxygenation and ozonation: clinical and biological implications of ozone therapy. *Redox Rep.* 2005,10:121-130.

Diamond JR, Karnovsky MJ. Non-anticoagulant protective effect of heparin in chronic nephrosis. *Renal Physiol.* 1986,9:366-374.

Differtshofer M, Hennerici M. Sonothrombolysis: experimental evidence. *Front Neurol Neurosci.* 2006,21:140-149.

Dijkgraaf LC, Zardeneta G, Cordewener FW, Liem RS, Schmitz JP, de Pont LG, Milam SB. Crosslinking of fibrinogen and fibronectin by free radicals: a possible initial step in adhesion formation in osteoarthritis of the temporomandibular joint. *J Oral Maxillofac Surg.* 2003, 61:101-11.

Dohlsten M, Lando PA, Bjork P. Immunotherapy of human colon cancer by antibody-targeted superantigens. *Cancer Immunol Immunother.* 1995,41:162-168.

Doi K, Suzuki Y, Nakao A, Fujita T, Noiri E. Radical scavenger edaravone developed for clinical use ameliorates ischemia/reperfusion in jury in rat kidney. *Kidney Int.* 2004,65:1714-1723.

Doronina AM, Lipinski B, Bokarev IN. Fibrinogen and their role in atherogenesis in diabetes mellitus. *Klin Med (Mosk).* 2007,85:52-55.

Duguid JB. Thrombosis as a factor in the pathogenesis of coronary atherosclerosis. *J Pathol Bacteriol.* 1946,58:207-212.

Egyud LG, Lipinski B. Significance of fibrin formation and dissolution in the pathogenesis and treatment of cancer. *Med Hypotheses,* 1991,36:336-340.

El-Sayed MS, Ali N, Al-Bayatti M. Aerobic power and the main determinants of blood rheology. *Blood Coagul Fibrinolysis,* 2009 (Sept.25).

Fang YZ, Yang S, Wu G. Free radicals, antioxidants, and nutrition. *Nutrition,* 2002,18:872-879.

Farbiszewski R, Rzeczycki W, Worowski K, Glowinski S. The arginine content of fibrin clots and fibrinolysis in neoplastic disease. *Neoplasma,* 1973,20:203-208.

Ferrucci LM, Cross Aj, Graubard BI, Brinton LA, McCarthy CA, Ziegler RG, Ma X, Mayne ST, Sinha R. Intake of meat and iron and the risk of breast cancer in the prostate, lung, colorectal and ovarian cancer screening trial. *Br J Cancer,* 2009,101:178-184.

Fiala, M, Liu, QN, Sayre, J, Popp, V, Brahmandam, V, Graves,MC,Vinters, HV. Cyclooxygenase-2-positive macrophage infiltrate the Alzheimers's disease brain and damage the blood-brain barrier. *Eur J Clin Invest.* 2002,32:360-371.

Finlayson JS, Mosesson MW. Heterogeneity of human fibrinogen. *Biochemistry,* 1963,2:42-46.

Flick MJ, LaJeunesse CM, Talmage KE, White P, Palumbo DP, Pinkerton MD, Thorton S, Degen JL. Fibrin(ogen) exacerbates inflammatory joint disease through a mechanism linked to the integrin alphaMbeta2 binding motif. *J Clin Invest.* 2007,117:3224-3235.

Forceville X. Effects of high doses of sodium selenite in septic shock patients: a placebo controlled, randomized double blind, multicenter phase II study: selenium and sepsis. *J Trace Elem Med Biol.* 2007,21,S1:62-65.

Frenkel GD, Falvey D, MacVicar C, Products of the reaction of selenite with intracellular sulhydryl groups. *Biol. Trace Elem Res.* 1991,30:9-18.

Fu S, Davies MJ, Stocker R, Dean RT. Evidence for roles of radicals in protein oxidation in advanced human athreosclerotic plaque. *Biochem J.* 1998,333:519-525.

Fukudome D, Matsuda M, Kawasaki T, Ago Y, Matsuda T. The radical scavenger edaravone counteracts diabetes in multiple low-dose streptozotocin-treated mice. *Eur J Pharmacol.* 2008,583:164-169.

Gabriel DA, Muga K, Boothroyd EM. The effect of fibrin structure on fibrinolysis. *J Biol Chem.* 1992,267:24259-24263.

Gaffney PJ. Heterogeneity of human fibrinogen. *Nature New Biol.* 1971,230:54-56.

Ghiselli A, Laurenti O, DeMattia G, Maiani G, Ferro-Luzzi A. Salicylate hydroxylation as an early marker of in vivo oxidative stress in diabetic patients. *Free Rad Biol Med.* 1992,13:621-626.

Gifford RG, Xu L, Zhao H, Carrico W, Ouyang Y, Qiao Y, Sapolsky R, Steinberg G, Hu B, Yenari MA. Chaperones, protein aggregation, and brain protection from hypoxic/ischemic injury. *J Exp Biol.* 2004, 207:3213-3220.

Gladyshev VN. The 15 kDa selenoproten: functional studies and a role in cancer etiology. In: Selenium: Its Molecular Biology and Roel in Human Health. pp.147-156 [DL Hatfield, ed.], Kluer Academic Publishers, 2001.

Gollwitzer R, Bode W, Karges HE. On the aggregation of fibrinogen molecules. *Thromb Res.* 1983,Suppl.V:41-53.

Goodnight SH. Bleeding and intravascular clotting in malignancy: a review. *Ann NY Acad Sci.* 1974,230:271-288.

Grant PJ. Diabetes mellitus as a prothrombotic condition. *J Intern Med.* 2007,262:157-172.

Green P, Glozman S, Weiner L, Yavin E. Enhanced free radical scavenging and decreased lipid peroxidation in the rat fetal brain after treatment with ethyl docosahexanoic acid. *Biochim Biophys Acta,* 2001,1532:203-208.

Groggel GC, Marindes GM, Hovinge P, Hammond E, Linker A. Inhibition of rat mesengial cell growth by heparan sulphate. *Am J Physiol.* 1990,258:F259-F265.

Guardado-Mendoza R, Jimenez-Ceja L, Pecheco-Carrasco MF, et al. Fibrinogen is associated with silent myocardial ischaemia in type 2 diabetes mellitus. *Acta Cardiol.* 2009,64:523-530.

Gum ET, Swanson RA, Alano C, Liu J, Hong S, Weistein PR, Panter S. Human serum albumin and its N-terminal tetrtapeptide block oxidant-induced neuronal death. *Stroke,* 2004,35:590-595.

Gupta A, Watkins A, Thomas P, majer R, Habubi N, Morris G, Pansari K. Coagulation and inflammatory markers in Alzheimer's and vascular dementia. *Int J Clin Pract.* 2005,59:52-57.

Gurewich V, Liu JN. Intra-arterial pro-urokinase in ischemic stroke. *Stroke,* 1998,29:1255-1256.

Gverie D, Hanemaaijer R, Newcombe J, van Lent NA, Sier CF, Cuzner ML. Plasminogen activators in multiple sclerosis lesions: implications for the inflammatory response and axonal damage. *Brain,* 2001,124:1978-1988.

Hall ED, Andrus PK, Yonkers PA, Smith SL, Zhang JR, Taylor BM, Sun FF. Generation and detection of hydroxyl radicals following experimental head injury. *Ann NY Acad Sci.* 1994,738:15-24.

Hall CE, Slayter HS. The fibrinogen molecule: its size, shape and mode of polymerization. *J Biophys Biochem Cytol.* 1959,5:11-16.

Halliwell B, Gutteridge JMC. Oxygen toxicity, oxygen radicals, transition metals and disease. *Biochem J.* 1984,219:1-14.

Hankey GJ, Eikelboom JW. What does the results of the PRoFESS trial teach us? *Lancet Neurol.* 2008,7:860-862.

Hartley RW, Waugh DR. Solubility, denaturation, and heterogeneity of bovine fibrinogen. *J Am Chem Soc.* 1960,82:978-986.

Hasday JD, Bachwich PR, Lynch JP, et al. Procoagulant and plasminogen activator activities of bronchoalveolar fluid in patients with pulmoary sarcoidosis. *Exp Lung Res.* 1988,14:261-278.

Hasselmark L, Malmgren R, Zetterstrom O, Unge G. Selenium supplementation in intrinsic asthma. *Allergy,* 1993,48:30-36.

Haust MD, Wyllie JC, More RH. Atherogenesis and plasma constituents. I. Demonstration of fibrin in the whole plaque by the fluorescent antibody technique. *Amer J Path.* 1964, 44:255-258.

Henschen AH. Human fibrinogen - structural variants and functional sites. *Thromb Haemost.*1993,70:42-47.

Hertig A, Rondeau E. Role of the coagulation/fibrinolysis system in fibrin-associated glomerular injury. *J Am Soc Nephrol.* 2004,15:844-853.

Ho E, Bray TM. Antioxidants, NFkB activation and diabetogenesis. *Proc Soc Exp Biol Med.* 1999,222:205-213.

Hoffman SW, Rzigalinski BA, Willoughby KA, Ellis EF. Astrocytes generate isoprostanes in response to trauma or oxygen radicals. *J Neurotrauma.* 2000,17:415-20.

Hold GL, El-Omar ME. Genetic aspects of inflammation and cancer. *Biochem J.* 2008,410:225-235.

Holmdahl I. The role of fibrinolysis in adhesion formation. *Eur J Surg. Suppl.* 1997, 577:24-27.

Horn RG. Evidence for participation of granulocytes in the pathogenesis of the generalized Shwartzman reaction: a review. *J Infect Dis.* 1973,128:S114-S121.

Hsia CH, Shen MC, Lin JS, Wen YK, Hwang KL, Cham TM, Yang NC. Nattokinase decreases plasma levels of fibrinogen, factor VII and VIII in human plama. *Nutr Res.* 2009,29:190-196.

Hsu RL, Lee KT, Wang JH, Lee LY, Chen RP. Amyloid-degrading ability of nattokinase from Bacillus subtilis natto. *J Agric Food Chem.* 2009,57:503-508.

Huang X. Iron overload and the association with cancer risk in humans: evidence for iron as a carcinogenic metal. *Mutat Res.* 2003,533:153-171.

Hu FB. Plant-based foods and prevention of cardiovascular disease: an overview. *Am J Clin Nutr.* 2003,78:544S-551S.

Husain SS, Lipinski B, Gurewich V. Rapid purification of a high-affinity plasminogen activator from human blood. *Proc Natl Acad Sci USA.* 1981,78:4265-4269.

Idell S. Coagulation, fibrinolysis, and fibrin deposition in acute lung injury. *Crit Care Med.* 2003,31:S213-220.

Inoue H, Hirobe M. Disulfide cleavage and insulin denaturation by active oxygen in copper(II)/ascorbic acid system. *Chem Pharm Bull.* 1986,34:1075-1079.

Inoue A, Koh CS, Yamazaki M, Yanagisawa N, Ishihara Y, Kim Bs. Fibrin deposition in the central nervous system correlates with the degree Theiler's murine encephamyelitis virus induced demyelination disease. *J Neuroimmunol.* 1997,77:185-194.

Ishikawa I, Yoshida Y, Fogo A, Purkerson ML, Klahr S. Effect of heparin on the glomerular structure and function on remnant nephrons. *Kidney Int.* 1988,34:638-644.

Jahangard T, Torkaman G, Ghoosheh B, Hedayati M, Dibaj A. The effect of short-term aerobic training on coagulation and fibrinolytic factors in sedentary healthy postmenopausal women. *Maturitas.* 2009,64:223-227.

Jakubowski H. Mechanism of the condensation of homocysteine thiolactone with aldehydes. *Chemistry,* 2006,12:8039-8043.

Jax TW, Peters AJ, Plehn G, Schoebel FC. Hemostatic risk factors in patients with coronary artery disease and type 2 diabetes - a two year follow-up of 243 patients. *Cardiovasc Diabetol.* 2009,8:48-53.

Jiang C, Jiang W, Ip C, Ganther H, Lu J. Selenium-induced inhibition of angiogenesis in mammary cancer chemopreventive levels of intake. *Mol Carcinog.* 1999,26-213-235.

Jiang XR, Macey MG, Lin HX, Newland AC. The anti-leukemic effect and mechanism of sodium selenite. *Leuk Res.* 1992,16:347-352.

Jung S-Y, Lim S-M, Albertorio F, Kim G, Gurau MC, Yang RD, Holden MA, Cremer PS. The Vroman effect: A molecular level description of fibrinogen replacement. *J Am Chem Soc.* 2003,125:12782-12786.

Kabat GC, Rohan TE. Does iron play a role in breast carcinogenesis? An unresolved hypothesis. *Cancer Causes Control.* 2007,18:1047-1053.

Kalaria RN. Vascular factors in Alzheimer's disease. *Int Psychogeriatr.* 2003, 15:S47-S52.

Kannel WB, Wolf PA, Castelli WP, D'Agnostino RB. Fibrinogen and risk of cardiovascular disease. The Framingham Study. *JAMA,* 1987,258:1183-1186.

Katsuyama M, Ichikawa H, Ogawa S, Ikezawa Z. A novel method to control the balance of skin microflora. Part 1. Attack on biofilm of Staphylococcus aureus without antibiotics. *J Dermatol Sci.* 2005,38:197-205.

Kaufman P, Huppertz B, Frank HG. The fibrinoids of human placenta: origin, composition and functional relevance. *Ann Anat.* 1996,178:485-501.

Kaur J, Zhao Z, Klein GM, Lo EH, Buchan AM. The neurotoxicity of tissue plasminogen activator? *J Cereb Blood Flow Metab.* 2004, 24:945-63.

Keaney JF, Simon DI, Freedman JE. Vitamin E and vascular homeostasis: implications for atherosclerosis. *FASEB J.* 1999,13:965-975.

Khansari N, Shakiba Y, Mahmoudi M. Chronic inflammation and oxidative stress as a major cause of age-related diseases and cancer. *Recent Pat Inflamm Allergy Drug Discov.* 2009,3:73-80.

Khodabandenhlou T, Le Devehat C. Hemorheological disturbances as a marker of diabetic foot syndrome deterioration. *Clin Hemorheol Microcirc.* 2004,30:219-23.

Kim YM, Chung SI, Lee SY. Roles of plasma proteins in the formation of silicotic nodules in rats. *Toxicol Lett.* 2005,158:1-9.

Kim KJ, Kim Y-J, Fillmore JJ, Chen Y, Moore L, Yuan M, Li ZW, Karin M, Perret P, Shoelson EE, Shulman GL Prevention of fat-induced insulin resistance by salicylate. *J Clin Invest.* 2001,108:437-446.

Kim MK, Park JH. Conference on "Multidiscilpinary approaches to nutritional problems". Symposium on "Nutrtion and health". Cruciferous vegetables intake and the risk of human cancer: epidemiological evidence. *Proc Nutr Soc.* 2009,68:103-110.

Kiremidjian-Schumacher L, Roy M, Wishe HI, Cohen MW, Stotzky G. Supplementation with selenium augments the function of natural killer cells. *Biol Trace Element Res.* 1996,52:227-239.

Kirchner HH, Anton P, Atzpodien J. Adjuvant treatment of locally advanced renal cancer with autologus virus-modified tumor vaccines. *World J Urol.* 1995,13:171-173.

Kirstein JM, Graham KC, Mackenzie LT, Johnston DE, Martin LJ, Tuck AB, MacDonald IC, Chambers AF. Effect of anti-fibrinolytic therapy on experimental melanoma metastasis. *Clin Exp Metastasis,*2009,26:121-131.

Klonowska M-T, Klonowski W. Aging, Alzheimer's disease and protein crosslinking. *J Bioelectricity,* 5:269-284,1986.

Kloczewiak M, Wegrzynowicz Z, Matthias FR, Heene DL, Zajdel M. Studies on chemically modified fibrinogen. *Thromb Haemost.* 1976,35:324-333.

Konstantinides S. Should thrombolytic therapy be used in patients with pulmonary embolism? *Am J Cardiovasc Drugs*, 2004,4:69-74.

Koopman I et al. Molecular basis for fibrinogen Dusart (Alpha 554Arg-->Cys) associated with abnormal fibrinogen polymerization and thrombophilia. *J Clin Invest.* 1993,91:1637-1643.

Kotani I, Sato A, Hayakawa h, et al. Increased procoagulant and antifibrinolytic activities in the lungs with idiopathic pulmonary fibrosis. *Thromb Res.* 1995,77:493-504.

Kourie JI, Henry CL. Protein aggregation and deposition: Implications for ion channel formation and membrane damage. *Croat Med* J 42:359-374,2001.

Kovac IB, Gorog DA, Yamamoto J. Enhanced sponateous thrombolysis: a new therapeutic challenge. *J Thromb Throbolysis*, 2006,21:221-227.

Kowalski E, Kopec M, Niewiarowski S. An evaluation of the euglobulin method for the determination of fibrinolysis. *J Clin Path.* 1959,12:215-218.

Kramer J, Ames BN. Mechanism of mutagenecity and toxicity of sodium selenite in Salmonella typhimorium. *Mutat Res.* 1988,201:169-180.

Kruszewski M. The role of labile iron pool in the cardiovascular disease. *Acta Biochem Pol.* 2004,51:471-480.

Kubo H, Nakayama K, Yanai M, et al. Anticoagulant therapy for idiopathic pulmonary fibrosis. *Chest,* 2005,128:1475-1482.

Kwan AH, Winefield RD, Sunde M et al. Structural basis for rodlet assembly in fungal hydrophobins. *Proc Natl Acad Sci USA,* 2006,103:3621-3626.

Kyselova Z, Rackova L, Stefek M. Pyroindole antioxidant stobadine protected bovine serum albumin against hydroxyl radical mediated cross-linking in vitro. *Arch Gerentol Geriatr* 2003,36:221-229.

Larson EB, Wang L, Bowen JD, McCormick WC, Teri L, Crane P, Kukull W. Exercise is associated with reduced risk of incident dementia among persons 65 years of age and older. *Ann Intern Med.* 2006,144:73-81.

Latallo ZS, Budzynski AZ, Lipinski B, Kowalski E. Inhibition of thrombin and of fibrin polymerization: two activities derived from plasmin-digested fibrinogen. *Nature,* 1964,203:1184-1185.

Ledesma MD, Da Silva JS, Crassaerts K, Delacourte A, De Strooper B, Dotti Cg. Brain plasmin enhances APP alpha-clevage and Abeta degradation and is reduced in Alzheimer's disease brains. *EMBO Rep.* 2000,1:530-535.

Levenson J, Giral P, Ravazian M, Gapieri J, Simon A. Fibrinogen and silent atherosclerosis in subjests with cardiovascular risk factors. *Arterioscler Thromb Vasc Biol.* 1995,15:1269-1279.

Levy DE, Del Zoppo GJ, Demaerschalk BM et al. Ancrod in acute ischemic stroke. Results of 500 subjects beginning treatment within 6 hours of stroke onset in the Ancrod Stroke Program. *Stroke,* 2009, (in press).

Leys D, Deplanque D. Thrombolysis beyond the three-hour time window. *Clin Exp Hypertens.* 2006,28:313-316.

Lima, de, MN, Polydoro M, Laranja DC, Bonatto F, Bromgerg E, Moreira JC, Dal-Pizzol F, Schroeder N. Recognition memory impairement and brain oxidative stress induced by postnatal iron administration. *Eur J Neurosci.* 2005,21:2521-2528.

Lins L, Brausseur R. The hydrophobic effect in protein folding. *FASEB J.* 1995,9:535-540.

Lipinska I, Lipinski B, Gurewich V. Fibrinogen heterogeneity in human plasma. Electrophoretic demonstration of two major firionogen components. *J Lab Clin Med.* 1974,84:503-508.

Lipinska I, Lipinski B, Gurewich V, Hoffmann KD. Fibrinogen heterogeneity in cancer, occlusive vascular disease and after surgery. *Amer J Clin Pathol.* 1976,66:958-964.

Lipinski B. Soluble fibrin monomer complexes. *Post Biochem.* 1968,14:373-378.

Lipinski B. Demonstration of antiparacoagulating activity of acid mucopolysaccharides and extracts of aortic wall. *Thrombos. Diathes Haemorrh.* 1969,22:401-402.

Lipinski B. Biological significance of piezoelectricity in relation to acupuncture, osteopathic medicine and action of air ions. *Med Hypotheses,* 1977,3:9-12.

Lipinski B. Bioelectrical theory of pathogenesis of atherosclerosis. *J Bioelectricity,* 1984,3:177-191.

Lipinski B. Effect of thiol-induced disulfide exchange in proteins on plasma clotting and fibrinolysis. *Thromb Haemost.* 1993,69:1260.

Lipinski, B. Hydrophobic interactions in plasma proteins and pathogenesis of atherosclerosis. *Arterosclerosis* 1995a,115:123.

Lipinski B. In vitro preparation and partial characterization of a novel complex of human fibrinogen with albumin. *J Prot Chem.* 1995b,14:259-262.

Lipinski B. Pathophysiology of oxidative stress in diabetes mellitus. *J Diabetes Complications,* 2001,15:203-209.

Lipinski B. Evidence in support of a concept of reductive stress. *Br J Nutr.* 2002,87:93-94.

Lipinski B. Modification of fibrin structure as a possible cause of thrombolytic resistance. *J Thromb Thrombolysis,* 2010,29:296-298.

Lipinski, B. Egyud, L.G. Thiol-induced crosslinking of human blood proteins. Implications for tumor immunity. *Bioorg. Med. Chem. Lett.* 1992,2:919-924.

Lipinski B, Egyud LG. Resistance of cancer cells to immune recognition and killing. *Med Hypotheses,* 2000,54:456-460.

Lipinski B, Federman SM, Krolewski AS. Plasma macromolecular protein complex: Interaction with fibrin and fibrinolysis. *Thromb Res.* 1995,78:461-465.

Lipinski B, Gurewich V. Non-clottable, protamine sulfate precipitable protein of blood. Studies on its in vitro generation and incorporation into the fibrin clot. *Thromb Res.* 1972,1:569-572.

Lipinski B, Hawiger J, Jeljaszewicz J. Staphylococcal clumping with soluble fibrin monomer. *J Exp Med.* 1967,126:979-984.

Lipinski B, Jeljaszewicz J. A hypothesis for the pathogenesis of the generalized Shwartzman reaction. *J Infect Dis.* 1969,120:160-168.

Lipinski B, Lewicki Z, Zajdel M, Miks B, Hagel E. Saline extractable acid acid mucopolysaccharides of human aorta in relation to age, sex and atherosclerosis. *Materia Med Polona,* 1072,10:1-6.

Lipinski B, Lipinska I, Nowak A, Gurewich V. Abnormal fibrinogen heterogeneity and fibrinolytic activity in advanced liver disease. *J Lab Clin Med.* 1977,90:187-194.

Lipinski B, Lipinska I. Effect of magnesium on fibrin formation from lower molecular weight (LMW) fibrinogen. *Magnes Res.* 2000,13:233-237.

Lipinski, B., Lipinska, I. Free radical-induced modification of human fibrinogen: Implication for arteriosclerosis. In: Arteriosclerosis, Risk Factors, Diagnosis and Treatment. Eds. M. Kostner and K.M. Kostner, 2002.

Lipinski B, Nowak A, Gurevich V. The organ distribution of I-125-fibrin in the generalized Shwartzman reaction and its relation to leukocytes. *Br J Haematol.* 1974, 28:221-231.

Lipinski, B., Nowak, A., Gurewich, V. Fibrinolysis versus fibrinogenolysis of man: resistance of fibrinogen to breakdown by fibrinolytic activity induced by venous occlusion. *Experientia,* 1974, 30:84-86.

Lipinski B, Lipinska J, Splawinski J. A photometric method for measurement of red blood cell aggregation (unpublished manuscript).

Lipinski B, Sajdel-Sulkowska EM. New insight into Alzheimer's disease: demonstration of fibrin(ogen)-serum albumin insoluble deposits in brain tissue. *Alzheimer Dis Assoc Disord.* 2006,20:324-326

Lipinski B, Wegrzynowicz Z, Budzynski AZ, Kopec M, Latallo ZS, Kowalski E. Soluble unclottable complexes formed in the presence of fibrinogen degradation products (FDP) during the fibrinogen-fibrin conversion and their potential significance in pathology. *Thromb Diath Haemorrh.* 1967,17:65-69.

Lipinski B, Worowski K. Detection of soluble fibrin monomer complexes in blood by means of protamine sulphate test. *Thromb Diathes Haemorrh.* 1968,20:44-48.

Lipinski B, Worowski K, Mysliwiec M, Farbiszewski R. Erythrocyte sedimentation and soluble fibrin monomer complexes. *Thromb Diathes Haemorrh.* 1969,21:198-202.

Liu H, Savaraj N , Priebe W, Lampidis TJ. Hypoxia increases tumor cell sensitivity to glycolytic inhibitors: a strategy for solid tumor therapy (Model C). *Biochem Pharmacol.* 2002,64:1745-1751.

Lonergan PE, Martin DS, Horrobin DF, Lynch MA. Neuroprotective effect of eicosapentanoic acid in hippocampus of rats exposed to gamma-radiation. *J Biol Chem.* 2002,277:20804-20811.

Lopaciuk S, Snigurowicz J, Rostkowska J, Pnieja-Olszynski W, Powiertowska-Rezmer M. Disorders in the conversion of fibrinogen to fibrin in patients with multiple myeloma. *Acta Haematol Pol.* 1978,9:157-164.

Lorand L, Ong HH, Lipinski B, Rule GG, Downey J, Jacobsen A. Lysine as a amine donor in fibrin crosslinking. *Biochem Biophys Res Comm.* 1966,25:625-629.

Loughrey CM, Young IS, Lightbody JH. Oxidative stress in hemodialysis. *Q J Med.* 1993,87:679-683.

Lowe GD. Virchows's triad revisited: abnormal flow. *Pathophysiol Haemost Thromb.* 2003,33:455-457.

Lu KT, Chiou RY, Chen LG, Chen MH, Tseng WT, Hsieh HT, Yang YL, Neuroprotective effects of resveratrol on cerebral ischemia-induced neuron loss mediated by free radical scavenging and cerebral blood flow elevation, *J Agric Food Chem.* 2006,54:3126-3131.

Maltais D, Desroches D, Aouffen M, Mateescu MA, Wang R, Paquin J. The blue copper ceruloplasmin induces aggregation of newly differentiated neurons: a potential modulator of nervous system organization. *Neurosci.* 2003, 121:73-82.

Mandel S, Weinreb O, Reznichenko L, Kaflon L, Amit T. Green tea catechins as brain-permeable iron chelators from the brain. J Neural Transm Suppl. 2006,71:249-257.

Manevich Y, Held KD, Biaglow JE. Coumarin-3-carboxylic acid as a detector for hydroxyl radicals generated chemically and by gamma radiation. *Radiat Res.* 1997,148:580-91.

Margaretten W, McKay DG. The role of the platelet in the Generalized Shwartzman reaction. *J Exp.Med.* 1969,129:585-589.

Markesbery WR, Carney JM. Oxidative alterations in Alzheimer's disease. *Brain Pathol.* 1999, 9:133-146.

Marsh N, Williams V. Practical applications of snake venom toxins in haemostasis. *Toxicon,* 2005,45:1171-1181.

Marchi R, Mirshahi SS, Soria C, Mirshahi M, Zohar M, Collet JP, de Bosch NB, Arocha-Pinango CL, Soria J. Thrombotic dysfibrinogemia. Fibrinogen "Caracas V" relation between very tight network and defective clot degradability. *Thromb Res.* 2000,99:187-193.

Marty I, Peclat V, Kirdaite G, Salvi R, So AK, Busso N. Amelioration of collagen-induced arthritis by thrombin inhibition. *J Clin Invest.* 2001,107:631-640.

Marx G, Chevion M. Fibrinogen coagulation without thrombin: reaction with vitamin C and copper(II). *Thromb Res.* 1985,40:11-18.

Matteucci E, Giampietro O. Oxidative stress in families of Type 1 diabetic patients. *Diabetes Care,* 2000,23:1182-1186.

McLennan, P. Howe, M. Abeywardena, R. Muggli, D. Readerstorff, The cardiovascular protective role of docosahexanoic acid. *Eur J Pharmacol.* 1996,300: 83-89.

Meairs S, Culp W. Microbubles for thrombolysis of acute ischemic stroke. *Cerebrovasc Dis.* 2009,27, S.2:55-65.

Medina J, Moreno-Otero R. Pathophysiological basis for antioxidant therapy in chronic liver disease. *Drugs,* 2005,65:2445-2461.

Melcher K. New chemical crosslinking methods for the identification of transient protein-protein interactions with multiprotein complexes. *Curr Protein Pept Sci.* 2004,5:287-296.

Menotti A, Conti S, Dima F, Giampaoli S, Giuli B, Rumi A, Seccareccia F, Signorettti P. Prediction of all causes of death as a function of some factors commonly measured in cardiovascular population surveys. *Prevent Med.* 1983,12: 318-325.

Merkle DL, Cheng CH, Castellino FJ, Chibber BA. Modulation of fibrin assembly and polymerization by beta-amyloid of Alzheimer's disease. *Blood Coagul Fibrinolysis.* 1996,7:650-658.

Michiels C. Physiological and pathological responses to hypoxia. *Am J Pathol.* 2004,164:1875-1882.

Min JY, Jang JY, Kim HY, Lee WY, Ghong HJ, Chung SK, Chung SC. A relationship between the obstructive sleep apnea syndrome and the erythrocyte sedimentation rate. *Clin Exp Otorhinolaryngol.* 2009,2:126-130.

Miyata T, van Ypersele de Strihou C, Kurokawa K, Baynes JW. Origin and significance of carbonyl stress in long-term uremic complications. *Kidney Int.* 1999,55:389-399.

Molina et a. Transcranial ultrasound in clinical thrombolysis (TUCSON) trial. *Ann Neurol.* 2009,66:28-38.

Monnier VM. Transition metals redox: reviving an old plot for diabetic vascular disease. *J Clin Invest.* 2001,107:799-801.

More RM, Movat HZ, Haust DM. Role of mural fibrin thrombi of the aorta in genesis of arteriosclerotic plaques. *Arch Pathol.* 1957,63:612-616.

Moreira PI, Oliveira CR, Santos MS, Nunomura A, Honda K, Zhu X, Smith MA, Perry G. A second look into the oxidant mechanism in Alzheimer's disease. *Curr Neurovasc Res.* 2005,2:179-184.

Moreno PR, Purushothaman KR, Purushothaman M. et al. Haptoglobin genotype is a major determinant of the amount of iron in the human atherosclerotic plaque. *J Am Coll Cardiol.* 2008,52:1049-1051.

Mori TA, Woodman RJ, Burke V, Puddey JB, Croft KD, Beili LJ. Effects of eicosapentanoic acid and docosahexanoic acid on oxidative stress and inflammatory markers in treated-hypertensive type 2 diabetic patients. *Free Rad Biol Med.* 2003,35:772-781.

Motojima M, Matsusaka T, Kon V, Ichikawa I. Fibrinogen that appears in Bowman's space of proteinuric kidneys in vivo activates podocyte toll-like receptors 2 and 4 in vitro. *Nephron Exp Nephrol.* 2009,114:e39-e47.

Muller-Berghaus G, Mann B. Precipitation of ancrod-induced soluble fibrin by Aprotinin and norepinephrine. *Thromb Res.* 1973,2:305-310.

Multhaup G, Schlicksupp A, Hesse L, Beher D, Rupert T, Masters CL, Beyreuther K. The amyloid precursor protein of Alzheimer's disease in the reduction of Copper(II) to Copper(I). *Science,* 1996, 217:1406-1409.

Nakajima Y, Masaoka N, Hayakawa Y, Watanabe M, Nagaishi M, Sakata H, Yamamoto T. The production of hydroxyl radicals in the fetal lamb brain resulting from occlusion of the umbilical circulation and the transpalcental effect of MCI-186 to inhibit hydroxyl radical production. *Pediatr Res.* 2006,59:216-220.

Nanjo K, Sanke T, Miyano M, Okai K, Sowa R, et al. Diabetes due to secretion of a structurally abnormal insulin (Insulin Wakayama). *Diabetologia,* 1987,30:87-92.

Nielsen VG, Kirklin JK, Holman WL et al. Mechanical circulatory device thrombosis: A new paradigm linking hypercoagulation and hypofibrinolysis. *ASAIO J.* 2008,54:351-358.

Niewiarowski S, Budzynski AZ, Lipinski B. Significance of the intact polypetide chains in human fibrinogen in ADP-induced platelet aggregation. *Blood,* 1977,49:635-644.

Ninomia T, Wang L, Kumar SR, Kim A, Zlokovic BV. Brain injury and cerebrovascular fibrin deposition correlate with reduced antithrombotic brain capillary functions in a hypertensive stroke model. *J Cereb Blood Flow Metab.* 2000,20:998-1009.

Nowak A, Lipinski B, Drzewiecki J. Soluble fibrin monomer complexes level in the course of myocardial infarction. *Br Heart J.* 1972,34:593-567.

Obata T. Role of hydroxyl radical formation in neurotoxicity as revealed by in vivo free radical trapping. *Toxicol Lett.* 2002,132:83-93.

O'Brian RC, Luo M, Balazs N, Mercuri J. In vitro and in vivo antioxidant properties of gliclazide. *J Diabetes Complicat.* 2000,14:201-206.

Olm E, Johnsson-Videsater K, Ribera-Cortada I, Fernandes AP, Eriksson LC, Lehmann S, Rundlof AK, Paul C, Bjornstedt M. Selenite is a potent cytotoxic agent for human primary AML cells. *Cancer Lett.* 2009,282:116-123.

Onogi H. et al. Edaravone reduces myocardial infarct size and improves cardiac function and remodeling in rabbits. *Clin Exp Pharmacol Physiol.* 2006,33:1035-1041.

Opatrny K Jr, Zemanova P, Opatrna S, Vit L. Fibrinolysis in chronic renal failure, dialysis and renal transplantation. *Ann Transplant.* 2002,7:34-43.

Packer L. Antioxidant properties of lipoic acid and its therapeutic effects in the prevention of diabetic complications and cataracts. *Ann NY Acad Sci.* 1994,738:257-264.

Pariza MW, Ha YL. Newly recognized anticarcinogenetic fatty acids. *Basic Life Sci.* 1990,52: 167-170.

Patterson C, Madamanchi NR, Runge MS. The oxidative paradox. Another piece in the puzzle. *Circ Res.* 2000,87:1074-1078.

Paul J, Strickland S, Melchor JP. Fibrin deposition accelerates neurovascular damage and neuroinflammation in mouse models of Alzheimer's disease. *J Exp Med.* 2007,204:1999-2008.

Plyakov NE, Leshina TV, Konovalova TA, Kispert LD. Carotenoids as scavengers of free radicals in Fenton reaction; Antioxidants or pro-oxidants? *Free Radic Biol Med.* 2001,31:398-404.

Pocker Y, Biswas SB. Self-association of insulin and the role of hydrophobic bonding: A thermodynamic model of insulin dimerization. *Biochemistry,* 1981,20;4354-4361.

Podhaisky H-P, Abate A, Polte T, Oberle S, Schroder H. Aspirin protects endothelial cells from oxidative stress - possible synergism with vitamin E. *FEBS Lett.* 1997:417:349-351.

Potter K, Hankey GJ, Green DJ, Eikelboom J, Jamrozik K, Arnolda LF. The effect of long-term homocysteine-lowering on carotid intima-media thickness and flow mediated vasodilatation in stroke patients: a randomized controlled tial and meta-analysis. *BCM Cardiovasc Disord.* 2008,20:8-24.

Qi X, Okuma Y, Hosoi T, Nomura Y. Edaravone protects against hypoxia/ischemia-induced endoplasmic reticulum dysfunction. *J Pharmacol Exp Ther.* 2004:311-393.

Quintana IL, Oberholzer MV, Kordich L, Lauricella AM. Impaired fibrin gel permeability by high homocysteine levels. *Thromb Res.* 2009 (in press).

Radin NS. Meta-analysis of anticancer drug structures - significance of their polar allylic moieties. *Anticancer Agents Med Chem.* 2007,7:209-222.

Ramokrishna G, Cooper LT. Iron and peripheral arterial disease: revisiting the iron hypothesis in a diferent light. *Vasc Med.* 2003,8:203-210.

Rayman MP. The argument for increasing selenium intake. *Proc Nutr Soc.* 2002,61:203-215.

Reis KA, Guz G, Ozdemir H, Erten Y, Atalay V, Bicik Z, Ozkurt ZN, Bali M, Sindel S. Intravenous iron therapy as a possible risk for atherosclerosis in end-stage renal disease. *Int Heart J.* 2005,46:255-264.

Reizenstein P. Iron, free radicals and cancer: a review. *Med Oncol Tumor Pharmacother.* 1991,8:229-233.

Riso P, Martini D, Visioli F, Martinetti A, Porrini M. Effect of broccoli intake on markers related to oxidative stress and cancer risk in healthy smoker and nonsmokers. *Nutr Cancer*, 2009,61:232-237.

Rockwell WB, Ehrlich HP. Fibrinolysis inhibition in human burn blister fluid. *J Burn Care Rehabil.* 1990,11:1-6.

Roher AE, Kokjohn TA, Beach TG. An association with great implications: vascular pathology and Alzheimer disease. *Alzheimer Dis Assoc Dosord.*2006,20:73-75.

Rokitansky C. Abnormal conditions of the arteries. In: A Manual of Pathological Anatomy. Vol.IV, Part II, Chapter 3, London, 1952.

Rotilio G, Carri MT, Rossi L, Ciriolo MR. Copper-dependent oxidative stress and neurodenegeneration. *IUMB Life* 2000,50:309-314.

Sahu SC. Dietary iron and cancer: a review. *Environ Carcino Ecotox Revs.* 1992,C10:205-237.

Saini AK, Kumar HSA, Sharma SS. Preventive and curative effect of edaravone on nerve function and oxidative stress in experimental neuropathy. *Eur J Pharmacol.* 2007,568:164-172.

Sanchez-Pernaute O, Largo R, Calvo E, Alvarez-Soria MA, Egido J, Herrero-Beaumont G. A fibrin based model for rheumatoid synovitis. *Ann Rheum Dis.* 2003,62:1135-1138.

Sauls DL, Lockhart E, Warren ME, Lenkowski A, Wilhelm SE, Hoffman M. Modification of fibrinogen by homocysteine thiolactone increases resistance to fibrinolysis: a potential mechanism of the thrombotic tendency in hyperhomocysteinemia. *Biochemistry,* 2006,45:2480-2487.

Schafer M, Werner S. Cancer as an overhealing wound: an old hypothesis revisited. *Nature Rev Molec Cell Biol.* 2008,9:628-638.

Schmidt E. n-3 Fatty acids and the risk of coronary heart disease. *Danish Med Bull.* 1997,14:1-22.

Schrauzer GN, Surai PF. Selenium in human and animal nutrition: resolved and unresolved issues. A partly historical treatise in commemoration of the fiftieth anniversary of the discovery of the biological essentiality of selenium. *Crit Rev Biotechnol.* 2009,29:2-9.

Sengoelge G, Sunder-Plassmann G, Horl WH. Potential risk for infection and atherosclerosis due to iron therapy. *J Ren Nutr.* 2005,15:105-110.

Serebruany VL, Atar D, Dalesandro MR, O'Connor CM, Gurbel PA. Changes in hemostasis after parental magnesium in myocardial ischemia-reperfusion: from animal studies to clinical trials. *Magnes Res.* 1998,11:133-140.

Shacter E, Willimas JA, Levine RL. Oxidative modification of fibrinogen inhibits thrombin-catalyzed clot formation. *Free Radic Biol Med.* 1995,18:815-821.

Shaheen SO, Sterne JAC, Thompson RL, Songhurst CE, Margetts BM, Burney PGJ. Dietary antioxidants and asthma in adults. *Am J Respir Crit Care Med.* 2001,164:1823-1828.

Shainoff JR, Page IH. Deposition of modified fibrinogen within the aortic intima. *Atherosclerosis,* 1972,16:287-290.

Sharma P, Radhavan SAV, Saini R, Dikshit M. Ascorbate-mediated enhancement of reactive oxygen species generation from polymorphonuclear leukocytes: modulatory effect of nitric oxide. *J Leukoc Biol* 2004,75:1070-1078.

Shulman S, Ferry JD. The conversion of fibrinogen to fibrin. II. The influence of pH and ionic strength on clotting time and clot opacity. *J Phys Colloid Chem.* 1950,54:76-79.

Sies H. Oxidative stress: oxidants and antioxidants. *Exp Physiol.* 1997,82:291-295.

Sinha R, Park Y, Graubard BI, Leitzmann MF, Hollenbeck A, Schatzkin A, Cross AJ. Meat and meat-related compounds and risk of prostate cancer in a large prospective cohort study in the United States. *Am J Epidemiol.* 2009,170:1165-1177.

Sjoland JA, Sidelmann JJ, Brabrand M et al. Fibrin clot structure in patients with end-stage renal disease. *Thromb Haemost.* 2007,98:339-345.

Skrha J, Hodinar A, Kvasnicka J, Hikgertova J. Relationship of oxidative stress and fibrinolysis in diabetes mellitus. *Diabetic Med.* 1996,13:800-805.

Smith EB. Fibrin deposition and fibrin degradationproducts in athersoclerotic plaques. *Thromb Res.* 1994,75:329-335.

Smith EB, Alexander KM, Massie IB. Insoluble fibrin in human aortic intima. Quantitattive studies on the relationship between insoluble fibrin, soluble fibrinogen and low density lipoprotein. *Athersoclerosis,* 1976,23:29-39.

So AK, Varisco P-A, Kemkes-Matthes B, Herkenne-Morard C, Chobaz-Peclat V, Gereser J-C, Busso N. Arthritis is linked to local and systemic activation of coagulation and fibrinolysis pathways. *J Thromb Haemost.* 2003,1:2510-2515.

Song C, Horrobin D. Omega-3 fatty acid ethyl-eicosapentaenoate, but not soybean oil, attenuated memory impairment induced by central IL-1beta administration, *J Lipid Res.* 2004,45:1112-1121.

Soreide J, Lea OA, Kvinnsland S. Cytosol albumin content in operable breast cancer. *Acta Oncol.* 1991,30:797-802.

Sorensen JD, Olsen SF, Secher NJ, Jespersen J. Effects of fish oil supplementation in late pregnacy on blood lipids, serum ureate, coagulation and fibrinolysis. *Fibrinolysis,* 1994,8:54-60.

Soria J, Soria C, Caen JP. A new type of congenital dysfibrinogenemia with defective fibrin lysis-Dusard syndrome: possible relationship to thrombosis. *Br J Haematol* 1983,53:575-586.

Spallholtz JE. On the nature of selenium toxicity and cancerostatic activity. *Free Radic Biol Med.* 1994,17:45-64.

Squier TC. Oxidative stress and protein aggregation during biological aging. *Exp Gerentol.* 2001, 36:1539-1550.

Srinivasan M, Sudheer AR, Menon VP. Ferulic acid: therapeutic potential through its antioxidant property. *J Clin Biochem Nutr.* 2007,40:92-100.

Stahl W, Sies H, Bioactivity and protective effect of natural carotenoids. *Biochim Biophys Acta,* 2005,1740:101-107.

Stankiewicz JM, Brass SD. Role of iron in neurotoxicity: a cause for concern in the elderly? *Curr Opin Clin Nutr Metab Care,* 2009,12:22-29.

Steinman C, Bogli C, Jungo M. et al. A new substitution, gamma 358Ser-->Cys in fibrinogen Milano. *Blood,* 1994,84:1874-1880.

Stern RA, Trojanowski JQ, Lee VM. Antibodies to the beta-amylod peptide cross-react with conformational epitopes in human fibrinogen subunits from peripheral blood. *FEBS Lett.*1990,264:43-47.

Stief TW. Nonradical excited oxygen species induce selective thrombolysis in vivo. *Thromb Res.*1991,62:147-163.

Stocklet JC, Chataigneau T, Ndiaye M, Oak MH, El Bedoui J, Chataigneau M, Schini-Kerth VB. Vascular protection by dietary polyphenols. *Eur J Pharmacol.* 2004,500:299-313.

Struck M, Watkins T, Tomeo A, Halley J, Birenbaum M, Jordan KL. Effect of red and white wine on serum lipids, platelet aggregation, oxidation products and antioxidants. *Nutr Res.* 1994,14:1811-1891.

Sullivan IL. Iron in arterial plaque: modifiable risk factor for atherosclerosis. *Biochim Biophys Acta,* 2009,1790:718-723.

Suzuki Y, Nakano T, Ohno T, Kato S, Niibe Y, Morita S, Tsujii H. Oxygenated and reoxygenated tumors show better local control in radiation therapy for cervical cancer. *Int J Gynecol Cancer.* 2006,16:306-311.

Sweet F, Kao MS, Lee SC, Hagar WL, Sweet WE. Ozone selectively inhibits growth of human cancer cells, *Science,* 1980,209:931-933.

Szczepanski M, Szostek P, Pypno W, Borowka A. The lack of effect of a prophylactic dose of enoxaparin on thrombin generation in patients subjected to nephrectomy because of kidney cancer. *Throm Res.* 2001,104:427-432.

Szpilman H, Stachurska J, Kossakowska M, Koroscik A, Kopec M. Soluble fibrin and fibrinogen degradation products in rat's blood in Freund's adjuvant-induced experimental polyarthritis. *Reumatologia,* 1972,10:297-302.

Szweda PA, Friguet B, Szeda LI. Proteolysis, free radicals and aging. *Free Radic Biol Med.* 2002,33:29-36.

Takemura T, Yoshika K, Akano N, Miyamoto H, Matsumoto K, Maki S. Glomerular deposition of cross-linked fibrin in human kidney disease. *Kidney Int.* 1987,32:102-111.

Tarumi T, Mrtincic D, Thomas A, Janco R, Hudson M, Baxter P, Gailani D. Familial thrombophilia associated with fibrinogen Paris V: Dusart syndrome. *Blood,* 2000,96:1191-1193.

Terada A, Yoshida M, Seko Y, Kobayashi T, Yoshida K, Nakada M et al. Active oxygen species generation and cellular damage by additives of parenteral preparation: selenium and sulfhydryl compounds. *Nutrition,* 1999,15:651-655.

The Edavarone Acute Brain Infarction Study Group. Effect of a novel free radical scavenger, edaravone (MCI-186), on acute brain infarction. *Cerebrovasc Dis.* 2003,15:222-229.

Thomas L, Good RA. Studies on the generalized Shwartzman reaction. I. General observations concerning the phenomenon. *J Exp Med.* 1952,96:605-609.

Thomes RD. Oral anticoagulat therapy of human cancer. *J Med.* 1974,5:83-91.

Thompson HJ. Selenium as anticarcinogen *J Agr Food Chem.* 1984,32:422-425.

Toyoda K, Fujii K, Kamouchi M, et al. Free radical scavenger, edaravone, in stroke with internal carotid artery occlusion. *J Neurol Sci.* 2004,221:11-17.

Toyokuni S, Okamoto K, Yodil J, Hiai H. Persistent oxidative stress in cancer. *FEBS Lett.* 1995,358:1-3.

Trousseau A. Phlegmasis Alba Dolen. *Clin Med del'Hotel de Paris*, 1895,3:654.

Tsivgoulis G, Culp WC, Alexandrow AV. Ultrasound enhanced thrombolysis in acute arterial ischemia. *Ultrasonics,* 2008,48:303-311.

Tuck KL, Freeman MP, Hayball PJ, Stretch GL, Stupans I. The in vitro fate of hydroxyl-tyrosol and tyrosol, antioxidant constituents of olive oil, after intravenous and oral dosing of labeled compounds in rats. *J Nutr.* 2001,131:1993-1996.

Ueno S, Kashimoto T, Susa N, Wada K, Ito N, Takeda-Homma NS, Nishimuta Y, Sugiyama M. Estimation of hydroxyl radical generation by salicylate hydroxylation method in multiple organs of mice exposed to whole-body X-ray irradiation. *Free Radic Res.* 2006,40:944-951.

Undas A, Brozek J, Jnakowski M, Siudak Z, Szczeklik A, Jakubowski H. Plasma homocysteine affects fibrin clots permeability and resistance to lysis in human subjects. *Arterioscler Thromb Vasc Biol.* 2006,26:1397-1404.

Undas A, Kolarz M, Kopec G, Tracz W. Altered fibrin clot properties on long-term haemodialysis: relation to cardiovascular mortality. *Nephrol Dial Transplant.* 2008,23:2010-2015.

Undas A, Szuldrzynski K, Stepien E, Zalewski J, Godlewski J, Tracz W, Pasowicz M, Zmudka K. Reduced clot permeability and susceptibility to lysis in patients with acute coronary syndrome: effects of inflammation and oxidative stress. *Athertosclerosis,* 2008a,196:551-557.

Undas A, Zawilska K, Ciesla-Dul M, Lehmann-Kopydlowska A, Skubiszak A, Ciepluch K, Tracz W. Altered fibrin clot structure/function in patients with idiopathic venous thromboembolism and their relatives. *Blood,* 2009,114:4227-4278.

Upchurch GR, Ramdev N, Walsh MT, Loscalzo J. Prothrombotic consequences of the oxidation of fibrinogen and their inhibition by aspirin. *J Thromb Thrombolysis,* 1998,5:9-14.

Vadseth C et al. Pre-thrombotic state by post-transational modification of fibrinogen by reactive nitrogen species. *J Biol Chem.* 2004,279:8820-8826.

Van Oijen, M, Witteman, JC, Hoffman, A et al. Fibrinogen is associated with an increased risk of Alzheimer disease and vascular dementia. *Stroke,* 2005,36:2637-2641.

Vazquez-Medina JP, Zenteno-Savin T, Elsner R. Antioxidant enzymes in ringed seal tissue: potential protection against dive-associated ischemia/reperfusion. *Comp Biochem Physiol C. Toxicol Pharmacol.* 2006,142:198-204.

Vincent JL, Forceville X. Critically elucidating the role of selenium. *Curr Opin Anaesthesiol.* 2008,21:148-154.

Visavadiya NP, Soni B, Dalwadi N. Free radical scavenging and antiatherogenic activities of Sesamus indicum seed extracts in chemical and biological model systems. *Food Chem Toxicol.* 2009,47:2507-2515.

Von Hutten H, Mihatsch M, Lobeck M, Rudolph B, Eriksson M, Rocken C. Prevalence and origin of amyloid in kidney biopsies. *Am J Surg Pathol.* 2009(in press).

Wallberg-Jonsson S, Cederfelt M, Rantapaa-Dahlqvist S. Hemostatic factors and cardiovascular disease in active rheumatoid arthritis: and 8 year followup study. *J Rheumatol.* 2000,27:71-75.

Ward NC, Croft KD. Hypertension and oxidative stress. *Clin Exp Pharmacol Physiol.* 2006,33:872-876.

Warketin TE et al. Heparin-induced thrombocytopenia in patients treated with low MW heparin or unfractionated heparin. *N Engl J Med.* 1995,332:1330-1335.

Wasiutynski A, Wiczynski GM, Morton M, Koperski L, Gornicka B, Ziarkiewicz-Wroblewska B. Fibrinogen/fibrin and albumin colocalize on the surface of placental villi: a novel element of feto-maternal barrier? *Ann Diagn Paediatr Pathol.* 2002,6:125-129.

Weinberg JB, Pippen AM, Greenberg CS. Extravascular fibrin formation and dissolution in synovial tissue of patients with osteoarthritis and rheumatoid arthritis. *Arthritis Rheum.* 1991,34:996-1005.

Weisel JW, Litvinov RI. The biochemical and physical process of fibrinolysis and effects of clot structure and stability on the lysis rate. *Cardiovasc Hematol Agents Med Chem.* 2008,6:161-80.

Westergren A. Sedimentation of erythrocyte test. *Acta Med Scand.* 1924,Suppl.7:102-105.

Whanger PD. Selenium and its relationship to cancer: an update. *Br J Nutr.* 2004,91:11-18.

Wintrobe MM, Landsberg JW. A standard technique for for sedimentation test. *Amer J Sci.* 1935,189:102-106.

Witko-Sarsat V, Friedlander M. Capeillere-Blandidn C et al. Advanced oxidation protein products as a novel marker of oxidative stress in uremia. *Kidney Int.* 1996,49:1304-1313.

Wieman B, Starnes CO. Coley's toxins, tumor necrosis factor and cancer research: a historical perspective. *Pharmac Ther.* 1994,64:529-564.

Wohner N. Role of cellular elements in thrombus formation and dissolution. *Cardiovasc Hematol Agents Med Chem.* 2008,6:224-228.

Woolf N. The distribution of fibrin within the aortic intima. An immunochemical study. *Am J Pathol.* 1961,39:521-525.

Worowski K, Farbiszewski R. Activity of aminotransferases and phosphatases in experimental intoxication of rabbits with mercuric chloride. *Acta Physiol Pol.* 1970,21:312-319.

Wygrecka M, Jablonska E, Guenther A, Preissner KT, Markart P. Current view on alveolar coagulation and fibrinolysis in acute inflammatory and chronic interstitial lung disease. *Thromb Haemost.* 2008,99:494-501.

Yamamoto T, Yuki S, Watanabe T, Mitsuoka M, Saito K, Kogure K. Delayed neuronal death prevented by inhibition of incereased hydroxyl radical formation in a transient cerebral ischemia. *Brain Res.* 1997,762:240-242.

Yan JJ, Cho JY, Kim HS, Kim KL, Jung JS, Huh SO, Suh HW, Kim YH, Song DK. Protection against beta-amyloid peptide toxicity in vivo with long-term administration of ferulic acid. *Br J Pharmacol.* 2001,133:89-96.

Yang YH, Carmeliet P, Hamilton JA. Tissue-type plasminogen activator deficiency exacerbate arthritis. *J Immunol.* 2001,167:1047-1052.

Yang ZJ, Xie Y, Bosco GM, Camporesi EM. Hyperbaric oxygenation allieviates MCAO-induced brain injury and reduces hydroxyl radical formation and glutamate release. *Eur J Appl Physiol.* 2009 (in press).

Yavin E, Glozman S, Green P. Docosahexanoic acid accumulation in the prenatal brain: prooxidant and antioxidant features. *J Mol Neurosci.* 2001,16:229-35.

Yoshida H, Yanai H, Namiki Y, Fukatsu-Sasaki K, Furutani N, Tada N. Neuroprotective effects of edaravone: a novel free radical scavenger in cerebrovascular injury. *CNS Drug Rev.* 2006,12:9-20.

Zanker KS, Kroczek R. In vitro synergic activity of 5-fluorouracil with low dose ozone against a chemoresistant tumor cell line and fresh human tumor cells. *Exp Chemother.* 1990,36:147-151.

Zhang Y, Cliff WJ, Schoefl GI, Higgins G. Immunochemical study of intimal microvessels in coronary atherosclerosis. *Am J Pathol.* 1993,143:164-172.

Zhang W, Sato K, Hayashi T, et. al. Extension of ischemic therapeutic window by a free radical scavenger, edaravone, reperfused with tPA in rat brain. *Neurol Res.*2004,26:342-348.

Zhang N, Komine-Kobayashi M, Tanaka R, Liu M, Mizuno Y, Urabe T. Edaravone reduces early accumulation of oxidative products and sequential inflammatory responses after transient focal ischemia in mice brain. *Stroke,* 2005,36:2220-2225.

Zielonka J, Gebicki J, Grynkiewicz G., Radical scavenging properties of Genistein. *Free Radic. Biol. Med.* 2003,35:958-965.

In: Thrombosis: Causes, Treatment and Prevention
Editor: D. G. Macri and L. D. Procaccini, pp. 53-92
ISBN 978-1-61668-696-3

Chapter II

THROMBOEMBOLIC COMPLICATIONS IN CHILDHOOD NEPHROPATHIES

Marco Zaffanello[1,*], Giuseppe Lippi[2], Milena Brugnara[1] and Massimo Franchini[2]

[1]University of Verona, Verona, Italy.
[2]University of Parma, Parma, Italy.

ABSTRACT

Several well-recognized glomerulopathies in children may result in nephrotic range proteinuria. A possible complication of nephrotic syndrome and its treatment is thromboembolic complications (TEC). Patients with membranous glomerulopathy with heavy proteinuria and lupus nephritis/antiphospholipid syndrome run the highest risk of thromboembolic complications. A lower incidence of TEC has been found in children with nephrotic syndrome as compared with adults with NS, although children had severe morbidity. Clinically silent thromboembolic complications may be much more common than previously reported in studies designed to collect data only from symptomatic events. Thus, this chapter covers the pathogenesis of thromboembolic complications in children with heavy proteinurias, either with acquired thrombophilia or associated with congenital hemostasis disorders. Moreover, the clinical features of patients experiencing venous and arterial thromboemolic complications in different areas of the body, such as the lungs, kidneys, brain and heart, will be described. The prevention of thromboembolism in patients at high risk, either through drugs or through appropriate management of the main condition, will be emphasized. In addition, treatment options after a thromboembolism has begun will be discussed. Patients with lupus nephritis/antiphospholipid syndrome run the highest risk of thromboembolic complications. Venous thrombosis is more frequent than arterial thrombosis. Systemic

* Correspondence concerning this article should be addressed to: Dr. Marco Zaffanello, MD, Department of Mother-Child and Biology-Genetics, University of Verona, Piazzale L. Scuro, 10, 37134 Verona, Italy. E-mail: marco.zaffanello@univr.it; Tel: +39 045 812 4469; Fax: +39 045 812 4790.

lupus eritematosus patients with nephritis are more prone to arterial thromboembolic complications than those without renal involvement. The chapter also covers the pathogenesis of TEC in lupus nephritis patients, with particular emphasis on antiphospholipid antibodies. However, we present the clinical features of patients with either thrombotic microangiopathy or vasal thrombosis and their treatment options. Finally, a concise overview of physiological hemostasis is given.

INTRODUCTION

Physiological hemostasis encompasses a faint balance between anti- and pro-thrombotic forces, which ultimately maintain blood in a fluid state within the blood vessels or which trigger the development of blood clots after an endothelial injury. Traditionally, hemostasis develops through three distinct but subsequent phases (primary hemostasis; blood coagulation or secondary hemostasis; and fibrinolysis) which actively interplay and tightly cooperate to repair vessel wounds, promote vascular healing and otherwise maintain vessel patency. The perturbation of this delicate balance between hemorrhagic and pro-thrombotic forces could trigger excessive haemorrhaging (when anti-thrombotic forces prevail) or undue thrombosis (when pro-thrombotic forces prevail) [1].

Although a definitive comprehension of all the puzzling phases of hemostasis is far from being achieved, recent scientific discoveries have allowed a satisfactory description of the mechanisms that regulate this challenging system. Primary hemostasis is thereby traditionally defined as the formation of a primary platelet plug that involves the active cooperation of platelets, blood vessel components and the von Willebrand factor (VWF). This initial step leads to the formation of a fragile platelet clot, which is, however, effective in stopping or limiting the bleeding immediately after a vessel injury. Immediately afterwards, secondary hemostasis (blood coagulation) begins, which is essential to ensure stability of the primary platelet plug. The complex model of blood coagulation was originally described by two independent groups in the early 1960s [2,3] and involves a broad series of coordinated and calcium-dependent conversions of proenzymes to the respective serine proteases. The goal of this complex model, which has some analogies with that of the complement system, is the conversion (activation) of prothrombin to thrombin. Basically, the single reactions are catalyzed by an enzymatic molecule which has the inherent potential to activate several specific substrates in sequence so that the huge amplificatory potential of blood coagulation is easily understandable. Nevertheless, activation, amplification and propagation of the coagulation cascade and stabilization of the blood clot are efficiently regulated by the activity of specific proteases (the protein C and protein S systems) and allosteric or enzymatic inhibitors (Tissue Factor Pathway Inhibitor and antithrombin). A major breakthrough in understanding physiological hemostasis was represented by the evidence that severe deficiencies of clotting factor XII (FXII), high-molecular-weight kininogen and prekallikrein are not associated with any clinically significant bleeding tendency [4]. This led to revolutionizing the traditional model of blood coagulation, classically divided between intrinsic and extrinsic pathways, since activation of the former pathway does not provide a substantial contribution to the initiation of the hemostatic process ex vivo. It is to mention here, however, that the activation of coagulation factor X (FX) by the extrinsic pathway appears to be still inefficient in boosting the thrombin burst and counteracting moderate to severe deficits of clotting factors VIII (FVIII) and IX (FIX), which are associated with traditional hemophilia A and B disorders. These observations paved the way for an innovative view of the blood coagulation system, placing thrombin generation at the centre of the whole hemostatic process. Accordingly, the system develops through sequential steps, in which the extrinsic pathway plays a predominant (exclusive) role in activation; whereas the factors of the intrinsic pathway enable the subsequent amplification and propagation of the so-called "hemostatic burst" [1]. The high concentrations of thrombin generated through this mechanism are also necessary for the activation of the thrombin activatable fibrinolysis inhibitor (TAFI), which is essential to prevent the lysis of the fibrin clot by attenuation of the plasmin-mediated fibrin degradation.

In synthesis, therefore, the blood coagulation cascade involves several sequential steps including (i) activation of the extrinsic pathway and initiation of blood coagulation by Tissue Factor (TF) exposure on specific surfaces; (ii) preliminary thrombin generation catalyzed by an enzymatically active complex between activated factor VII (FVIIa) and TF; (iii) propagation and amplification of the enzymatic reactions (the "thrombin burst") promoted by the small amount of thrombin generated during the initial step, which in turn enables a feedback activation of the intrinsic pathway characterized by generation of numerous active enzymatic complexes; (iv) conversion of fibrinogen to fibrin; (v) fibrin polymerization and stabilization by coagulation factor XIII (FXIII) and TAFI; (vi) attenuation and termination of blood coagulation by natural inhibitors, which regulate the blood clot-growing process; and (vii) dissolution and elimination of the blood clot by a highly regulated enzymatic cascade (fibrinolysis) (Figure 1). The fibrinolytic process is then mediated by activation of the tissue-type plasminogen activator (tPA) and conversion of fibrin- bound plasminogen to plasmin. Fibrinolysis is also modulated by specific inhibitors including plasminogen activator inhibitor (PAI-1), plasminogen activator inhibitor-2 (PAI-2), a2-antiplasmin and a2-macroglobulin and TAFI [1].

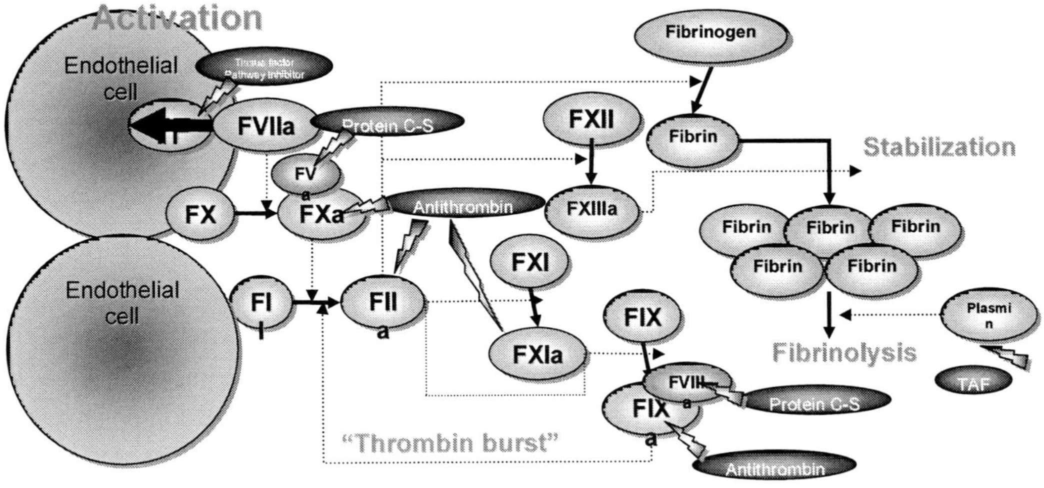

Figure 1.

NEPHROTIC SYNDROME

1. Introduction

1.1. Definition of Nephrotic Syndrome:

Proteinuria can occur in association with primary or secondary glomerular disorders and glomerulonephritis. The most severe form of proteinuria is nephrotic syndrome. The main clinical features of nephrotic syndrome are heavy proteinuria (at least 3.5 grams per day per 1.73m2 body surface area), hypoalbuminemia, hyperlipidemia and edema. Nephrotic syndrome is most commonly idiopathic in nature, resulting from any of several well-described primary glomerulopathies defined by histopathology and clinical criteria. Idiopathic nephrotic syndrome has an incidence of 2-7 per 100,000 children and a prevalence of about 16 cases per 100,000 children per year. However, several well-recognized secondary glomerulopathies may result in nephrotic range proteinuria [5].

Common complications of nephrotic syndrome and its treatment include infection, cardiovascular disease, bone mineral loss, acute renal failure and thromboembolic complications [5]. In particular, thromboembolic complications in patients with nephrotic syndrome result from acquired or congenital coagulopathy (Table 1) or disturbances in hemostasis [6].

Table 1. Acquired and inherited thrombophilia in children with nephrotic syndrome

Acquired thrombophilia	***Conditions***	***Pathophysiology***
AT III	Serum reduction	Urinary loss
Protein S	Serum reduction	Urinary loss
Protein S	Raised activity	Increased hepatic synthesis
Protein C	Raised activity	Increased hepatic synthesis
Fibrin network	Hypofibrinolysis	Abnormal conformation
Proteins S and C levels	Serum reduction	Increased binding proteins
Platelets	Dysfunctional, Increased activation	Increased number, increased synthesis of thromboxane
t-PA, PAI-1	Increased concentration	Cyclosporine A
Inherited thrombophilia		
Protein-C, protein-S, ATIII		Defect
Lipoprotein (a)		Raised
Coagulation factors V and II		Gene mutations
Factor V Leiden		Presence
Prothrombin variant (20210G>A)		Presence
MTHFR gene		Gene mutation

1.2. Thromboembolic Complications in Nephrotic Syndrome

The incidence of thromboembolic complications (arterial or venous thrombosis, pulmonary embolism) is approximately 35% in all patients [7]. In pediatric ages, the incidence of thromboembolic complications appears to peak in infancy, with a secondary adolescent peak at approximately 12 years of age. From the Canadian Paediatric Thrombophilia Registry, the overall mortality rate caused by deep venous thrombosis/pulmonary embolism was 2.2% (9 out of 405 children) [8,9].

However, several studies have reported an incidence of thromboembolic complications in children with idiopathic nephrotic syndrome ranging from 1.8%-5%, and an estimated higher incidence in adults ranging from 20% to 30% [5,10-13]. A retrospective study of 16 children with steroid responsive minimal change nephrotic syndrome reported that 27.9% of them showed evidence of previous thromboembolic complications assessed by combined scintigraphic pulmonary ventilation and perfusion studies. Thus, the authors suggested that clinically silent thromboembolic complications might be much more common than previously estimated [14]. Patients with membranous glomerulopathy and heavy proteinuria showed the highest risk of thromboembolic complications. Renal venous thrombosis was found in 13 out of 27 patients with membranous glomerulopathy [15]. Moreover, there was platelet hyperaggregability in 31.5% of 64 nephrotic patients, although thromboembolic complications occurred in six of these subjects [16]. However, Louis et al reported two pediatric cases of membranous nephropathy with thromboembolic complications with no evidence of predisposing factors or coagulation abnormalities [17].

Although thromboembolic complications are reported to be less common in children than in adults, the consequences are more severe [11,18,19]. In a recent cohort study, the authors investigated the occurrence of thromboembolic complications in children with primary nephrotic syndrome (steroid-sensitive nephrotic syndrome, minimal-change nephrotic syndrome, focal segmental glomerulosclerosis, mesangial proliferative glomerulonephritis, membranous nephropathy) and secondary nephrotic syndrome (lupus erytematosus, crescentic glomerulonephritis, IgA nephropathy, Henoch-Shoenlein purpura nephritis). Thromboembolic complications were found in 6.6% of patients with primary nephrotic syndrome, a percentage similar to previous reports for primary nephrotic syndrome, and in 17.1% of those with secondary nephrotic syndrome. Nearly 10% of the children developed symptomatic thromboembolic complications during treatment, and more than 20% of these were life- or limb-threatening [20].

2. Pathogenesis

Maintenance of hemostasis involves a number of processes including formation of platelet plugs through platelet activation and aggregation, activation of the clotting cascade initiated by exposure of the tissue factor at sites of vessel wall injury, termination of the clotting cascade through a variety of inhibitors, and dissolution of the formed clot via plasmin (fibrinolysis).

Thrombosis in nephrotic syndrome may arise from a preferential loss of proteins involved in the inhibition of systemic hemostasis, an increased synthesis of factors promoting thrombosis, or from local activation of the glomerular hemostasis system [7]. Massive proteinuria and severe hypoalbuminemia play a predictive role in high thrombotic risk [18,21]. The classical risk factors for thrombosis during nephrotic syndrome are severe hypoalbuminemia (<20 g/L), proteinuria over 3g/24h, low plasma antithrombin III levels and fibrinogen levels above 6g/L [22]. Predisposing factors, personal and family history of thromboembolic complications and the evolution of the disease should always be investigated in any child with nephrotic syndrome. Other co-existing factors not specific to nephrotic syndrome, such as venous stasis associated with immobility or venous injury related to catheterization procedures, may also play a role [22].

The pathogenesis of hypercoagulable states can be classified as acquired if it is a consequence of heavy proteinuria, whether congenital or genetic, only if causally associated with nephrotic syndrome.

2.1. Acquired Thrombophilia

There are usually multiple abnormalities in the coagulation pathways in nephrotic syndrome (Table 2); in fact, a number of hemostatic abnormalities have been described in nephrotic syndrome. The increased synthesis of coagulation factors (fibrinogen and factors II, V, VII, VIII, X, and XIII), platelet anomalies (thrombocytosis and increased platelet aggregation), hypofibrinolysis, hyperviscosity and hyperlipidemia facilitate thromboembolic complications in nephrotic syndrome. Other factors, such as an acute reduction of plasma volume due to the use of diuretics or from intercurrent episodes of gastroenteritis, can increase the risk of thrombosis in patients with nephrotic syndrome [12,23-26].

Table 2. Leading causes of hypercoagulable states and tromboembolic complications in nephrotis syndrome

Increased in platelet aggregability	-
Increase in fibrinogen and factor I, II, V, VII, VIII, X and XIII	Increased hepatic synthesis
Decreased levels of antithrombin III (heparin cofactor), protein C and S, and factors XI and XII	Loss in the urine An increase in C-protein activity in nephrotic syndrome patients represents a protective mechanism against thrombosis.
Increase in fibrinolytic system components (e.g. tissue plasminogen activator and plasminogen activator inhibitor-1)	The fibrinolytic system also plays an important role in preventing the thrombotic activity in these patients

2.1.1. Platelet Activation and Aggregation

Enhanced platelet reactivity may play a significant role in the genesis of the hypercoagulable state of nephrotic syndrome [27]. However, platelets are dysfunctional and often more numerous in nephrotic syndrome patients. The increased activation of blood platelets may be an independent risk factor of thromboembolic complications in the early stages of a nephrotic syndrome relapse [28-34]. Studies on intrinsic platelet abnormality have shown a reduced negative surface charge of isolated nephrotic platelets with possible increased binding of VWF to glycoprotein Ib [35].

A study of 18 patients with nephrotic syndrome evaluated platelet function using a variety of methods [36]. Platelet hyperaggregability was seen in 72% of patients;

reproducible markers of platelet activation, including plasma P-selectin levels and circulating CD62P-positive platelets, were higher in nephrotic patients than in healthy controls. Another study on pediatric patients also found increased CD62P expression present during early relapse of nephrotic syndrome but not during remission [33]. Hyperaggregability has a multifactorial pathogenesis and is associated with low serum albumin, hypercholesterolemia and hyperfibrinogenemia [37].

Hypolabuminemia

Hypoalbuminemia leads to an increased availability of free arachidonic acid resulting in the increased formation of the proaggregatory agent thromboxane A2 in platelets [30,32], which sustains platelet aggregation [30,38-40]. Platelet hyperaggregability from other stimuli, such as ADP, collagen and ristocetin, could not be related to hypoalbuminemia. This suggests that the presence of additional plasma factors could be involved in platelet hyperaggregability [32,37].

Hypercholesterolemia

Remarkably high levels of LDL cholesterol in the nephrotic patient [41] may increase in vitro platelet aggregation, as has been observed in patients with familial hypercholesterolemia [42]. In agreement with this hypothesis, 12 weeks of lipid lowering treatment resulted in the disappearance of spontaneous hyperaggregability in nephrotic syndrome. However, the increased aggregation when exposed to arachidonic acid persisted in these experiments [43].

Nephrotic patients have high levels of LDLs, which are probably enriched with lysolecithin [41,44]. Such modified LDL is toxic, particularly for the endothelium, and leads to impaired production of nitric oxide [45]. Since nitric oxide has been advocated as an inhibitor of platelet adhesion [46], it is possible that some patients with nephrotic syndrome produce less nitric oxide.

Amelioration of hypercholesterolemia by HMG-CoA reductase inhibitor (Pravastatin) improved platelet hyperaggregability in nephrotic patients [47].

Hyperfibrinogenemia

Hyperfibrinogenemia is invariably present in nephrotic patients. Platelet aggregability has beencorrelated with plasmatic fibrinogen in nephrotic subjects [32]. Hyperfibrinogenemia may contribute to the procoagulant state by providing more substrate for the formation of fibrin and by promoting increased blood viscosity and red blood cell aggregation [43]. Furthermore, augmented concentrations of fibrinogen, a ligand of glyeoprotein IIb-IIIa receptors on activated platelets, enhanced spontaneous platelet aggregation in platelet-rich suspensions [28]. Increased fibrin deposits, however, may also occur due to the increased formation of thrombin, in turn due to the high levels of factors V and VIII [48]. Fibrinogen is also known to be a risk factor for venous thromboembolism in patients without nephrotic syndrome [49,50]. Moreover, abnormal fibrin network conformation may be involved in hypofibrinolysis. Therefore, albumin supplementation partially restored normal fibrin architecture and increased the rate of fibrinolysis [51].

Increased platelet release product thromboglobulin

The presence of increased in vivo platelet activation is supported by levels of the platelet-released product thromboglobulin [32,46,52-56]. Activation of the coagulation cascade was confirmed by higher serum concentrations of prothrombin fragments during follow-up [33]. Levels of plasma β-thromboglobulin, plasma P-selectin and CD62P/CD63-positive platelets were significantly higher in nephrotic syndrome patients than in healthy controls [36].

2.1.2. Hyperthrombocitemia

Nephrotic syndrome without clinical thromboembolic complications had a higher number of platelets of reduced volume and greater size diversity, but with normal total mass; they also showed a greater release of PDGF into the blood [34].

2.1.3. Increased Thrombomodulin, Plasminogen Activator Inhibitor-1 and von Willebrand Factor

Plasma thrombomodulin, plasminogen activator inhibitor-1 (PAI-1) and von Willebrand factor (VWF) activity were found to be greater in nephrotic children (aged 2-18 years) with early NS relapse. However, VWF persisted to be higher in drug-free remission [28,57].

2.1.4. Increaed Platelet-vessel wall Interaction

The expected increase in platelet adherence by high VWF, decreased red blood cell deformation and platelet hyperaggregation are possibly neutralized by fibrinogen binding to glycoprotein IIb-IIIa, thereby interfering with VWF-glycoprotein IIb-IIIa mediated adhesive processes [28]. However, the increased risk of acute thromboembolic complications in nephrosis was not adequately explained by a strongly enhanced platelet-vessel wall interaction. Therefore, the main determinant of in vivo platelet-vessel wall interaction is blood flow. Thus, the models of injured vessel walls used in perfusion studies do not take into account modifications of the vessel wall that may occur in in vivo nephrotic syndrome [43].

2.1.5. Increased Fibrin Formation

Increased formation of fibrin may also cause the pre-thrombotic state of nephrotic syndrome. In in vitro studies [28], nephrotic blood forms extensive fibrin deposits, even at high flow rates, whereas control blood tends to form substantial fibrin networks only at lower venous flow rates [28]. The increased fibrin generation has not been associated with increased fragment 1.2 formation, which is cleaved from prothrombin during its activation [28]. This suggests that activation of the coagulation cascade was not enhanced in these patients. Therefore, in these patients a more effective fibrinogen-fibrin transition seems to be an explanation for the massive fibrin deposits. The obvious cause is availability of a greater substrate. A strong correlation between fibrin deposits and hyperfibibrinogenemia constitutes an important risk factor for thrombus formation. In agreement, the addition of fibrinogen to control perfusate also resulted in greater fibrin deposits [28]. Increased fibrin deposits in these studies were associated with decreased platelet adhesion directly to the subendothelium, illustrating the more clotting-dependent hemostasis in nephrotic patients.

Accelerated fibrinogen-induced fibrin formation contributes to the thrombotic risk of these patients. In vivo fibrin deposits in nephrotic subjects are also explained by high levels of circulating fibrinopeptide A and high-molecular-weight fibrin complexes [58,59]. Fibrin networks promote the inclusion of red blood cells and other cellular elements, and thus the formation of a mixed thrombus [60]. Furthermore, fibrin deposits are also present in atherosclerotic lesions and seem to contribute to atherosclerosis by causing disorganization of endothelial cells by stimulating the proliferation of vascular smooth muscle cells and by providing an adsorptive surface for accumulation of LDL [61,62]. However, high fibrinogen in renal vein blood correlates with intraglomerular fibrin deposits and may contribute to the development of glomerular injury [63]. Finally, in nephrosis, hyperfibrinogemia increases blood viscosity [64] and red blood cell aggregation [65,66]. These changes decrease organ blood flow and also contribute to the formation of a mixed thrombus.

2.1.6. Increased Thrombin Formation

An accepted cause of increased thromboembolic risk is the less effective inhibition of the coagulation cascade that stimulates thrombin formation. Although data on increased thrombin formation and thrombin activity are sometimes conflicting in nephrosis, it is very likely that these mechanisms do occur in a subset of nephrotic patients. A greater formation of thrombin may be caused by increased levels of clotting factors V and VIII, which are often found in NS [27,67].

2.1.7. Decreased Fibrinolytic Activity

The thrombotic risk of nephrosis is enhanced by decreased fibrinolytic activity. Most studies have focused on plasminogen, the precursor of plasmin.

Decreased plasminogen levels

Decreased fibrinolysis in nephrotic patients may be caused by lower levels of plasminogen [68], which has been shown to correlate with the magnitude of the proteinuria [69]. Albumin appears to be a co-factor for the binding of plasminogen to fibrin and the subsequent interaction with tissue plasminogen activator (tPA) [70].

Increased levels of α2-antiplasmin

High levels of α2-antiplasmin in some patients will further contribute to the hypofibrinolytic state by inhibiting plasmin and interfering with its binding to fibrin [71].

Elevated levels of Lp(a)

Patients with nephrotic syndrome have high levels of Lp(a) [72-74], which has a close structural similarity to plasminogen [75]. In vitro studies have shown that Lp(a) can compete with plasminogen in binding to fibrinogen or fibrin and may inhibit the fibrin-dependent enhancement of plasminogen activation by tissue plasminogen activator (t-PA) [76,77].

2.1.8. Increased Factor XIII, Fibronectin and Fibrinogen

Plasma and urine concentrations of factor XIII and its circulating substrates (fibronectin, fibrinogen, and alpha 2-antiplasmin) are found to be high in nephrotic syndrome and are considered to be the result of a combination of increased synthesis and possibly contracted intravascular distribution of these macromolecular proteins in light of their negligible loss in the urine [78].

2.1.9. Antithrombin III, Protein C and S Deficiency

Several studies have reported lower levels of plasma antithrombin III in nephrotic patients [79] due to gross proteinuria, hypoalbuminemia [80,81] and excess thrombin generation [14]. However, normal or high levels of antithrombin III have also been found in patients with nephrotic syndrome [27,68,82].

The thrombotic risk is most evident at the onset of NS when serum ATIII levels are low. Antithrombin III deficiency leads to less effective inhibition of thrombin that results in increased coagulant activity and subsequent fibrin formation [80,83,84]. Several children with very low plasma antithrombin III levels and fibrinogen levels above 750 mg/dl were at risk for deep vein thrombosis [7].

High levels of plasma protein C, which inactivates factors V and VIII and its co-factor S, have been reported in several studies. Low levels of protein S have also been observed [85-88]. Low free protein S levels in the serum are associated with a reduction of antithrombin III in nephrotic syndrome. Peripheral arterial thrombosis was observed in a child with longstanding nephrotic syndrome with both low acquired serum antithrombin III and protein S levels [89]. The levels of protein S, protein C and antithrombin III are frequently low in nephrotic syndrome because they are lost in the urine. Thromboembolic complications in patients with nephrotic syndrome could be due to combined low plasma antithrombin III, protein S and protein C deficiency, albumin, high fibrinogen and cholesterol levels [18,90]. Furthermore, anticoagulant proteins S and C in the serum may also remain functionally inactive because of an increase in the hepatic synthesis of binding proteins for protein S and protein C [19]. Ozkayyn et al found a significant decline in ATIII levels in patients with NS and a significant increase in protein C, thrombin antithrombin complex and D-Dimer levels in the same study group. The significant increase in protein C activity could be an intrinsic protective mechanism against thrombosis. A marked increase in proteins C and S may counterbalance the reduction of ATIII [25].

2.1.10. Low Protein Z Levels

Protein Z (PZ) is a single-chain vitamin K-dependent glycoprotein that is synthesized by the liver. Its structure is very similar to vitamin K-dependent coagulation factors such as factors XII, IX, X and protein C [90-93]. Several authors have shown that low levels of protein Z is a risk factor for thromboembolic complications [94,95]. Protein Z plays an important role in inhibiting coagulation since it serves as cofactor for the inactivation of activated factor X by forming a complex with the plasma protein Z-dependent protease inhibitor. It was found to promote the bonding of thrombin with phospholipid vesicles in a Ca-dependent fashion, which could promote coagulation [96].

Low plasma PZ has been reported to be associated with a prothrombotic state. Several papers suggested that low PZ levels increased the frequency of ischemic stroke [94,95,97]. A significant decrease in plasma protein Z was found in proteinuric patients when compared with patients in remission or healthy controls. A negative correlation between proteinuria and

PZ levels and a positive correlation with serum albumin levels and PZ levels suggest the possibility of renal PZ loss, although this has not been proven by urinary tests [98].

2.1.11. Antiphospholipid Antibodies

Potential underlying prothrombotic conditions in children with NS include acquired antiphospholipid antibodies or the lupus anticoagulant.

2.1.12. Membranous Nephropathy

Membranous nephropathy is inherently thrombogenic, for poorly inderstood reasons. However, TEC are more frequent when the NS is due to membranous nephropathy rather than other causes of NS [22].

2.1.13. Medical Interventions

Central venous access device

A central venous access device is a well-known risk factor for TEC in children [8]. More than half of the TEC that develop within months of a NS diagnosis and nearly half of the children who develop symptomatic TEC during treatment were associated with the use of central venous access devices [20]. In a cohort study, the authors concluded that a central venous access device should be avoided whenever possible and particular vigilance should be maintained when the use of a central venous access device is deemed necessary for supportive care of patients with NS [20].

Medications

Certain medication (including steroids and diuretics) as well as immobilization may increase the risk of TEC in children with NS [5,99]. The risk of TEC in NS is increased by hyperviscosity of the blood caused by hyperfibrinogenemia and intravascular volume depletion resulting from an inappropriate use of diuretics [23]. Thus, a very important cause of thrombosis in NS that should always be kept in mind is volume depletion, especially when iatrogenic through over vigorous diuresis [7].

2.2. Inherited Thrombophilia

Genetic prothrombotic defects in protein C, protein S and ATIII deficiency, mutations of coagulation factors II and V and high lipoprotein (a) are established risk factors for TEC [13]. In NS, acquired hypercoagulability (ATIII deficiency, increased concentrations of fibrinogen, factors V and VIII and platelet hyperaggregability) could coincide with the underlying inherited thrombophilia [100,101]. In fact, screening for inherited thrombophilia failed to identify inherited risk factors although TEC occured in 11% of children with NS [100]. These data support the hypothesis that there is a low incidence of inherited thombogenic factors in NS patients with thrombosis. Likewise, only one child has been reported with steroid-dependent NS and a homozygous mutation of the MTHFR gene, who developed thrombosis in the superior mesenteric artery [102]. In addition, in a young man with concomitant deep vein thrombosis, idiopathic NS and resistance to activated protein C, the factor V Leiden was found to increase the risk of thrombosis [103]. Moreover, Martinez and co-workers found an increased prevalence of heterozygous factor V Leiden in patients with glomerulonephritis and a history of thrombotic events [104].

Potential inherited thrombophilia could be due to factor V Arg506>Gln mutation (factor V Leiden), prothrombin variant (20210G>A) and homozygosity of Ala677>Val in the methylenetetrahydrofolate reductase gene (MTHFR). Other potential prothrombotic conditions in childhood may include abnormalities of protein C, protein S and ATIII. Moreover, abnormalities could result in increased lipoprotein (a) and hyperprothrombinemia due to the prothrombin G20210A mutation [105,106].

3. Clinical Features

Venous thromboembolic complications in nephrotic syndrome include venous and artery thrombosis, pulmonary embolism and renal vein thrombosis (Table 3). Although deep vein thrombosis, pulmonary embolism and renal venous thrombosis occur most often, thrombosis of peripheral and coronary arteries has been described [6,7,15,27,55,107]. Of 326 patients with nephrotic syndrome evaluated retrospectively, the Midwest Pediatric Nephrology Consortium study reported that 13.3% of 38 patients with thromboembolic complications were diagnosed simultaneously with nephrotic syndrome. Thromboembolic complications included 76.3% of patients with deep venous thrombosis, 21.1% with pulmonary embolism, only 1 patient with arterial thrombus, and 1 with thrombosed arteriovenous fistula. Out of all the cases of pulmonary embolism and arterial thrombus, 23.7% were considered potentially life- or limb-threatening, an incidence of 6.1 life- or limb-threatening thromboembolic complications per 1000 patient-years [20].

Table 3. Clinical syndromes and risk factors of thromboembolic complications in nephrotic patients

Clinical syndrome	*Risk factor*
Pulmonary emboli	Hypovolemia
Pulmonary artery thrombosis	Hyperviscosity
Cerebral venous thrombosis	Low antithrombin III
Renal vein thrombosis	High fibrinogen
Peripheral venous and artery thrombosis	Platelet hyperaggregability, hyperlipemia

3.1. Pulmonary Embolism

Basis of the Problem

An uncommon, but known and severe complication of nephrotic syndrome is pulmonary embolism, which was the second most frequent thromboembolic complication found in 27.9% of the 26 children with nephrotic syndrome studied with systematic ventilation-perfusion scintigraphy [14]. Of 20 young nephrotic patients evaluated, Huang et al reported 8 cases (aged 5 to 12 years) with pulmonary embolism. Most of them (7/8 patients) did not present clinical signs or symptoms [108]. In another series, Cherng et al investigated 89 patients with nephrotic syndrome and found that 21% had a high probability of pulmonary embolism, based on positive pulmonary angiograms and on high-probability lung scans. However, pulmonary angiography found that 10 (11%) other patients had pulmonary embolism despite having lung scan findings categorized as intermediate or having a low probability of pulmonary embolism [109]. Finally, the relative risk of pulmonary embolism for patients (all ages) hospitalized with nephrotic syndrome was 1.39 (1.35-1.43) times greater than those patients without nephrotic syndrome [110].

Symptoms

All physicians should be aware of the possible complications of pulmonary embolism when treating nephrotic patients. Pulmonary embolism may be a complication of deep vein thrombosis involving the lower extremities, inferior vena cava or renal venous thrombosis. Pulmonary thrombosis may have subtle symptoms in children [111,112] but requires prompt diagnosis and treatment to prevent fatal outcomes [113]. In particular, a pulmonary embolism should be kept in mind for children with tachypnea [114], whether intermittent or persistent, especially when other venous thromboembolic risk factors are present, in order to avoid delay in starting anticoagulant treatment and a fatal outcome [115]. Moreover, tachycardia and shortness of breath might be the only signs indicating pulmonary thrombosis [116]. The potential severity of pulmonary embolism requires that this diagnosis must be systematically ruled out in patients with nephrotic syndrome who suffer from chest pain or isolated dyspnea [113].

Radiology

Pulmonary embolism should be suspected in cases of pulmonary or cardiovascular symptoms and can be ruled out with angiography or angioscintigraphy. Pulmonary embolism is not a rare complication in patients with NS and is usually clinically silent. Coagulation disturbances in children are no less severe than in adults with nephrotic syndrome. In fact, Hoyer et al suggested that scintigraphic pulmonary ventilation and perfusion studies are valuable tools to diagnose subclinical pulmonary embolism in nephrotic children [14]. A significant incidence of abnormal ventilation/perfusion scans was found in adult nephrotic patients who had no clinical evidence of pulmonary thrombosis, suggesting that the real incidence of thromboembolism in nephrotic syndrome may be even higher. Cheng et al suggested that "serial" ventilation/perfusion lung scans in 29 adult patients with nephrotic syndrome proved to be a valuable follow-up practice. With the exception of plasma fibrinogen and antithrombin III levels, clinical symptoms and signs, electrocardiogram findings, chest x-rays and results of hematochemical testing were not consistent with the occurrence of pulmonary embolism [109]. In 8 out of 20 nephrotic children with high plasma D-Dimer, Huang et al identified a thromboembolic lung complication through pulmonary perfusion imaging and chest radiography [108]. Deshpande et al confirmed pulmonary thrombosis and thromboembolism in two young girls aged 12 years with CT pulmonary angiography scans [115].

Treatment

Possible pulmonary embolism should be kept in mind for children with tachypnea, especially when other venous thromboembolic risk factors are present, in order to avoid delaying anticoagulant treatment and possible death [117]. Pulmonary thrombosis in two tachypneic young girls presenting with severe edema in NS relapse was diagnosed by CT pulmonary angiography. They were treated with continuous heparin infusion with resolution of the pulmonary thromboembolism [118]. The risk of death for nephrotic syndrome patients with lung thromboembolic complications could increase if treatment is delayed. Lung perfusion scans, thrombolytic therapy (streptokinase, heparin and warfarin) and follow-up therapy are very important [114].

Prognosis

The mortality rate of nephrotic patients with lung theromboembolic complications could go up if they are not treated in time. Lung perfusion scans, thrombolytic therapy, for instance streptokinase (2000 IU/kg as bolus followed by 2000 IU/kg/h for 12 h), heparin and warfarin, and follow-up therapy are essential [114].

3.2. Renal Venous Thrombosis

Basis of the problem

Advanced roentgenographic techniques and renal vein catheterization have made it clear that renal venous thrombosis is a consequence of nephrotic syndrome [67,119,120]. More than 80% of cases of renal venous thrombosis in adults occur within the context of nephrotic syndrome from membranous nephropathy. In particular, in 12 out of 36 patients with renal vein thrombosis, the renal pathology was membranous glomerulonephritis in 10 and membranoproliferative glomerulonephritis in 2 [121]. From another study, of 33 patients with renal vein thrombosis, 20 had membranous nephropathy [119]. Several studies reported that the prevalence of renal venous thrombosis was 6.8%-48.1% in patients with primary glomerular diseases, the highest percentage for patients with membranoproliferative glomerulonephritis and minimal change disease [15,120]. A large prospective study of 151 adult patients with nephrotic syndrome showed that 22% of cases developed renal venous thrombosis. However, acute renal venous thrombosis tended to be present in young adults, whereas chronic renal venous thrombosis occurred more frequently in the older patients [119]. Renal venous thrombosis was the most frequently detected form of thromboembolic complications (42.3%) in 26 adult patients with idiopathic nephrotic syndrome, although it was asymptomatic in more than 90% of cases [122]. The relative risk for deep venous thrombosis in hospitalized patients of all ages with nephrotic syndrome was 1.72 (1.70-1.75) times that of non-nephrotic patients [110].

Necropsy analysis showed that 8 out of 21 (38%) children with renal vein thrombosis had some connection with nephrotic syndrome [123]. Finally, systematic investigations have shown that renal venous thrombosis was present in three out of 38 children with nephrotic syndrome [20].

Clinical features

Renal venous thrombosis is probably asymptomatic in most cases, but it may present with side pain, sudden macroscopic hematuria or by unexplained rapid deterioration of renal function [6,7,15]. However, Doppler ultrasonography may show an enlarged kidney and an absence of blood flow in the renal vein [119]. Generally, hematuria is rare in membranous glomerulopathy. Thus, hematuria in patients with membranous glomerulopathy would be a clinical sign suggesting renal vein thrombosis [15].

3.3. Cerebral Venous Thrombosis

The Canadian Pediatric Ischemic Stroke Registry (Toronto Site) between 1992 and 2004 identified a total of 85 children aged 2.5 to 8.5 years with cerebral sinovenous thrombosis. The most consistent biological risk factors were severe hypoalbuminemia (n=14) and, to a lesser extent, decreased antithrombin III levels (n=9/16) [124]. Appenzeller and co-workers, investigating 24 patients with a mean age of 29.5 years (range 3-48 years), showed that the etiology of cerebral venous thrombosis could be determined in 88 % of these patients but only 1 patient had nephrotic syndrome [125]. Thus, cerebral venous thrombosis is a rare complication of NS.

Clinical features

Obviously, the main clinical features have neurological patterns varying from mild to severe. In a 7-year-old Chinese boy with steroid-resistant nephrotic syndrome, the main clinical pattern was status epilepticus and coma [117]. Another 7-year-old child with secondary steroid-resistant nephrotic syndrome had headaches and facial palsies [126]. An 8.5-year-old female child with steroid- resistant nephrotic syndrome had recurrent vomiting, headaches and impaired consciousness [127]; a 5-year-old boy with FV-Leiden heterozygous for the G1691A mutation suffered swelling of the eyelids and legs [128]. Therefore, even subtle symptoms can be alerting manifestations. A young boy with nephrotic syndrome and dehydration had vague neurological symptoms and seizures. Subsequently, he had seizures and cerebral sinovenous thrombosis [118]. From a large 12-year study, a total of 85 children were found to have cerebral sinovenous thrombosis, but only four children had nephrotic syndrome. In general, in the majority of cases clinical manifestations included seizures and signs of high intracranial pressure such as headache, vomiting, lethargy and irritability. Papilloedema was observed in half of the patients. Focal neurological deficits including cranial nerve palsy and hemiparesis were reported less frequently [124].

Imaging

Sinovenous thrombosis may be documented either by computer tomography with venography and/or magnetic resonance imaging with or without magnetic resonance venography. Magnetic resonance imaging with venography was important in the early diagnosis of a cerebral sinus thrombosis [117] in a 5-year-old boy; cranial MRI angiography revealed thromboses in the superior sagittal sinus and right transverse sinus [128]. From a large review study, the most frequently used technique was neuroimaging with CT scans with contrast enhancement followed by magnetic resonance imaging with venography [124].

Treatment

A young child with thalamic stroke secondary to straight sinus thrombosis was treated successfully with low-molecular-weight heparin at 90 U/kg/day (subcutaneously and continuously for 2 weeks) and warfarin at an initial dose of 0.125 mg/kg/day and titrated by monitoring PT levels for the next 3 months [117]. Two young children, one with steroid-responsive nephrotic syndrome and the other with steroid-resistant nephrotic syndrome, who developed thrombosis of the superior sagittal sinus, were successfully treated without anticoagulant therapy [129] or with subcutaneous low-molecular-weight heparin (2 mg/kg /day) [127], respectively. Duration of treatment with heparin therapy at a dose of 6 mg/kg/day was 3–6 months in the case of a 7-year-old boy suffering from secondary steroid-resistant nephrotic syndrome [126]. Another 5-year-old boy received unfractioned heparin (starting with 20 U/kg/hour) for 10 days as the initial anticoagulant therapy followed by low-molecular-weight heparin for the following 2 months [128]. From one large study, of the 21 patients discussed, 20 received anticoagulant therapy- initial low-molecular-weight heparin (seven patients) and standard unfractioned heparin (13 patients). Duration of treatment varied and ranged from 3 to 5 months in the Toronto patients. No bleeding complications were reported [124]. Current recommendations are either unfractioned heparin or low-molecular-weight heparin for 5 to 7 days followed by low-molecular-weight heparin or vitamin K antagonists for 3 to 6 months [130].

Since efficient heparin therapy requires adequate levels of antithrombin, which is often low in nephrotic patients, direct replacement or addition of antithrombin III from fresh frozen plasma could be necessary [131]. To ensure an optimal outcome in cerebral sinovenous thrombosis, it is essential to begin anticoagulant therapy with heparin and fresh frozen plasma to correct antithrombin III levels [132]. Thromboses of the superior sagittal and straight sinuses, which led to thalamic stoke, were successfully treated with subcutaneous low-molecular-weight heparin and warfarin in children with steroid-resistant nephrotic syndrome [127,129,133].

Prophylactic treatment with warfarin was prescribed for a 6-year-old boy suffering from secondary steroid-resistant nephrotic syndrome because he had very low serum albumin levels following the first event of thromboembolic complications [126]. No prospective or randomized trial studies are available on the effectiveness of prophylactic treatment in these patients.

3.4. Venous and Arterial Thrombosis

Basis of the problem

In a prospective study on 151 patients of all ages with nephrotic syndrome, deep venous thrombosis was found to be associated with renal venous thrombosis in 33 patients [119]. A prospective study on 44 patients (12-65 years) with nephrotic syndrome found renal venous thrombosis in a deceased patient which extended beyond the renal veins to involve the inferior vena cava [120]. In a retrospective large study of 447 children with nephrotic syndrome, the incidence of thromboembolic complications was 2%; thromboembolic complications were predominantly venous (81%) and less frequently arterial (19%). The most commonly affected vessels were deep leg veins followed by the inferior vena cava. Rare locations of thromboembolic complications were also observed, such as the superior vena cava, the mesenteric artery and hepatic veins with the development of Budd-Chiari syndrome [134].

Arterial thromboembolism warrants attention in patients with nephrotic syndrome. In one case report and in an extensive review of the literature, 44 patients with nephrotic syndrome were reported to have arterial thromboembolic complications- thrombosis in aortic, renal, femoral, mesenteric, cerebral and brachial sites. The most common site in pediatric patients was the femoral artery [135]. Acute subclavian and brachial artery thromboses were reported as very rare complications of nephrotic syndrome in an adult patient [136].

Pathogenesis

The predisposition of patients with nephrotic syndrome to arterial thromboembolism has been only partially explained. Low serum levels of albuminemia and antithrombin III could be involved [80,135,137], although the latter has not been consistently found to be predictive of thromboembolism [11,16]. However, deep venous thrombosis and pulmonary embolism were found to be associated with acquired protein S deficiency in a pediatric case of nephrotic syndrome [138]. Two pediatric patients, 9 and 16 years old, with idiopathic membranous nephropathy and nephrotic syndrome, respectively, developed venous thromboses without the presence of known predisposing factors or coagulation abnormalities [17]. In a large cohort study including 30 patients between 1 and 21.6 years (mean 15.2 yrs), the majority of thromboembolic complications were deep venous thromboses (76.3%); the use of a central venous access device was associated with nearly half (44.8%) of these events [20].

Risk factors

Iatrogenic vessel trauma, dehydration and corticosteroid therapy are accepted as predisposing factors for thromboses. In a pediatric case of brachial artery thrombosis, arterial puncture was assumed to be the cause [135]. A large retrospective study on 447 children found that the major risk factors were iatrogenic, such as the administration of furosemide, which was responsible for thromboembolic complications in 7 out of 9 children. In some patients, additional predisposing factors were infections, trauma, venepuncture and immobilization [99]. Deep venous thrombosis was the most common thromboembolic complication associated with the use of a central venous catheter in 45% of patients with primary and secondary nephrotic syndrome [20].

Treatment

Therapy for thromboembolic complications in children with nephrotic syndrome has been reviewed in the literature [26]. The therapeutic approach to thrombosis in children employs anticoagulants (low-molecular-weight heparin) and/or fibrinolytic agents such as streptokinase, urokinase or tPA [104]. One retrospective study reports the therapeutic protocol for 9 children with thromboembolic complications. These children were treated with continuous infusions of heparin for 7–14 days with fresh-frozen plasma given at dosages that varied from 500 to 1,000 IU/kg per 24h. The partial thromboplastin time was maintained at twice the level of controls. Streptokinase was administered at a loading dosage of 2,000–3,300 U/kg followed by maintenance dosages of between 1,000 and 1,330 U/kg/hour for 3 consecutive days. The dosages were adjusted according to indicators of fibrinolysis. An indirect oral anticoagulant –4-oxycoumarin (Sintrom)– was administered for 6 months according to the prothrombin time with loading dosages varying between 6 and 10 mg/24 h, followed by maintenance dosages of 1–2 mg/24 h. However, prophylaxis with heparin in dosages between 150 and 200 IU/kg per 24h in 3 patients was unable to prevent new thromboembolic complications. No new thromboembolic complications occurred under oral anticoagulant prophylaxis [99]. Satisfactory thrombolysis of an arterial leg thrombosis with continuous catheter-directed low-dose rt-PA (alteplase; dose of 0.014-0.016 mg/kg/hr and continued for 4-5 days, with D-Dimer assessment) was achieved in two patients with recurring nephrotic syndrome. Subsequently, anticoagulation therapy was changed to low-molecular-weight heparin (150 IU/kg/ddat) and warfarin. [139]. Therefore, the most widely used thrombolytic agent for many years has been rTPA [140]. rTPA treatment in newborns was first reported in 1990 [141]. A caval thrombosis developed during the first days of life in a 10-day-old newborn with congenital nephrotic syndrome. After a trial of heparin (up to 20 IU/kg/hr) over a period of 24 hours and treatment with antithrombin III (2 x 250 IU/day) proved to be ineffective, systemic thrombolytic therapy with rTPA was started. An initial bolus of 0.4 mg/kg during 1 hour was followed by an infusion of 0.5 mg/kg/d rTPA over a period of 36 hours. Low-dose heparin (5 IU/kg/hour) was given simultaneously [142]. Although rTPA has proven to be effective in thrombolysis in pediatric patients and has no counter-indications in cases of nephrotic syndrome, to date there are no studies assessing its efficacy and safety in children [143].

3.5. Cardiac and Coronarial Thrombosis

Acute anterior myocardial infarction was found in a young man with nephrotic syndrome secondary to minimal change glomerulonephritis [144]. Also, a 7-year-old boy with a 5-year history of steroid-unresponsive nephrotic syndrome due to minimal change disease presented with acute myocardial infarction [145]. A hypercoagulable state resulting from nephrotic syndrome was suggested to be the cause of acute myocardial infarction in a 16-year-old boy with nephrotic syndrome secondary to membranoproliferative glomerulonephritis from the age of 8 years [146]. Finally, Weisz et al reported an asymptomatic intracardiac thrombus in a 6.5-year-old child with frequently relapsing steroid-sensitive NS and a ventricular septal defect [132].

4. Prevention

From a study of 64 nephrotic patients, neither platelet aggregation nor levels of antithrombin III, clotting factors or even fibrinogen had clear predictive value in identifying patients at risk for thromboembolic complications [16] who would be eligible for treatment. Another report advocated the importance of coagulation profiling in a study on 41 children (between 2 and 14 years) with relapse of nephrosis and 48 children (3 to 14 years) in remission. Doctors should be highly suspicious of thromboembolic complications in children with thrombocytosis, hyperfibrinogenemia, low levels of antithrombin III, increases in proteins C and S, and serum albumin levels below 2 g/dl [147]. Thus, anticoagulant therapy is recommended to prevent thromboemolic complications when such abnormalities are observed [24].

A previous history of thromboembolism in newly-diagnosed patients with nephrotic syndrome appears to be a particularly strong risk factor for additional thromboembolic complications after the development of nephrotic syndrome. Thus, these patients should be the object of preventive strategies [20]. Generally, prevention through mobilization, the avoidance of hemoconcentrations and treatment for early sepsis or volume depletion are highly recommended. Preventive strategies such as overaggressive diuresis should be avoided and the use of indwelling catheters should be limited because these practices may increase the likelihood of clotting complications. Since several compensatory mechanisms have explained the frequent absence of thrombotic incidents in children, the benefit of preventive antithrombotic treatment is often considered to be unsuitable. Finally, there are no randomized trials that support prophylactic anticoagulation therapy in the management of nephrotic syndrome. In general, prophylactic anticoagulation therapy is not recommended in children unless they have had previous thromboembolic events.

Prophylaxis with Heparin and Warfarin

There are no randomized clinical trials in the literature that support prophylactic anticoagulation for the management of nephrotic syndrome [22]. Oral anticoagulant prophylaxis (warfarin) requires careful case-by-case analysis of the risks for thromboembolic events in consideration of the risks for anticoagulant-induced bleeding [148,149]. In view of the higher risk of thromboembolic complications in patients with membranous glomerulonephritis [16], prophylactic anticoagulation therapy has been suggested for these patients in the setting of nephrotic syndrome [150,151].

Low levels of antithrombin III were counterbalanced, as a compensatory mechanism, by increased α2-macroglobulin and antithrombin activity, making the benefit of prophylactic heparin therapy questionable in 28 children with nephrotic syndrome [84]. Therefore, a pilot study on 10 adult nephrotic patients with biological markers of thrombosis risk prescribed enoxaparin 4,000 U daily for 3-12 months as preventive anticoagulation therapy; the clinicians found no obvious side effects and no thromboses were observed in the long term [152].

Prophylactic warfarin (0.125 mg/kg/day, titrated by monitoring PT levels for the next 3 months) has been suggested for patients with steroid-resistant nephrotic syndrome. In these patients, plasma albumin concentrations were below 20g/L, fibrinogen levels were over 6g/L, and antithrombin III levels were 70% less than normal values [117,153,154].

Prophylaxis with Antithrombin III

Thromboembolic complications in nephrotic syndrome have been associated with thrombophilic states (antithrombin III 37, normal 80–120%; D-Dimer 979, normal <500 μg/l) and/or use of diuretics. Still, prophylactic treatment with an intravenous infusion of highly purified, human, blood-derived antithrombin III (1,000 units, the same treatment was repeated 2 days later), before administering albumin infusion and diuretics, was given to a high-risk 7-year-old girl characterized by an altered coagulation profile [79]. The correction of diminished serum antithrombin III levels, by substituting antithrombin III concentrates, may be beneficial in cases when it is necessary to interrupt an enhanced coagulatory process during nephrotic syndrome. However, there are no structured studies in support of antithrombin III prophylaxis in patients with nephrotic syndrome and low levels of antithrombin III in serum. Theoretically, low-dose aspirin therapy should compensate for the low antithrombin III levels, although controlled trials of aspirin therapy are also lacking in regards to nephrotic patients.

5. Treatment

Treatment with antithrombotic agents usually begins after a thromboembolic incident [18], also in those patients with previously known risk factors. In the absence of trials that prospectively examined the efficacy of various therapeutic modalities, the choice of therapy for thromboembolic complications in nephrotic syndrome will continue to depend on the extent and type of underlying disease, renal function and the overall clinical situation [22].

In most cases, therapy should be directed at coagulation, such as enhancement of thrombin inhibition, a reduction of thrombin formation, reduction of fibrinogen or by improving fibrinolysis, rather than inhibition of platelet aggregation. Optimal therapy to treat thromboembolic complications should include drugs that have a maximum effect on the thrombus with only minimal systemic effects. The therapeutic approach to thrombosis in two children included anticoagulants- for example, long-term intravenous heparin (loading dose 5,000 IU, infusion after a loading dose of 16 U/kg/hour, and APTR of 2.5), warfarin for 6 months [115], and/or thrombolytic agents, such as streptokinase, urokinase, or rTPA [26,104,114].

5.1. Enhancement of Thrombin Inhibition

Heparin alone or in association with thrombolytic agents may be given if thrombosis occurs. When therapy with heparin followed by warfarin is begun early in the course of acute renal vein thrombosis, renal function and other symptoms of renal vein thrombosis have been shown to improve significantly in diopathic membranous glomerulopathy [15,119]. Warfarin should be continued for the duration of nephrotic range proteinuria [6] as renal venous thrombosis can recur in the setting of ongoing nephrosis after withdrawal of anticoagulation therapy [155].

Heparin causes rapid anticoagulation in patients with manifest thromboembolic complications, exerting its anticoagulant effect by forming a complex with antithrombin III and increasing the rate at which antithrombin III inactivates thrombin. Therefore, higher dosages of heparin are needed to achieve adequate anticoagulation in nephrotic patients in conditions of high plasma α2-macroglobulin levels and reduced antithrombin III concentrations [156,157]. High dosage heparinization might be necessary in children with deep vein thrombosis. A case of Budd-Chiari syndrome was resolved after immediate heparin infusion in a very young boy with nephrotic syndrome due to hepatic vein and inferior vena cava thrombosis [99]. Therefore, although higher than usual doses of heparin may be required in nephrotic syndrome because of decreased levels of antithrombin III [156], treatment with heparin in such patients should incorporate a standard heparin dosing nomogram, because of compensation mechanisms, with dose adjustments based on activated partial thromboplastin levels [158].

The use of low-molecular-weight heparin for the treatment of renal venous thrombosis has been described, and appears to have a reasonably safe profile [152,159,160]. Therefore, low-molecular-weight heparins should be used with caution in patients with renal insufficiency due to the risk of drug accumulation, excessive anticoagulant activity and potential increased risk of bleeding [161]. Finally, just how long anticoagulation therapy should be continued is not clear. For practical purposes, it seems wise to anticoagulate a nephrotic patient after a thromboembolic event for as long as proteinuria persists [6].

5.2. Improving Thrombolisis

The use of thrombolytic agents is widely advocated for patients with thromboembolism in the setting of nephrotic syndrome [162-165]. For many years rTPA has been the most widely used thrombolytic agent in various thromboembolic disorders [140,142]. Use of rTPA treatment for children was first reported in 1990 [141]. rTPA has been shown to be effective for thrombolysis in pediatric patients but it was not counter-indicated in cases of nephrotic syndrome [143]. Satisfactory thrombolysis of an arterial leg thrombosis was achieved in two children with relapsing nephrotic syndrome after four days of continuous catheter-directed low-dose rTPA (alteplase) [139]. Therefore, there are no advantages to thrombectomy or to fibrinolytic therapy in most cases of renal venous thrombosis. A case report described a mechanical thrombectomy for renal venous thrombosis that complicated membranous glomerulopathy [166].

The risk of bleeding due to thrombolytic therapy should also include the potential for hemorrhagic transformation of ischemic renal parenchyma, particularly in patients with acute renal venous thrombosis [162]. In the absence of randomized trials that compare thrombolytic with conventional anticoagulant therapy in patients with renal venous thrombosis, a reasonable approach is to reserve thrombolytic agents for massive renal venous thrombosis associated with acute and marked deterioration of renal function and to use conventional anticoagulant therapy in all other cases [163]. Patients treated with rTPA typically had an abrupt onset of acute renal failure, extensive thrombosis with bilateral renal venous thrombosis or renal venous thrombosis involving the inferior vena cava. However, no studies assessing the effectiveness and safety of rTPA in children are available [167].

5.3. Decreasing Thrombin Formation

Coumarin derivatives interfere with the formation of factor VII-activated thrombin. Since protein binding of these drugs is >99%, coumarin derivatives may have different pharmacokinetics in the presence of hypoalbuminemia [107]. Wagoner et al reported patients with renal venous thrombosis who received anticoagulant drugs for a minimum of 1 year, and who suffered no further thromboembolic events. The authors concluded that there is no advantage to thrombectomy or fibrinolytic therapy over the administration of coumarins [15].

5.4. Decreasing Fibrinogen Levels

Fibrates have been shown to decrease fibrinogen by 20% to 40% in hyperlipidemic subjects [168]; but whether this is also the case in nephrotic subjects remains to be determined. Moreover, three cases of severe nephrotic syndrome associated with hyperfibrinogenemia, hypercholesterolemia and thromboembolic disease, which showed poor response to therapy with warfarin, improved their coagulation profile upon concomitant administration of bezafibrate [169].

Lupus Nephritis

Systemic lupus erithematosus (SLE) is a known risk factor for thrombosis. Lupus nephritis develops in up to 60 % of patients with SLE during the course of the disease [170]. The most severe form of nephritis or lupus membranous nephropathy (Class V lupus glomerulonephritis) represents 10% to 20% of cases of lupus nephropathy [171]. Nathanson et al found that 18% of the 81 children with SLE with renal involvement presented histological features of membranous nephritis. On the first kidney biopsy, 12 of 15 pediatric patients had histological features of proliferative membranous nephropathy, which was observed secondarily in three of these patients [171]. Proteinuria is present at diagnosis in 80% of cases of lupus nephritis. The proteinuria is often nephrotic and can be associated with high arterial pressure and hematuria. Alternatively, it can be asymptomatic with no edema.

Thrombosis is a common complication of SLE. Eleven out of 120 children (9%) with SLE had thrombotic episodes [172]. Increasing age increased the risk of thromboembolic complications independently of SLE status, with no detectable racial predilection. However, a recent analysis of the risks for thrombosis in patients with SLE found that a younger age was a protective factor. In fact, a large study on 1,930 subjects with SLE found that a younger age at diagnosis was a protection against thrombosis [173]. Thromboembolic complication frequency did not differ significantly between patients with class V SLE and those with non–class V SLE histology (27.3% vs 11.5%) [20].

Pathogenesis

The risk factors for thromboembolic complications in SLE include the presence of antiphospholipid antibodies (aPL) [174]. However, decreased levels of plasminogen activator, decreased levels of protein S, and in some patients, the additional risks related to the nephrotic syndrome have also been reported [175-180].

Antiphospholipid Antibodies

Thrombosis and SLE

The ability of aPL to activate endothelial cells in vitro and in vivo, to induce platelet activation and its interaction with elements of the coagulation cascade has been well established [181]. These findings indicate that aPL seems to play an important role in the initial phase of a cascade that will lead to thrombotic events. The principal aPLs are anticardiolipin antibodies (aCL), β2-glycoprotein I (β2-GPI) antibodies and the lupus anticoagulant (LAC) - all responsible for thrombosis [182]. In children and adolescents with SLE, the prevalence of aPL ranged from 12% to 30% for aCL and 15%-34% for LAC [183].

In a cross-sectional cohort study of 59 pediatric patients (aged 4-19 years) with SLE, 13 thrombotic events occurred in 10 of the 59 patients (17%). There was a direct relationship between the presence of a LAC and a thrombotic event [184].

Thrombosis and lupus nephritis

Patients with SLE and lupus nephritis with positive aPL should be considered at high risk for developing arterial or venous thrombosis. A direct relationship between the presence of a LAC and a thrombotic event was reported in a retrospective study on 36 children with lupus nephritis [185]. Moroni et al screened for aPL in 111 subjects with lupus nephritis followed up for a mean of 173 ± 100 months. They found that those with positive aPL were more likely to have thrombosis than those with negative aPL. In particular, the authors found that 79% of lupus nephritis patients who were aPL positive experienced thrombotic events [186]. The cumulative 10-year risk of arterial thrombosis in patients with primary glomerulonephritis with positive aPL antibodies was higher (hazard ratio 3.57) than that of patients without antiphospholipid antibodies [187].

Thrombotic microangiopathy

Renal thrombotic microangiopathy was typically associated with the presence of aPL, both aCL and LAC, in SLE patients [188-191]. Therefore, thrombotic microangiopathy never develops in many patients with high aPL titlers. Conversely, thrombotic microangiopathy has been reported also in several SLE patients without aPL [188,192]. In renal biopsy specimens obtained from SLE patients, evidence of a thrombotic microangiopathy was found in 3% of them. Thus, other factors are necessary to trigger the endothelial damage that leads to thrombotic events. Altered fibrinolysis, secondary to an increase in the inhibitor of the plasminigen activator and a decrease in protein S, has also been described in patients with SLE [192-195].

Antiphospholipid syndrome

The association of aPL and thrombosis is known as antiphospholipid syndrome (APS). During follow up of patients with aPL positive nephropathy, manifestations of APS (especially arterial thromboses) developed more frequently in the SLE/non-APS patients with APS nephropathy than in those without APS nephropathy [190].

Complement

Complement and LES

Many studies have shown complement activation to be essential in aPL-induced thrombosis. The detrimental role of complement has been pointed out in experimental studies, such as that by Nangaku et al, who showed that thrombotic microangiopathy can be prevented if C5b-9 (the membrane attack complex) is temporarily inhibited [196]. However, Pierangeli et al showed that activation of the complement cascade is necessary for aPL-mediated thrombophilia. Mice deficient in complement components C3 and C5 were resistant to enhanced thrombosis and endothelial cell activation that was induced by aPL. The inhibition of C5 activation using anti-C5 monoclonal antibodies prevented thrombophilia induced by aPL [197,198]. APL-induced complement activation and down-stream signalling via C5a receptors in neutrophils, leading to induction of tissue factor, is a key initiating component of the blood coagulation cascade. Tissue factor expression by neutrophils was associated with enhanced procoagulant activity, as verified by a modified prothrombin time assay inhibited by anti-tissue factor antibodies [199]. Navratil et al reported that plateled-bound C4d, a sensitive marker for the classical pathway of complement activation, is highly specific (not sensitive) for the presence of aPL in SLE patients. Platelet C4d was detected in 18% of 105 patients with SLE, and was 100% specific for a diagnosis of SLE compared with healthy controls, and 98% specific for SLE compared with patients with other diseases. Platelet-bound C4d may be a biomarker for SLE, providing a clue to the pathogenic mechanism responsible for the myriad thrombotic and vascular complications of lupus associated with aPL [200].

Complement and lupus nephritis

A striking relationship has been detected between the quantity of the deposits of glomerular C4d and the presence of renal microthrombi in lupus nephritis [201]. Thus, it is likely that activation of the classical pathway of complement is a crucial pathogenic intermediary in the development of thrombosis in lupus nephritis, even in absence of aPL [201]. It seems wise to look at complement deposits, and deposits of C4d in particular, in all patients with lupus nephritis. Because activation of the classical pathway of complement is likely to be a marker of endothelial damage leading to thrombotic microangiopathy in lupus nephritis, C4d immunodetection may be a useful tool in determining whether patients are at risk of this complication [200,201].

Circulating Endothelial Cells

Several studies have shown greater numbers of circulating endothelial cells in cardiovascular diseases whose risk factors are unstable angina, acute myocardial infarction and stroke. Renal thrombotic microangiopathy is an uncommon vascular complication of SLE, but with deleterious effects on long-term renal function and overall survival of patients. Microvascular endothelial damage, which means the endothelium is usually swollen or denuded, is the histopathological hallmark of trombothic microangiopathy. Sometimes there is marked luminal narrowing or total occlusion due to intraluminal, subendothelial or medical accumulation of eosinophilic, fuchsinophilic material [202]. Damaged endothelial cells detach from the base membrane and become detectable in peripheral blood in patients with thrombotic microangiopathy. The number of these circulating endothelial cells in patients with thrombotic microangiopathy was higher in these patients than in those without thrombotic microangiopathy [203].

Clinical Features

APS is common among patients with SLE. The clinical hallmark of SLE and APS is the presence of vascular thrombosis. APS is characterized by recurrent arterial or venous thromboembolism and thrombocytopenia in association with aPL [204]. The presence of aPL in the serum of patients with SLE has been identified as an independent risk factor for thrombosis [205]. Although the majority of patients with APS develop venous or arterial thrombosis at a single anatomical site, a minority presents with multiorgan involvement of rapid onset. This dramatic event, called "catastrophic" antiphospholipid syndrome (CAPS), is characterized by the acute involvement of small-calibre blood vessels in multiple organs, including the kidneys, lungs, central nervous system, heart and skin. Thus, its clinical presentation often has several similarities with thrombotic microangiopathies. CAPS, which may be complicated by disseminated intravascular coagulation in up to 25% of cases, is associated with a high mortality rate as a consequence of multiorgan failure [206].

Thrombotic Microangiopathy

In renal biopsy specimens obtained from SLE patients, evidence of a thrombotic microangiopathy was found in 3% of them. In its most fulminant form, thrombotic microangiopathy presents with multiple fibrin thrombi in glomeruli and/or arterioles and capillaries and is accompanied by a severe decline in renal function [192-195]. SLE patients with thrombotic microangiopathy also exhibit extrarenal complications, including thrombocytopenia, microangiopathic hemolytic anemia, neurologic manifestations, and even multiple organ failure [188]. Not all patients with SLE and aPL develop thrombotic microangiopathy. Infection and trauma are necessary to trigger thrombosis at the vessel site where aPL have deposited. Conversely, not all patients with SLE and thrombotic microangiopathy have aPL [207].

Venous Thrombosis

The most common clinical manifestation of APS is venous thrombosis [208], especially deep venous thrombosis of the legs, which is complicated by pulmonary embolism in up to 50% of cases [182]. Involvement of small vessels, particularly in the kidneys, can mimic hemolytic-uremic syndrome or thrombotic thrombocytopenic purpura.

Arterial Thromboembolism

SLE was an independent risk factor for arterial thromboembolism, after adjustment for demographic variables and traditional risk factors. Other significant risk factors for arterial thrombosis were increasing age, LDL-hyperlipidemia and renal insufficiency [209]. In a prospective cohort study, the 5-year cumulative risk of an arterial thrombotic event was 8.5% in 258 Chinese patients with newly-onset SLE [210]. Arterial thromboembolic events referred to signs and symptoms caused by partial or complete stenosis of major arteries. These included cerebrovascular accident (stroke), transient ischemic attack, angina pectoris, claudication, amaurosis fugax and retinal artery occlusion [187].

The brain is the most common site of arterial thrombosis, with strokes and transient ischemic attacks accounting for nearly half of arterial occlusions. Arterial thromboses most often involving cerebral arteries are observed in lupus patients with aPL [211]. Other anatomical sites for arterial thrombosis are the heart (coronary occlusions), the eyes (retinal occlusions), the kidneys and peripheral arteries. Cardiac valvular abnormalities (i.e., nonbacterial vegetations on the mitral and aortic valves) are frequently seen, especially in patients with SLE-associated APS, and may serve as sources of emboli in the brain [212].

SLE patients with nephritis are more prone to arterial thromboembolic complications than those without renal involvement [209]. The absolute incidence of myocardial infarction and cerebovascular accidents is higher in patients with primary glomerulonephritis than that in patients with lupus nephritis. Therefore, amaurosis fugax and retinal artery thrombosis occurred exclusively in patients with lupus nephritis, for unknown reasons. These events were diagnosed and ascertained with the collaboration of cardiologists and neurologists, based on symptoms, clinical signs and investigations such as CT scans, magnetic resonance imaging, radionuclide heart perfusion scans, exercise stress tests and cardiac catheterization [187].

Deep Venous Thrombosis and Pulmonary Embolism

Deep venous thrombosis in the lower extremities is the most common manifestation of APS, occurring in 29% to 55% of patients during follow-up of less than 6 years, with as many as half of these patients having pulmonary emboli [213]. Up to 20% of cases of deep vein thrombosis, with or without pulmonary embolism, may be associated with aPL [214].

Pulmonary conditions such as dyspnea and respiratory distress syndrome are common in patients with catastrophic APS. Pulmonary embolism may be complicated by pulmonary hypertension. In a 14-year-old boy, pulmonary embolism was the first clinical sign of nephrotic syndrome due to lupus membranous nephropathy [215]. Therefore, patients with APS may have spontaneous thrombosis in pulmonary vessels, pulmonary hypertension and noninflammatory pulmonary vasculopathy [213].

Treatment

Therapy for SLE-aPL patients with lupus nephritis should include a combination of immunosuppressants (to induce remission in the kidneys) and prophylactic therapy to prevent thrombosis. For vascular thromboses, anticoagulation therapy should be initiated in the standard manner with heparin (either intravenous or subcutaneous low-molecular-weight heparin). Oral anticoagulation with warfarin is usually started simultaneously. For those patients with a positive LA test that raises baseline aPTT, monitoring heparin dosages to ensure adequate anticoagulation can be accomplished by monitoring activated factor Xa levels drawn 6-8 hours after the start of the heparin infusion. The use of non-aspirin antiplatelet agents (dipyridamole, dipyridamole/aspirin, or clopidogrel) in APS is anecdotal (no controlled studies on this are available) [216].

Prophylactic treatment with aspirin alone had controversial benefits in patients with primary and secondary APS [217]. Retrospective or cross-sectional studies have suggested that low-dose aspirin is protective against the first thrombosis in aPL-positive patients [218-220]. In the APLASA study, a randomized double-blind placebo-controlled trial of asymptomatic aPL-positive patients, 98 patients were chosen at random to receive either low-dose aspirin or the placebo; no difference was found in the acute thrombosis rate between the 2 groups after approximately 2.5 years of follow-up [221].

Because anticoagulation treatment without any anticomplement effect might not be protective, C4d staining could guide the therapeutic strategy, such as the earlier and prolonged use of immunosuppressants or anticoagulant therapy [201].

REFERENCES

[1] Lippi, G; Franchini, M; Guidi, GC. Diagnostic approach to inherited bleeding disorders. *Clin Chem Lab Med,* 2007 45, 2-12.

[2] Macfarlane, RG. An enzyme cascade in the blood clotting mechanism, and its function as a biochemical amplifier. *Nature,* 1964 202, 498-499.

[3] Davie, EW; Ratnoff OD. Waterfall sequence for intrinsic blood clotting. *Science,* 1964 145, 1310-1312.

[4] Monroe, DM; Hoffman, M; Roberts, HR. Platelets and thrombin generation. *Arterioscler Thromb Vasc Biol,* 2002 22, 1381-1389.

[5] Eddy, AA; Symons, JM. Nephrotic syndrome in childhood. *Lancet,* 2003 362, 629-639.

[6] Cameron, JS. Coagulation and thromboembolic complications in the nephrotic syndrome. *Adv Nephrol,* 1984 13,75-114.

[7] Llach, F. Hypercoagulability, renal vein thrombosis, and other thrombotic complications of nephrotic syndrome. *Kidney Int,* 1985 28, 429-439.

[8] Andrew, M; David, M; Adams, M; Ali, K; Anderson, R; Barnard, D; Bernstein, M; Brisson, L; Cairney, B; DeSai, D et al. Venous thromboembolic complications (VTE) in children: first analyses of the Canadian Registry of VTE. *Blood,* 1994 83, 1251-1257.

[9] Monagle, P; Adams, M; Mahoney, M; Ali, K; Barnard, D; Bernstein, M; Brisson, L; David, M; Desai, S; Scully, MF; Halton, J; Israels, S; Jardine, L; Leaker, M; McCusker, P; Silva, M; Wu, J; Anderson, R; Andrew, M; Massicotte, MP. Outcome of pediatric thromboembolic disease: a report from the Canadian Childhood Thrombophilia Registry. *Pediatr Res,* 2000 47, 763-766.

[10] Abella, EM. Hemostatic problems associated with renal disease. *Int J Pediatr Hematol Oncol,* 1994 1,43-51.

[11] Mehls, O; Andrassy, K; Koderisch, J; Herzog, U; Ritz, E. Hemostasis and thromboembolism in children with nephrotic syndrome: differences from adults. *J Pediatr,* 1987 110, 862-867.

[12] Orth, SR; Ritz, E. The nephrotic syndrome. *N Engl J Med,* 1998 338, 1202-1211.

[13] Nowak-Göttl, U; Kosch, A; Schlegel, N. Neonatal thromboembolism. *Semin Thromb Hemost,* 2003 29, 227-234.

[14] Hoyer, PF; Gonda, S; Barthels, M; Krohn, HP; Brodehl, J. Thromboembolic complications in children with nephrotic syndrome. Risk and incidence. *Acta Paediatr Scand,* 1986 75, 804-810.

[15] Wagoner, RD; Stanson, AW; Holley, KE; Winter, CS. Renal vein thrombosis in idiopathic membranous glomerulopathy and nephrotic syndrome: incidence and significance. *Kidney Int,* 1983 23, 368-374.

[16] Robert, A; Olmer, M; Sampol, J; Gugliotta, JE; Casanova, P. Clinical correlation between hypercoagulability and thrombo-embolic phenomena. *Kidney Int,* 1987 31, 830-835.

[17] Louis, CU; Morgenstern, BZ; Butani, L. Thrombotic complications in childhood-onset idiopathic membranous nephropathy. *Pediatr Nephrol,* 2003 18, 1298-1300.

[18] Citak, A; Emre, S; Sairin, A; Bilge, I; Nayir, A. Hemostatic problems and thromboembolic complications in nephrotic children. *Pediatr Nephrol,* 2000 14, 138-142.

[19] Harris, RC; Ismail, N. Extrarenal complications of the nephrotic syndrome. *Am J Kidney Dis,* 1994 23, 477-497.

[20] Kerlin, BA; Blatt, NB; Fuh, B; Zhao, S; Lehman, A; Blanchong, C; Mahan, JD; Smoyer, WE. Epidemiology and risk factors for thromboembolic complications of childhood nephrotic syndrome: a Midwest Pediatric Nephrology Consortium (MWPNC) study. *J Pediatr,* 2009 155, 105-110.

[21] Kanfer, A. Coagulation factors in nephrotic syndrome. *Am J Nephrol,* 1990 10, 63-68.

[22] Singhal, R; Brimble, KS. Thromboembolic complications in the nephrotic syndrome: pathophysiology and clinical management. *Thromb Res,* 2006 118, 397-407.

[23] Andrew, M; Brooker, LA. Hemostatic complications in renal disorders of the young. *Pediatr Nephrol,* 1996 10, 88-99.

[24] Kaizu, K; Etoh, S. Nephrotic syndrome and anticoagulant therapy. *Intern Med,* 1998 37, 210-212.

[25] Ozkayin, N; Mir, S; Kavakli, K. Hypercoagulability risk factors in children with minimal change disease and the protective role of protein-C activity. *Int Urol Nephrol,* 2004 36, 599-603.

[26] Zaffanello, M; Franchini, M. Thromboembolism in childhood nephrotic syndrome: a rare but serious complication. *Hematology,* 2007 12, 69-73.

[27] Kanfer, A; Kleinknecht, D; Broyer, M; Josso, F. Coagulation studies in 45 cases of nephrotic syndrome without uremia. *Thromb Diath Haemorrh,* 1970 24, 562-571.

[28] Zwaginga, JJ; Koomans, HA; Sixma, JJ; Rabelink, TJ. Thrombus formation and platelet-vessel wall interaction in the nephrotic syndrome under flow conditions. *J Clin Invest,* 1994 93, 204-211.

[29] Remuzzi, G; Mecca, G; Marchesi, D; Livio, M; de Gaetano, G; Donati, MB; Silver, MJ. Platelet hyperaggregability and the nephrotic syndrome. *Thromb Res,* 1979 16, 345-354.

[30] Yoshida, N; Aoki, N. Release of arachidonic acid from human platelets. A key role for the potentiation of platelet aggregability in normal subjects as well as in those with nephrotic syndrome. *Blood,* 1978 52, 969-977.

[31] Bennet, A; Sie, P; Caron, P; Boneu, B; Bazex, J; Pontonnier, F; Barret, A; Louvet, JP. Plasma fibrinolytic activity in a group of hypogonadic men. *Scand J Clin Lab Invest,* 1987 47, 23-27.

[32] Machleidt, C; Mettang, T; Stärz, E; Weber, J; Risler, T; Kuhlmann, U. Multifactorial genesis of enhanced platelet aggregability in patients with nephrotic syndrome. *Kidney Int,* 1989 36, 1119-1124.

[33] Tkaczyk, M; Baj, Z. Surface markers of platelet function in idiopathic nephrotic syndrome in children. *Pediatr Nephrol,* 2002 17, 673-677.

[34] Wasilewska, AM; Zoch-Zwierz, WM; Tomaszewska, B; Biernacka, A. Platelet-derived growth factor and platelet profiles in childhood nephrotic syndrome. *Pediatr Nephrol,* 2005 20, 36-41.

[35] Taira, K; Kamitsuji, H; Okajima, C; Fujimura, Y. Enhanced ristocetin-induced von Willebrand factor binding to platelet glycoprotein Ib in patients with steroid-responsive nephrotic syndrome. *Haemostasis,* 1990 20, 219-228.

[36] Sirolli, V; Ballone, E; Garofalo, D; Merciaro, G; Settefrati, N; Di Mascio, R; Di Gregorio, P; Bonomini, M. Platelet activation markers in patients with nephrotic syndrome. A comparative study of different platelet function tests. *Nephron,* 2002 91, 424-430.

[37] Bennett, A; Cameron, JS. Platelet hyperaggregability in the nephrotic syndrome which is not dependent on arachidonic acid metabolism or on plasma albumin concentration. *Clin Nephrol,* 1987 27, 182-188.

[38] Remuzzi, G; Marchesi, D; Mecca, G; de Gaetano, G; Silver, M. Platelet hypersensitivity in the nephrotic syndrome. *Proc Eur Dial Transplant Assoc,* 1979 16, 487-494.

[39] Jackson, CA; Greaves, M; Patterson, AD; Brown, CB; Preston, FE. Relationship between platelet aggregation, thromboxane synthesis and albumin concentration in nephrotic syndrome. *Br J Haematol,* 1982 52, 69-77.

[40] Schieppati, A; Dodesini, P; Benigni, A; Massazza, M; Mecca, G; Remuzzi, G; Livio, M; de Gaetano, G; Rossi, EC. The metabolism of arachidonic acid by platelets in nephrotic syndrome. *Kidney Int,* 1984 25, 671-676.

[41] Rabelink, AJ; Hené, RJ; Erkelens, DW; Joles, JA; Koomans, HA. Effects of simvastatin and cholestyramine on lipoprotein profile in hyperlipidaemia of nephrotic syndrome. *Lancet,* 1988 2, 1335-1338.

[42] Carvalho, AC; Colman, RW; Lees, RS. Platelet function in hyperlipoproteinemia. *N Engl J Med,* 1974 290, 434-438.

[43] Rabelink, TJ; Zwaginga, JJ; Koomans, HA; Sixma, JJ. Thrombosis and hemostasis in renal disease. *Kidney Int,* 1994 46, 287-296.

[44] Joles, JA; Willekes-Koolschijn, N; Scheek, LM; Koomans, HA; Rabelink, TJ; van Tol, A. Lipoprotein phospholipid composition and LCAT activity in nephrotic and analbuminemic rats. *Kidney Int,* 1994 46, 97-104.

[45] Kugiyama, K; Kerns, SA; Morrisett, JD; Roberts, R; Henry, PD. Impairment of endothelium-dependent arterial relaxation by lysolecithin in modified low-density lipoproteins. *Nature,* 1990 344, 160-162.

[46] de Graaf, JC; Banga, JD; Moncada, S; Palmer, RM; de Groot, PG; Sixma JJ. Nitric oxide functions as an inhibitor of platelet adhesion under flow conditions. *Circulation,* 1992 85, 2284-2290.

[47] Yashiro, M; Muso, E; Shio, H; Sasayama, S. Amelioration of hypercholesterolaemia by HMG-CoA reductase inhibitor (Pravastatin) improved platelet hyperaggregability in nephrotic patients. *Nephrol Dial Transplant,* 1994 9, 1842-1843.

[48] de Sain-van der Velden, MG; Kaysen, GA; de Meer, K; Stellaard, F; Voorbij, HA; Reijngoud, DJ; Rabelink, TJ; Koomans, HA. Proportionate increase of fibrinogen and albumin synthesis in nephrotic patients: measurements with stable isotopes. *Kidney Int,* 1998 53, 181-188.

[49] van Hylckama Vlieg, A; Rosendaal, FR. High levels of fibrinogen are associated with the risk of deep venous thrombosis mainly in the elderly. *J Thromb Haemost,* 2003 1, 2677-2678.

[50] Vayá, A; Mira, Y; Martínez, M; Villa, P; Ferrando, F; Estellés, A; Corella, D; Aznar, J. Biological risk factors for deep vein trombosis. *Clin Hemorheol Microcirc,* 2002 26, 41-53.

[51] Colle, JP; Mishal, Z; Lesty, C; Mirshahi, M; Peyne, J; Baumelou, A; Bensman, A; Soria, J; Soria, C. Abnormal fibrin clot architecture in nephrotic patients is related to hypofibrinolysis: influence of plasma biochemical modifications: a possible mechanism for the high thrombotic tendency? *Thromb Haemost,* 1999 82, 1482-1489.

[52] Kuhlmann, U; Steurer, J; Rhyner, K; von Felten, A; Briner, J; Siegenthaler, W. Platelet aggregation and beta-thromboglobulin levels in nephrotic patients with thrombosis. *Clin Nephrol,* 1981 15, 229-235.

[53] Adler, AJ; Lundin, AP; Feinroth, MV; Friedman, EA; Berlyne GM. Beta-thromboglobulin levels in the nephrotic syndrome. *Am J Med,* 1980 69, 551-554.

[54] Canavese, C; Stratta, P; Salomone, M; Priasca, GC; Muscolo, G; Vercellone, A. Platelet activation in nephrotic syndrome. *Clin Nephrol,* 1982 17, 268-269.

[55] Andrassy, K; Ritz, E; Bommer, J. Hypercoagulability in the Nephrotic syndrome. *Klin Wochenschr,* 1980 58, 1029-1036.

[56] Sagripanti, A; Cupisti, A; Ferdeghini, M; Pinori, E; Barsotti, G. Molecular markers of hemostasis activation in nephrotic syndrome. *Nephron,* 1989 51, 25-28.

[57] Tkaczyk, M; Czupryniak, A; Owczarek, D; Lukamowicz, J; Nowicki, M. Markers of endothelial dysfunction in children with idiopathic nephrotic syndrome. *Am J Nephrol,* 2008 28, 197-202.

[58] Alkjaersig, N; Fletcher, AP; Narayanan, M; Robson, AM. Course and resolution of the coagulopathy in nephrotic children. *Kidney Int,* 1987 31, 772-780.

[59] Tomura, S; Oono, Y; Kuriyama, R; Takeuchi, J. Plasma concentrations of fibrinopeptide A and fibrinopeptide B beta 15-42 in glomerulonephritis and the nephrotic syndrome. *Arch Intern Med,* 1985 145, 1033-1035.

[60] Baumgartner, HR. The role of blood flow in platelet adhesion, fibrin deposition, and formation of mural thrombi. *Microvasc Res,* 1973 5, 167-179.

[61] Thompson, WD; Smith, EB. Atherosclerosis and the coagulation system. *J Pathol,* 1989 159, 97-106.

[62] Tanaka, K; Sueishi, K. The coagulation and fibrinolysis systems and atherosclerosis. *Lab Invest,* 1993 69, 5-18.

[63] Tomura, S; Ideura, T; Ida, T; Osaka, Y; Kuriyama, R; Abe, T; Takeuchi, J. Renal vein fibrin degradation products (FDP's) in glomerulonephritis. *Clin Nephrol,* 1979 12, 248-253.

[64] McGinley, E; Lowe, GD; Boulton-Jones, M; Forbes, CD; Prentice, CR. Blood viscosity and haemostasis in the nephrotic syndrome.*Thromb Haemost,* 1983 49, 155-157.

[65] Ozanne, P; Francis, RB; Meiselman, HJ. Red blood cell aggregation in nephrotic syndrome. *Kidney Int,* 1983 23, 519-525.

[66] Böhler, T; Leo, A; Stadler, A; Linderkamp, O. Mechanical fragility of erythrocyte membrane in neonates and adults. *Pediatr Res,* 1992 32, 92-96.

[67] Kendall, AG; Lohmann, RC; Dossetor, JB. Nephrotic syndrome. A hypercoagulable state. *Arch Intern Med,* 1971 127, 1021-1027.

[68] Thomson, C; Forbes, CD; Prentice, CR; Kennedy, AC. Changes in blood coagulation and fibrinolysis in the nephrotic syndrome. *Q J Med,* 1974 43, 399-407.

[69] Edward, N; Young, DP; Macleod, M. Fibrinolytic activity in plasma and urine in chronic renal disease. *J Clin Pathol,* 1964 17, 365-368.

[70] Gandrille, S; Aiach, M. Albumin concentration influences fibrinolytic activity in plasma and purified systems. *Fibrinolysis,* 1990 4, 225-232.

[71] Du, XH; Glas-Greenwalt, P; Kant, KS; Allen, CM; Hayes, S; Pollak, VE. Nephrotic syndrome with renal vein thrombosis: pathogenetic importance of a plasmin inhibitor (alpha 2-antiplasmin). *Clin Nephrol,* 1985 24, 186-191.

[72] Karádi, I; Romics, L; Pálos, G; Domán, J; Kaszás, I; Hesz, A; Kostner, GM. Lp(a) lipoprotein concentration in serum of patients with heavy proteinuria of different origin. *Clin Chem,* 1989 35, 2121-2123.

[73] Thomas, ME; Freestone, A; Varghese, Z; Persaud, JW; Moorhead, JF. Lipoprotein(a) in patients with proteinuria. *Nephrol Dial Transplant,* 1992 7, 597-601.

[74] Wanner, C; Rader, D; Bartens, W; Krämer, J; Brewer, HB; Schollmeyer, P; Wieland, H. Elevated plasma lipoprotein(a) in patients with the nephrotic syndrome. *Ann Intern Med,* 1993 119, 263-269.

[75] McLean, JW; Tomlinson, JE; Kuang, WJ; Eaton, DL; Chen, EY; Fless, GM; Scanu, AM; Lawn, RM. cDNA sequence of human apolipoprotein(a) is homologous to plasminogen. *Nature,* 1987 330, 132-137.

[76] Rouy, D; Koschinsky, ML; Fleury, V; Chapman, J; Anglés-Cano, E. Apolipoprotein(a) and plasminogen interactions with fibrin: a study with recombinant apolipoprotein(a) and isolated plasminogen fragments. *Biochemistry,* 1992 31, 6333-6339.

[77] Loscalzo, J. Lipoprotein(a). A unique risk factor for atherothrombotic disease. *Arteriosclerosis,* 1990 10, 672-679.

[78] Vaziri, ND; Gonzales, E; Barton, CH; Chen, HT; Nguyen, Q; Arquilla, M. Factor XIII and its substrates, fibronectin, fibrinogen, and alpha 2-antiplasmin, in plasma and urine of patients with nephrosis. *J Lab Clin Med,* 1991 117, 152-156.

[79] Zaffanello, M; Brugnara, M; Fanos, V; Franchini, M. Prophylaxis with AT III for thromboembolism in nephrotic syndrome: why should it be done? *Int Urol Nephrol,* 2009 41, 713-716.

[80] Kauffmann, RH; Veltkamp, JJ; Van Tilburg, NH; Van Es LA. Acquired antithrombin III deficiency and thrombosis in the nephrotic syndrome. *Am J Med,* 1978 65, 607-13.

[81] Lau, SO; Tkachuck, JY; Hasegawa, DK; Edson, JR. Plasminogen and antithrombin III deficiencies in the childhood nephrotic syndrome associated with plasminogenuria and antithrombinuria. *J Pediatr,* 1980 96, 390-392.

[82] Rydzewski, A; Myśliwiec, M; Soszka, J. Concentration of three thrombin inhibitors in the nephrotic syndrome in adults. *Nephron,* 1986 42, 200-203.

[83] Vaziri, ND; Paule, P; Toohey, J; Hung, E; Alikhani, S; Darwish, R; Pahl, MV. Acquired deficiency and urinary excretion of antithrombin III in nephrotic syndrome. *Arch Intern Med,* 1984 144, 1802-1803.

[84] Boneu, B; Bouissou, F; Abbal, M; Sie, P; Caranobe, C; Barthe, P. Comparison of progressive antithrombin activity and the concentration of three thrombin inhibitors in nephrotic syndrome. *Thromb Haemost,* 1981 46, 623-625.

[85] Cosio, FG; Harker, C; Batard, MA; Brandt, JT; Griffin, JH. Plasma concentrations of the natural anticoagulants protein C and protein S in patients with proteinuria. *J Lab Clin Med,* 1985 106, 218-222.

[86] Vigano-D'Angelo, S; D'Angelo, A; Kaufman, CE Jr; Sholer, C; Esmon, CT; Comp, PC. Protein S deficiency occurs in the nephrotic syndrome. *Ann Intern Med,* 1987 107, 42-47.

[87] Gouault-Heilmann, M; Gadelha-Parente, T; Levent, M; Intrator, L; Rostoker, G; Lagrue, G. Total and free protein S in nephrotic syndrome. *Thromb Res,* 1988 49, 37-42.

[88] Pabinger-Fasching, I; Lechner, K; Niessner, H; Schmidt, P; Balzar, E; Mannhalter, C. High levels of plasma protein C in nephrotic syndrome. *Thromb Haemost,* 1985 53, 5-7.

[89] Hanevold, CD; Lazarchick, J; Constantin, MA; Hiott, KL; Orak, JK. Acquired free protein S deficiency in children with steroid resistant nephrosis. *Ann Clin Lab Sci,* 1996 26, 279-282.

[90] Kemkes-Matthes, B. Acquired protein S deficiency. *Clin Investig,* 1992 70, 529-534.

[91] Han, X; Fiehler, R; Broze, GJ Jr. Characterization of the protein Z-dependent protease inhibitor. *Blood,* 2000 96, 3049-3055.

[92] Han, X; Huang, ZF; Fiehler, R; Broze, GJ Jr. The protein Z-dependent protease inhibitor is a serpin. *Biochemistry,* 1999 38, 11073-11078.

[93] Broze, GJ Jr. Protein Z-dependent regulation of coagulation. *Thromb Haemost,* 2001 86, 8-13.

[94] Al-Shanqeeti, A; van Hylckama Vlieg, A; Berntorp, E; Rosendaal, FR; Broze, GJ Jr. Protein Z and protein Z-dependent protease inhibitor. Determinants of levels and risk of venous thrombosis. *Thromb Haemost,* 2005 93, 411-413.

[95] Vasse, M; Guegan-Massardier, E; Borg, JY; Woimant, F; Soria, C. Frequency of protein Z deficiency in patients with ischaemic stroke. *Lancet,* 2001 357, 933-934.

[96] Hogg, PJ; Stenflo, J. Interaction of vitamin K-dependent protein Z with thrombin. Consequences for the amidolytic activity of thrombin and the interaction of thrombin with phospholipid vesicles. *J Biol Chem,* 1991 266, 10953-10958.

[97] Kobelt, K; Biasiutti, FD; Mattle, HP; Lämmle, B; Wuillemin, WA. Protein Z in ischaemic stroke. *Br J Haematol,* 2001 114, 169-173.

[98] Ozkaya, O; Bek, K; Fişgin, T; Aliyazicioğlu, Y; Sultansuyu, S; Açikgöz, Y; Albayrak, D; Baysal, K. Low protein Z levels in children with nephrotic syndrome. *Pediatr Nephrol,* 2006 21, 1122-1126.

[99] Lilova, MI; Velkovski, IG; Topalov, IB. Thromboembolic complications in children with nephrotic syndrome in Bulgaria (1974-1996). *Pediatr Nephrol,* 2000 15, 74-78.

[100] Fabri, D; Belangero, VM; Annichino-Bizzacchi, JM; Arruda, VR. Inherited risk factors for thrombophilia in children with nephrotic syndrome. *Eur J Pediatr,* 1998 157, 939-942.

[101] Crew, RJ; Radhakrishnan, J; Appel, G. Complications of the nephrotic syndrome and their treatment. *Clin Nephrol,* 2004 62, 245-259.

[102] Ulinski, T; Guigonis, V; Baudet-Bonneville, V; Auber, F; Garcette, K; Bensman, A. Mesenteric thrombosis causing short bowel syndrome in nephrotic syndrome. *Pediatr Nephrol,* 2003 18, 1295-1297.

[103] Campisi, S; Cavatorta, F. A case of deep vein thrombosis in idiopathic nephrotic syndrome with resistance to activated protein C. *J Nephrol* 1998 11, 76-77.

[104] Martínez Ara, J; Gómez Rioja, R; Riñón, C; García Muñoz, MS; Ruiz Caravaca, ML; Miguel, JL. Prevalence of genetic prothrombotic factors (factor V Leiden and II20210 prothrombin mutation) in glomerular nephropathies with or without thrombosis. *Nefrologia,* 2000 20, 139-144.

[105] Segel, GB; Francis, CA. Anticoagulant proteins in childhood venous and arterial thrombosis: a review. *Blood Cells Mol Dis,* 2000 26, 540-560.

[106] Hoppe, C; Matsunaga, A. Pediatric thrombosis. *Pediatr Clin North Am,* 2002 49, 1257-1283.

[107] Llach, F; Pederson, JA. Acute joint syndrome (AJS) and maintenance hemodialysis (HD). *Proc Clin Dial Transplant Forum,* 1979 9, 17-22.

[108] Huang, J; Yang, J; Ding, J. Pulmonary embolism associated with nephrotic syndrome in children: a preliminary report of 8 cases. *Chin Med J,* 2000 113, 251-253.

[109] Cherng, SC; Huang, WS; Wang, YF; Yang, SP; Lin, YF. The role of lung scintigraphy in the diagnosis of nephrotic syndrome with pulmonary embolism. *Clin Nucl Med,* 2000 25, 167-172.

[110] Kayali, F; Najjar, R; Aswad, F; Matta, F; Stein, PD. Venous thromboembolism in patients hospitalized with nephrotic syndrome. *Am J Med,* 2008 121, 226-230.

[111] Jones, CL; Hébert, D. Pulmonary thrombo-embolism in the nephrotic syndrome. *Pediatr Nephrol,* 1991 5, 56-58.

[112] Reid, CJ; Segal, T. Pulmonary thrombo-embolism in nephrotic syndrome treated with tissue plasminogen activator. *Eur J Pediatr,* 1997 156, 647-649.

[113] Zimmerman, RL; Novek, S; Chen, JT; Roggli, V. Pulmonary thrombosis in a 10-year-old child with minimal change disease and nephrotic syndrome. A clinical, radiologic, and pathologic correlation with literature review. *Am J Clin Pathol,* 1994 101, 230-236.

[114] Rai Mittal, B; Singh, S; Bhattacharya, A; Prasad, V; Singh, B. Lung scintigraphy in the diagnosis and follow-up of pulmonary thromboembolism in children with nephrotic syndrome. *Clin Imaging,* 2005 29, 313-316.

[115] Deshpande, PV; Griffiths, M. Pulmonary thrombosis in steroid-sensitive nephrotic syndrome. *Pediatr Nephrol,* 2005 20, 665-669.

[116] van Ommen, CH; Heyboer, H; Groothoff, JW; Teeuw, R; Aronson, DC; Peters, M. Persistent tachypnea in children: keep pulmonary embolism in mind. *J Pediatr Hematol Oncol,* 1998 20, 570-573.

[117] Lin, CC; Lui, CC; Tain, YL. Thalamic stroke secondary to straight sinus thrombosis in a nephrotic child. *Pediatr Nephrol,* 2002 17, 184-186.

[118] Gangakhedkar, A; Wong, W; Pitcher, LA. Cerebral thrombosis in childhood nephrosis. *J Paediatr Child Health,* 2005 41, 221-224.

[119] Llach, F; Papper, S; Massry, SG. The clinical spectrum of renal vein thrombosis: acute and chronic. *Am J Med,* 1980 69, 819-827.

[120] Chugh, KS; Malik, N; Uberoi, HS; Gupta, VK; Aggarwal, ML; Singhal, PC; Suri, S; Jain, SK. Renal vein thrombosis in nephrotic syndrome-a prospective study and review. *Postgrad Med J,* 1981 57, 566-570.

[121] Llach, F; Arieff, AI; Massry, SG. Renal vein thrombosis and nephrotic syndrome. A prospective study of 36 adult patients. *Ann Intern Med,* 1975 83, 8-14.

[122] Velasquez Forero, F; Garcia Prugue, N; Ruiz Morales, N. Idiopathic nephrotic syndrome of the adult with asymptomatic thrombosis of the renal vein. *Am J Nephrol,* 1988 8, 457-462.

[123] Tinaztepe, K; Buyan, N; Tinaztepe, B; Akkok, N. The association of nephrotic syndrome and renal vein thrombosis: a clinicopathological analysis of eight pediatric patients. *Turk J Pediatr,* 1989 31, 1-18.

[124] Fluss, J; Geary, D; deVeber, G. Cerebral sinovenous thrombosis and idiopathic nephrotic syndrome in childhood: report of four new cases and review of the literature. *Eur J Pediatr,* 2006 165, 709-716.

[125] Appenzeller, S; Zeller, CB; Annichino-Bizzachi, JM; Costallat, LT; Deus-Silva, L; Voetsch, B; Faria, AV; Zanardi, VA; Damasceno, BP; Cendes, F. Cerebral venous thrombosis: influence of risk factors and imaging findings on prognosis. *Clin Neurol Neurosurg,* 2005 107, 371-378.

[126] Palcoux, JB; Gaspard, F; Campagne, D. Cerebral sinus thrombosis in a child with steroid-resistant nephrotic syndrome. *Pediatr Nephrol,* 2003 18, 610-611.

[127] Papachristou, FT; Petridou, SH; Printza, NG; Zafeiriou, DI; Gompakis, NP. Superior sagittal sinus thrombosis in steroid-resistant nephrotic syndrome. *Pediatr Neurol,* 2005 32, 282-284.

[128] Balci, YI; Tavil, B; Fidan, G; Ozaltin, F. Cerebral sinovenous thrombosis in a child with steroid sensitive nephrotic syndrome. *Eur J Pediatr,* 2007 166, 757-758.

[129] Tullu, MS; Deshmukh, CT; Save, SU; Bhoite, BK; Bharucha, BA. Superior sagittal sinus thrombosis: a rare complication of nephrotic syndrome. *J Postgrad Med,* 1999 45, 120-122.

[130] Monagle, P; Chan, A; Massicotte, P; Chalmers, E; Michelson, AD. Antithrombotic therapy in children: the Seventh ACCP Conference on Antithrombotic and Thrombolytic Therapy. *Chest,* 2004 126 Suppl 3, 645S-687S.

[131] Akatsu, H; Vaysburd, M; Fervenza, F; Peterson, J; Jacobs, M. Cerebral venous thrombosis in nephrotic syndrome. *Clin Nephrol,* 1997 48, 317-320.

[132] Weisz, W; Kemper, MJ; Weil, J; Muller-Wiefel, DE. Asymptomatic intracardiac thrombus in steroid-sensitive nephrotic syndrome. *Pediatr Nephrol,* 2002 17, 287-289.

[133] Passos, EM; Legallicier, B; Godin, M. Membranous nephropathy. *Rev Prat,* 2003 53, 2033-2038.

[134] Lilova, MI; Velkovski, IG; Velichkov, NI. Budd-Chiari syndrome and inferior vena cava thrombosis in a nephrotic child. *Pediatr Nephrol,* 2000 14, 412-415.

[135] Tarry, WC; Moser, AJ; Makhoul, RG. Peripheral arterial thrombosis in the nephrotic syndrome. *Surgery,* 1993 114, 618-23.

[136] Witz, M; Lehman, J; Shnaker, A; Korzets, Z. Acute subclavian and brachial artery thrombosis as a complication of the nephrotic syndrome. *Isr Med Assoc J,* 2004 6, 441-442.

[137] Kauffmann, RH ; de Graeff, J ; de la Rivière, GB ; van Es, LA. Unilateral renal vein thrombosis and nephrotic syndrome. Report of a case with protein selectivity and antithrombin III clearance studies. *Am J Med,* 1976 60, 1048-1054.

[138] Garbrecht, F; Gardner, S; Johnson, V; Grabowski, E. Deep venous thrombosis in a child with nephrotic syndrome associated with a circulating anticoagulant and acquired protein S deficiency. *Am J Pediatr Hematol Oncol,* 1991 13, 330-333.

[139] Ruud, E; Holmstrøm, H; Aagenaes, I; Hafsahl, G; Handeland, M; Kyte, A; Brosstad, F. Successful thrombolysis by prolonged low-dose alteplase in catheter-directed infusion. *Acta Paediatr,* 2003 92, 973-976.

[140] Crabbe, SJ; Cloninger, CC. Tissue plasminogen activator: a new thrombolytic agent. *Clin Pharm,* 1987 6, 373-386.

[141] Kennedy, LA; Drummond, WH; Knight, ME; Millsaps, MM; Williams JL. Successful treatment of neonatal aortic thrombosis with tissue plasminogen activator. *J Pediatr,* 1990 116, 798-801.

[142] Kändler, C; Ries, M; Rupprecht, T; Ruder, H; Harms, D. Successful systemic low-dose lysis of a caval thrombus by rt-PA in a neonate with congenital nephrotic syndrome. *J Pediatr Hematol Oncol,* 1997 19, 348-50.

[143] Manco-Johnson, MJ; Grabowski, EF; Hellgreen, M; Kemahli, AS; Massicotte, MP; Muntean, W; Peters, M; Schlegel, N; Wang, M; Nowak-Gottl, U. Recommendations for tPA thrombolysis in children. On behalf of the Scientific Subcommittee on Perinatal and Pediatric Thrombosis of the Scientific and Standardization Committee of the International Society of Thrombosis and Haemostasis. *Thromb Haemost,* 2002 88, 157-158.

[144] Lip, GY; Tean, KN; Dunn, FG. Acute myocardial infarction: a rare complication of the thrombotic tendency in nephrotic syndrome. *Br J Clin Pract,* 1994 48, 218-220.

[145] Hopp, L; Gilboa, N; Kurland, G; Weichler, N; Orchard, TJ. Acute myocardial infarction in a young boy with nephrotic syndrome: a case report and review of the literature. *Pediatr Nephrol,* 1994 8, 290-294.

[146] Osula, S; Bell, GM; Hornung, RS. Acute myocardial infarction in young adults: causes and management. *Postgrad Med J,* 2002 78, 27-30.

[147] al-Mugeiren, MM; Gader, AM; al-Rasheed, SA; Bahakim, HM; al-Momen, AK; al-Salloum, A. Coagulopathy of childhood nephrotic syndrome-a reappraisal of the role of natural anticoagulants and fibrinolysis. *Haemostasis,* 1996 26, 304-310.

[148] Palareti, G; Leali, N; Coccheri, S; Poggi, M; Manotti, C; D'Angelo, A; Pengo, V; Erba, N; Moia, M; Ciavarella, N; Devoto, G; Berrettini, M; Musolesi, S. Bleeding complications of oral anticoagulant treatment: an inception-cohort, prospective collaborative study (ISCOAT). Italian Study on Complications of Oral Anticoagulant Therapy. *Lancet,* 1996 348, 423-428.

[149] Glassock, RJ. Prophylactic anticoagulation in nephrotic syndrome: a clinical conundrum. *J Am Soc Nephrol,* 2007 18, 2221-2225.

[150] Bellomo, R; Atkins, RC. Membranous nephropathy and thromboembolism: is prophylactic anticoagulation warranted? *Nephron,* 1993 63, 249-254.

[151] Sarasin, FP; Schifferli, JA. Prophylactic oral anticoagulation in nephrotic patients with idiopathic membranous nephropathy. *Kidney Int,* 1994 45, 578-585.

[152] Rostoker, G; Durand-Zaleski, I; Petit-Phar, M; Ben Maadi, A; Jazaerli, N; Radier, C; Rahmouni, A; Mathieu, D; Vasile, N; Rosso, J et al. Prevention of thrombotic complications of the nephrotic syndrome by the low-molecular-weight heparin enoxaparin. *Nephron,* 1995 69, 20-28.

[153] Malik, GH; al-Wakeel, JS; al-Mohaya, S; Wasfy, I; Kechrid, MS; el-Gamal, HH. Intraventricular and brachial artery thrombosis in nephrotic syndrome. *Am J Nephrol,* 1998 18, 142-145.

[154] Skalova, S; Lukes, A; Vanicek, H; Klein, T; Hak, J; Dedek, P; Ocenaskova, E. Intracardiac thrombus-a rare complication of the steroid resistant nephrotic syndrome. *Bratisl Lek Listy,* 2008 109, 573-575.

[155] Briefel, GR; Manis, T; Gordon, DH; Nicastri, AD; Friedman, EA. Recurrent renal vein thrombosis consequent to membranous glomerulonephritis. *Clin Nephrol,* 1978 10, 32-37.

[156] Fischer, AM; Tapon-Bretaudiere, J; Bros, A; Josso, F. Respective roles of antithrombin III and alpha 2 macroglobulin in thrombin inactivation. *Thromb Haemost,* 1981 45, 51-54.

[157] Vermylen, CG; Levin, M; Lanham, JG; Hardisty, RM; Barratt, TM. Decreased sensitivity to heparin in vitro in steroid-responsive nephrotic syndrome. *Kidney Int,* 1987 31, 1396-1401.

[158] Hirsh, J; Raschke, R. Heparin and low-molecular-weight heparin: the Seventh ACCP Conference on Antithrombotic and Thrombolytic Therapy. *Chest,* 2004 126 Suppl 3, 188S-203S.

[159] Yang, SH; Lee, CH; Ko, SF; Chen, JB; Chung, FR; Hsu KT. The successful treatment of renal-vein thrombosis by low-molecular-weight heparin in a steroid-sensitive nephrotic patient. *Nephrol Dial Transplant,* 2002 17, 2017-2019.

[160] Alhenc-Gelas, M; Rossert, J; Jacquot, C; Aiach, M. Pharmacokinetic study of the low-molecular-weight heparin fraxiparin in patients with nephrotic syndrome. *Nephron,* 1995 71, 149-152.

[161] Farooq, V; Hegarty, J; Chandrasekar, T; Lamerton, EH; Mitra, S; Houghton, JB; Kalra, PA; Waldek, S; O'Donoghue, DJ; Wood, GN. Serious adverse incidents with the usage of low molecular weight heparins in patients with chronic kidney disease. *Am J Kidney Dis,* 2004 43, 531-537.

[162] Laville, M; Aguilera, D; Maillet, PJ; Labeeuw, M; Madonna, O; Zech, P. The prognosis of renal vein thrombosis: a re-evaluation of 27 cases. *Nephrol Dial Transplant,* 1988 3, 247-256.

[163] Markowitz, GS; Brignol, F; Burns, ER; Koenigsberg, M; Folkert, VW. Renal vein thrombosis treated with thrombolytic therapy: case report and brief review. *Am J Kidney Dis,* 1995 25, 801-806.

[164] Crowley, JP; Matarese, RA; Quevedo, SF; Garella, S. Fibrinolytic therapy for bilateral renal vein thrombosis. *Arch Intern Med,* 1984 144, 159-160.
[165] Lam, KK; Lui, CC. Successful treatment of acute inferior vena cava and unilateral renal vein thrombosis by local infusion of recombinant tissue plasminogen activator. *Am J Kidney Dis,* 1998 32, 1075-1079.
[166] Jaar, BG; Kim, HS; Samaniego, MD; Lund, GB; Atta, MG. Percutaneous mechanical thrombectomy: a new approach in the treatment of acute renal-vein thrombosis. *Nephrol Dial Transplant,* 2002 17, 1122-1125.
[167] Parasuraman, S; Goldhaber, SZ. Venous thromboembolism in children. *Circulation,* 2006 113, e12-16.
[168] Cook, NS; Ubben, D. Fibrinogen as a major risk factor in cardiovascular disease. *Trends Pharmacol Sci,* 1990 11, 444-451.
[169] Al-Momen, AK; Al-Abdul-Kareem, H. Potentiation of the action of warfarin by bezafibrate in patients with the nephrotic syndrome. *Saudi J Kidney Dis Transpl,* 1994 5, 12-16.
[170] Cameron, JS. Lupus nephritis: an historical perspective 1968-1998. *J Nephrol,* 1999 12 Suppl 2, S29-41.
[171] Nathanson, S; Salomon, R; Ranchin, B; Macher, MA; Lavocat, MP; Krier, MJ; Baudouin, V; Azéma, C; Bader-Meunier, B; Deschênes, G. Prognosis of lupus membranous nephropathy in children. *Pediatr Nephrol,* 2006 21, 1113-1116.
[172] Montes de Oca, MA; Babron, MC; Blétry, O; Broyer, M; Courtecuisse, V; Fontaine, JL; Loirat, C; Méry, JP; Reinert, P; Wechsler, B et al. Thrombosis in systemic lupus erythematosus: a French collaborative study. *Arch Dis Child,* 1991 66, 713-717.
[173] Kaiser, R; Cleveland, CM; Criswell, LA. Risk and protective factors for thrombosis in systemic lupus erythematosus: results from a large, multi-ethnic cohort. *Ann Rheum Dis,* 2009 68, 238-241.
[174] Calvo-Alén, J; Toloza, SM; Fernández, M; Bastian, HM; Fessler, BJ; Roseman, JM; McGwin, G Jr; Vilá, LM; Reveille, JD; Alarcón, GS; LUMINA Study Group. Systemic lupus erythematosus in a multiethnic US cohort (LUMINA). XXV. Smoking, older age, disease activity, lupus anticoagulant, and glucocorticoid dose as risk factors for the occurrence of venous thrombosis in lupus patients. *Arthritis Rheum,* 2005 52, 2060-2068.
[175] Qushmaq, K; Esdaile, J; Devine, DV. Thrombosis in systemic lupus erythematosus: the role of antiphospholipid antibody. *Arthritis Care Res,* 1999 12, 212-219.
[176] Esmon, NL; Smirnov, MD; Safa, O; Esmon, CT. Lupus anticoagulants, thrombosis and the protein C system. *Haematologica,* 1999 84, 446-451.
[177] Galli, M; Finazzi, G; Norbis, F; Marziali, S; Marchioli, R; Barbui, T. The risk of thrombosis in patients with lupus anticoagulants is predicted by their specific coagulation profile. *Thromb Haemost,* 1999 81, 695-700.
[178] Male, C; Lechner, K; Eichinger, S; Kyrle, PA; Kapiotis, S; Wank, H; Kaider, A; Pabinger, I. Clinical significance of lupus anticoagulants in children. *J Pediatr,* 1999 134, 199-205.

[179] Angles-Cano, E ; Sultan, Y ; Clauvel, JP. Predisposing factors to thrombosis in systemic lupus erythematosus: possible relation to endothelial cell damage. *J Lab Clin Med,* 1979 94, 312-23.

[180] Hasselaar, P; Derksen, RH; Blokzijl, L; Hessing, M; Nieuwenhuis, HK; Bouma, BN; De Groot, PG. Risk factors for thrombosis in lupus patients. *Ann Rheum Dis,* 1989 48, 933-940.

[181] Pierangeli, SS; Colden-Stanfield, M; Liu, X; Barker, JH; Anderson, GL; Harris, EN. Antiphospholipid antibodies from antiphospholipid syndrome patients activate endothelial cells in vitro and in vivo. *Circulation,* 1999 99, 1997-2002.

[182] Vianna, JL; Khamashta, MA; Ordi-Ros, J; Font, J; Cervera, R; Lopez-Soto, A; Tolosa, C; Franz, J; Selva, A; Ingelmo, M et al. Comparison of the primary and secondary antiphospholipid syndrome: a European Multicenter Study of 114 patients. *Am J Med,* 1994 96, 3-9.

[183] Lee, T; von Scheven, E; Sandborg, C. Systemic lupus erythematosus and antiphospholipid syndrome in children and adolescents. *Curr Opin Rheumatol,* 2001 13, 415-421.

[184] Berube, C; Mitchell, L; Silverman, E; David, M; Saint Cyr, C; Laxer, R; Adams, M; Vegh, P; Andrew, M. The relationship of antiphospholipid antibodies to thromboembolic events in pediatric patients with systemic lupus erythematosus: a cross-sectional study. *Pediatr Res,* 1998 44, 351-356.

[185] Massengill, SF; Hedrick, C; Ayoub, EM; Sleasman, JW; Kao, KJ. Antiphospholipid antibodies in pediatric lupus nephritis. *Am J Kidney Dis,* 1997 29, 355-361.

[186] Moroni, G; Ventura, D; Riva, P; Panzeri, P; Quaglini, S; Banfi, G; Simonini, P; Bader, R; Meroni, PL; Ponticelli, C. Antiphospholipid antibodies are associated with an increased risk for chronic renal insufficiency in patients with lupus nephritis. *Am J Kidney Dis,* 2004 43, 28-36.

[187] Mok, CC; Tong, KH; To, CH; Siu, YP; Ho, LY; Au, TC. Risk and predictors of arterial thrombosis in lupus and non-lupus primary glomerulonephritis: a comparative study. *Medicine,* 2007 86, 203-209.

[188] Jain, R; Chartash, E; Susin, M; Furie, R. Systemic lupus erythematosus complicated by thrombotic microangiopathy. *Semin Arthritis Rheum,* 1994 24, 173-82.

[189] Hughson, MD; Nadasdy, T; McCarty, GA; Sholer, C; Min, KW; Silva, F. Renal thrombotic microangiopathy in patients with systemic lupus erythematosus and the antiphospholipid syndrome. *Am J Kidney Dis,* 1992 20, 150-158.

[190] Tektonidou, MG; Sotsiou, F; Nakopoulou, L; Vlachoyiannopoulos, PG; Moutsopoulos, HM. Antiphospholipid syndrome nephropathy in patients with systemic lupus erythematosus and antiphospholipid antibodies: prevalence, clinical associations, and long-term outcome. *Arthritis Rheum,* 2004 50, 2569-2579.

[191] Nochy D, Daugas E, Huong DL, Piette JC, Hill G. Kidney involvement in the antiphospholipid syndrome. *J Autoimmun,* 2000 15, 127-132.

[192] Appel, GB, Pirani, CL ; D'Agati, V. Renal vascular complications of systemic lupus erythematosus. *J Am Soc Nephrol,* 1994 4, 1499-1515.

[193] Descombes, E; Droz, D; Drouet, L; Grünfeld, JP; Lesavre, P. Renal vascular lesions in lupus nephritis. *Medicine,* 1997 76, 355-368.

[194] Grishman, E; Venkataseshan, VS. Vascular lesions in lupus nephritis. *Mod Pathol,* 1988 1, 235-41.

[195] Magil, AB; McFadden, D; Rae, A. Lupus glomerulonephritis with thrombotic microangiopathy. *Hum Pathol,* 1986 17, 192-194.

[196] Nangaku, M; Alpers, CE; Pippin, J; Shankland, SJ; Kurokawa, K; Adler, S; Johnson, RJ; Couser, WG. Renal microvascular injury induced by antibody to glomerular endothelial cells is mediated by C5b-9. *Kidney Int,* 1997 52, 1570-1578.

[197] Pierangeli, SS; Girardi, G; Vega-Ostertag, M; Liu, X; Espinola, RG; Salmon, J. Requirement of activation of complement C3 and C5 for antiphospholipid antibody-mediated thrombophilia. *Arthritis Rheum,* 2005 52, 2120-2124.

[198] Pierangeli, SS; Chen, PP; González, EB. Antiphospholipid antibodies and the antiphospholipid syndrome: an update on treatment and pathogenic mechanisms. *Curr Opin Hematol,* 2006 13, 366-375.

[199] Ritis, K; Doumas, M; Mastellos, D; Micheli, A; Giaglis, S; Magotti, P; Rafail, S; Kartalis, G; Sideras, P; Lambris, JD. A novel C5a receptor-tissue factor cross-talk in neutrophils links innate immunity to coagulation pathways. *J Immunol,* 2006 177, 4794-4802.

[200] Navratil, JS; Manzi, S; Kao, AH; Krishnaswami, S; Liu, CC; Ruffing, MJ; Shaw, PS; Nilson, AC; Dryden, ER; Johnson, JJ; Ahearn, JM. Platelet C4d is highly specific for systemic lupus erythematosus. *Arthritis Rheum,* 2006 54, 670-674.

[201] Cohen, D; Koopmans, M; Kremer Hovinga, IC; Berger, SP; Roos van Groningen, M; Steup-Beekman, GM; de Heer, E; Bruijn, JA; Bajema, IM. Potential for glomerular C4d as an indicator of thrombotic microangiopathy in lupus nephritis. *Arthritis Rheum,* 2008 58, 2460-2469.

[202] Bridoux, F; Vrtovsnik, F; Noël, C; Saunier, P; Mougenot, B; Lemaitre, V; Dracon, M; Lelièvre, G; Vanhille, P. Renal thrombotic microangiopathy in systemic lupus erythematosus: clinical correlations and long-term renal survival. *Nephrol Dial Transplant,* 1998 13, 298-304.

[203] Yao, G; Liu, ZH; Zheng, C; Zhang, X; Chen, H; Zeng, C; Li, LS. Evaluation of renal vascular lesions using circulating endothelial cells in patients with lupus nephritis. *Rheumatology,* 2008 47, 432-436.

[204] Vianna, JL; Haga, HJ; Tripathi, P; Cervera, R; Khamashta, MA; Hughes, GR. Reassessing the status of antiphospholipid syndrome in systemic lupus erythematosus. *Ann Rheum Dis,* 1992 51, 160-161.

[205] Drenkard, C; Villa, AR; Alarcón-Segovia, D; Pérez-Vázquez, ME. Influence of the antiphospholipid syndrome in the survival of patients with systemic lupus erythematosus. *J Rheumatol,* 1994 21, 1067-1072.

[206] Asherson, RA; Cervera, R. Catastrophic antiphospholipid syndrome. *Curr Rheumatol Rep,* 2003 5, 395-400.

[207] Harris, EN; Pierangeli, SS. Primary, Secondary, Catastrophic Antiphospholipid Syndrome: is there a difference? *Thromb Res,* 2004 114, 357-361.

[208] Appel, GB; Williams, GS; Meltzer, JI; Pirani, CL. Renal vein thrombosis, nephrotic syndrome, and systemic lupus erythematosus: an association in four cases. *Ann Intern Med,* 1976 85, 310-317.

[209] Esdaile, JM; Abrahamowicz, M; Grodzicky, T; Li, Y; Panaritis, C; du Berger, R; Côte, R; Grover, SA; Fortin, PR; Clarke, AE; Senécal, JL. Traditional Framingham risk factors fail to fully account for accelerated atherosclerosis in systemic lupus erythematosus. *Arthritis Rheum,* 2001 44, 2331-2337.

[210] Mok, CC; Tang, SS; To, CH; Petri, M. Incidence and risk factors of thromboembolism in systemic lupus erythematosus: a comparison of three ethnic groups. *Arthritis Rheum,* 2005 52, 2774-2782.

[211] Asherson, RA; Khamashta, MA; Gil, A; Vazquez, JJ; Chan, O; Baguley, E; Hughes, GR. Cerebrovascular disease and antiphospholipid antibodies in systemic lupus erythematosus, lupus-like disease, and the primary antiphospholipid syndrome. *Am J Med,* 1989 86, 391-399.

[212] Franchini, M. The antiphospholipid syndrome: an update. *Clin Lab,* 2006 52, 11-17.

[213] Gezer, S. Antiphospholipid syndrome. *Dis Mon,* 2003 49, 696-741.

[214] Farmer-Boatwright, MK; Roubey, RA. Venous thrombosis in the antiphospholipid syndrome. *Arterioscler Thromb Vasc Biol,* 2009 29, 321-325.

[215] Harroche, A; Remus, N; Gaubicher, S; Dunand, O; Colombat, M; Delacourt, C; Madhi, F. Pulmonary thrombosis as the first manifestation of systemic lupus erythematosus in a 14-year-old boy. *Pediatr Nephrol,* 2009 24, 857-861.

[216] George, D; Erkan, D. Antiphospholipid syndrome. *Prog Cardiovasc Dis,* 2009 52, 115-125.

[217] Alarcón-Segovia, D; Boffa, MC; Branch, W; Cervera, R; Gharavi, A; Khamashta, M; Shoenfeld, Y; Wilson, W; Roubey, R. Prophylaxis of the antiphospholipid syndrome: a consensus report. *Lupus,* 2003 12, 499-503.

[218] Erkan, D; Yazici, Y; Peterson, MG; Sammaritano, L; Lockshin, MD. A cross-sectional study of clinical thrombotic risk factors and preventive treatments in antiphospholipid syndrome. *Rheumatology,* 2002 41, 924-929.

[219] Hereng, T; Lambert, M; Hachulla, E; Samor, M; Dubucquoi, S; Caron, C; Launay, D; Morell-Dubois, S; Queyrel, V; Hatron, PY. Influence of aspirin on the clinical outcomes of 103 anti-phospholipid antibodies-positive patients. *Lupus,* 2008 17, 11-15.

[220] Tektonidou, MG; Laskari, K; Panagiotakos, DB; Moutsopoulos, HM. Risk factors for thrombosis and primary thrombosis prevention in patients with systemic lupus erythematosus with or without antiphospholipid antibodies. *Arthritis Rheum,* 2009 61, 29-36.

[221] Erkan, D; Harrison, MJ; Levy, R; Peterson, M; Petri, M; Sammaritano, L; Unalp-Arida, A; Vilela, V; Yazici, Y; Lockshin, MD. Aspirin for primary thrombosis prevention in the antiphospholipid syndrome: a randomized, double-blind, placebo-controlled trial in asymptomatic antiphospholipid antibody-positive individuals. *Arthritis Rheum,* 2007 56, 2382-2391.

In: Thrombosis: Causes, Treatment and Prevention
Editor: D. G. Macri and L. D. Procaccini, pp. 93-118
ISBN 978-1-61668-696-3

Chapter III

RENAL VEIN AND ARTERY THROBOSIS IN NEWBORN AND CHILDREN

Marco Zaffanello[1,*], Vassilios Fanos[2], Bruna Franchi[1] and Massimo Franchini[3]
[1]University of Verona, Verona, Italy;
[2]University of Cagliari, Cagliari, Italy;
[3]University Hospital of Parma, Parma, Italy.

ABSTRACT

In newborns, renal thromboembolism has been associated most frequently with umbilical artery catheters. In children, the most common renal disorder associated with hemostatic complications is renal vein thrombosis. The main causes are severe dehydration secondary to sepsis, nephrotic syndrome and related glomerulonephropathy and congenital disorders of hemostasis. Clinical features of the condition in newborns and young children include enlarged kidneys, gross hematuria, thrombocytopenia, hypertension and kidney failure. The severity of the condition depends on whether one or both kidneys are involved. Clinical evaluation is feasible with ultrasound and scintigraphy as well as with other imaging tecniques. The treatment, either pharmacological or surgical, presents both benefits and risks. The prognosis, which is generally poor, champions the need for prevention of thromboembolism and a prompt diagnosis is essential in order to begin appropriate therapy and relative follow-up. Late sequelae include impairment of renal function, shrunken hypoplastic kidney, arterial hypertension and tubular defects. In this chapter, conditions concerning venous or arterial thrombosis associated with terminal renal failure, renal transplantation or tumors are not covered.

* Correspondence concerning this article should be addressed to: Dr. Marco Zaffanello, MD, Department of Mother-Child and Biology-Genetics, University of Verona, Piazzale L. Scuro, 10, 37134 Verona, Italy. E-mail: marco.zaffanello@univr.it; Tel: +39 045 812 4469; Fax: +39 045 812 4790.

INTRODUCTION

During fetal life, the coagulative system undergoes progressive maturation. In plasma, fibrinolytic activity, platelets and whole blood clotting are detectable at around 10 weeks of gestational age; measurable levels of all coagulation proteins are detectable at around 20 weeks of gestational age. Postnatal maturation of the coagulative system is characterized by 50% more aduls of K-dependent factors (II, VII, IX and X) and contact factors (XII, XI, precallicrein and HMWK), but also by a reduction of inhibitors of the thrombin system (antrithrombin, heparin cofactor II) and indirect inhibitors (protein C and S). However, α2-macroglobulin is increased. The capacity of newborn plasma to generate thrombin is quite low (50%). However, low levels of plasminogen, and increased tissue plasminogen activator (t-PA) and plasminogen activator inhibitor (PAI) lead to hypofibrinolytic states. This coagulative system develops progressively during the first weeks of life reaching adult values at 6 months of postnatal life. Factors V, VIII, XIII, and fibrinogen have similar concentrations as those of adults. The Von Willebrand factor is normal or increased, as are thrombin-AT complex, thrombomodulin and D-Dimer. These characteristics are dependent on gestational age and are more important in premature infants [1-3]. The conventional coagulative tests known as prothrombin time (PT) and activated partial thromboplastin time (aPTT) are physiologically higher in the newborn.

An increased risk of thrombosis has been reported during the neonatal period. A survey conducted in Germany reported an incidence for thrombosis of 5.1:100,000 live births [4] and a Canadian survey reported an incidence of 2.4:1,000 newborns in intensive care units [5]. A second peak of increased risk of thrombosis has been reported during puberty [6]. In 70% of cases of venous thrombosis, the risk factors are a central venous catheter, sepsis, asphyxia, dehydratation, congenital cardiopathy and maternal diabetes.

The most common sites of neonatal thrombosis are renal veins, cava, cerebral veins, portal and mesenteric veins, the aorta, and femoral and succlavian veins. In a review of the literature, Andrew et al reported renal vein thrombosis (RVT) as the most common renal disorder associated with hemostatic complications, followed by hemolytic-uremic syndrome, nephrotic syndrome, renal transplants, glomerulonephritis and finally end-stage kidney disease and dialysis [7]. Renal artery thrombosis (RAT) and RVT develop when a blood clot forms in the renal artery or vein, respectively. Both RAT and RVT occur most commonly in newborns and small children. RVT has been observed more frequently in at-term male newborns. No differences between sexes have been observed for RAT [6]. A retrospective revision of 15 years of medical literature on neonatal RVT enrolled 271 patients from 13 case series. The authors reported a majority of males (67.2%) suffering from neonatal RVT. More than 70% of these patients had unilateral RVT, which was more prevalent on the left side (63.6%). Of the cases of thrombus, 43.7% involved the inferior vena cava and 14.8% was associated with adrenal hemorrhage [8].

Renal Venous Thrombofilia

The true incidence and prevalence of people suffering from RVT is difficult to determine because many patients do not have symptoms and require specific tests. Approximately 90% of pediatric cases of RVT occur in infants under 1 year of age and 75% occur in infants under 1 month of age. However, the minimum incidence of symptomatic neonatal RVT evaluated between 1992 and 1994 in Germany was 2.2 per 100,000 live births (95% confidence interval 1.4-3.3) [4]. Out of 35 documented cases, RVT occurred in 15 premature babies with an incidence of 13 per 100,000 live births (95% confidence interval 5.9-24.8). Ten babies also had a caval occlusion [9]. RVT represents 22%-44% of neonatal thrombosis, causing renal scarring in 58%-100% of cases and leading to long-term sequels in 30% of cases [9,10]. A retrospective study reported 53 patients with neonatal RVT, which was unilateral in 56% of patients and associated with thrombi at other sites in 74% of patients [11].

Renal Artery Thrombofilia

Renal artery thrombosis is rarely found in the pediatric population. Therefore, the literature associates its occurrence with the use of umbilical artery catheterization. RAT that developed a few weeks after birth was reported in two patients with severe cardiac disease [12]. Moreover, RAT and ischemia were observed in a premature baby following umbilical arterial and venous catheterization which led to severe neonatal hypertension [13].

PATHOGENESIS

In young children, thrombophilia can be either acquired or inherited, or both. The main causes of inherited and acquired thrombophilia are summarized in Table 1 [14].

Newborn and Infants

Acquired Thrombofilia

In newborns and infants, RVT is commonly associated with asphyxia, dehydration [15], diminished vascular blood flow associated with septic shock, congenital hyper-coagulable states, mother with diabetes mellitus, and intra-vascular sledging due to polycythemia. Thrombus formation is mediated by endothelial cell injury resulting from hypoxia, endotoxin or contrast media.

RAT is strongly associated with an umbilical artery line [16] and patent ductus arteriosus. In a review of the literature, Kasaragod et al reported a 9-month-old male infant with systemic hypertension. RAT was usually a consequence of umbilical arterial catheterization, which can also lead to embolization of the renal artery [17]. Ellis et al reported a newborn with acute renal failure who developed extensive aortic and bilateral RAT from inadequate breastfeeding and severe dehydration. Renal function recovery began

11 days after the onset of anuria [18]. However, a 1-year-old baby suffering from Netherton syndrome with severe generalized erythrodermia developed acute renal failure from bilateral RVT after a short episode of enteritis [19]. Rare cases of RVT in infancy have been associated with congenital nephrotic syndrome [20,21].

Congenital Thrombofilia

The inherited risk factors for neonatal thrombophilia are shown in Table 1. Two newborns with severe cardiac disease developed RAT a few weeks after birth. Umbilical artery catheterization was not done at the time of vascular occlusion, which upholds the role of congenital thrombophilia [12]. In a survey of 28 newborns with thrombosis, only one mother had antiphospholipid syndrome (APS). Eleven newborns out of 28 studied had congenital thrombophilia, but only one carried the factor V Leiden mutation [22]. Procoagulant abnormalities were investigated in 23 newborns and 44% of them showed renal thrombophilia. Of these, 22.2% carried factor V Leiden mutations [23].

Table 1

Acquire thrombofilia	Inherited thrombofilia	
• Central venous catheter • Polycitemia • Postpartum asphyxia • Dehidratatation • Sepsis • Acute respiratory distress syndrome	Common • Factor V G1691A Leiden • Factor II G20210A • Increased lipoprotein(a) • Hyperhomocysteinemia • NTHFR, 677C>T, 1298A>C	Rare • Protein C deficiency • Protein S deficiency • Antithrombin deficiency • Eparinic factor II deficiency • ACE 1 deletion
• Cardiopathy • Necroziting entherocolitis • Maternal diabetes • Acute renal failure	Probably inherited • Increased FVIII • Increased FIX • Reduced FXII	Very rare • Disfibrinogenemia • Dis/hypoplasminemia • Homozigous homocystinuria

Children

Acquired Thrombofilia

RVT may occur in one or both kidneys, be associated with maternal diabetes, diarrhea and dehydration [24], congenital heart disease, acute blood loss, sepsis, asphyxia, or shock and may follow exposure to angiographic contrast agents [25]. Kauffmann et al investigated the occurrence of thromboembolism in 48 patients with various degrees of proteinuria. Thrombosis in patients with severe proteinuria was associated with a deficiency of antithrombin III, a protein lost through urination [26]. RVT is more common in patients with nephrotic syndrome [27], although studies have shown a high variability among these patients, with rates varying between 5% and 62 %. In particular, of 48 patients with nephrotic syndrome, 4 developed RVT [26]. However, thrombosis of the renal veins and inferior vena cava classically present with nephrotic range proteinuria and has also been described in aPL-positive patients with lupus nephritis. In fact, positive aPL was found in four out of six lupus patients with RVT [28] as well as in patients with primary antiphospholipid syndrome [29]. Patients with membranous nephropathy appeared to be at the greatest risk for developing RVT [30]. RVT developed in 11 out of 280 patients with either biopsy-proved membranous nephropathy or systemic lupus erythematosus with nephritis. Ten of the 11 patients also had pulmonary emboli at or near the time of RVT [31]. A 13-year-old Japanese boy with an 11-month history of systemic lupus erithematosus without a-PL suddenly developed severe hypertension from RVT [32]. Two cases of RVT have been reported in the course of Henoch-Schoenlein purpura in a woman and of polyarthritis nodosa in a 16-year-old girl, respectively [33].

Reuben et al investigated 18 out of 57 patients (31.6%) with nephrotic syndrome suffering from Familial Mediterranean Fever. Seven of them probably developed RVT. The authors advocated RVT as the major cause of kidney failure in Familial Mediterranean Fever from amyloidosis, associating nephrotic syndrome with kidney failure [34].

Finally, a calcified large renal artery aneurysm containing thrombus was associated with fibromuscular dysplasia in a 6-year-old girl who presented with hypertension [35].

Congenital Thrombofilia

Congenital deficiencies in the proteins of the coagulation cascade (protein C, protein S, antithrombin III and plasminogen) have been involved in RVT and RAT [15,36]. However, the presence of the factor V Leiden mutation, prothrombin variants, methylentetrahydrofolate reductase variants, and increased levels of lipoprotein(a) have been reported in patients with renal thrombosis [37-40]. A newborn infant carrying the heterozygous mutation of the gene encoding for clotting factor V, which causes resistance to activated protein C, showed bilateral RVT and adrenal hemorrhage [41]. One patient out of 30 (aged 14 to 58 years) with sickle cell disease investigated for abdominal pain and/or fever of uncertain cause developed RVT [42].

Clinical Features

The kidneys clear the body of wastes by filtering these wastes into the bladder where they exit the body through the urine. When one or more blood vessels in the kidneys become narrowed (renal artery stenosis) because of debris and plaque build-up, or blocked because of a blood clot (RVT), the kidneys are unable to function properly.

The diagnosis of RVT is based on the presence of symptoms, results of a medical examination and diagnostic tests. There is usually a rise in blood pressure, and kidney failure can occur if the patient does not receive prompt treatment. The onset of RVT can be rapid (acute) or gradual. Blood clots in the renal arteries are uncommon, but when they do occur, there is a risk of pulmonary embolism. There is also an increased risk of congestive heart failure. Acute renal failure may occur if there are large vessel insults such as in bilateral RAT and RVT or if they occur in a solitary kidney.

Newborn

RVT is the most frequently occurring vascular condition in the neonatal kidney. RVT may present clinically with a flank mass, hematuria, hypertension and/or thrombocytopenia or renal failure and edemas [19]. Adrenal hemorrhage and death may occur soon after onset. Hypertension and irreversible renal atrophy are late complications of RVT. Unilateral involvement was observed in 89% of 28 newborns with RVT, and bilateral involvement was found in 11%. Unilateral RVT affected mostly at-term infants, whereas 2 out of 3 infants with bilateral RVT were born before 32 weeks of gestation [22]. In addition, secondary hypertension from renal hypoperfusion is a typical feature in RAT.

Ante-natal Thrombosis

There are eleven cases in the literature of prenatal thrombosis of the inferior vena cava and the renal veins presenting as hydrops fetalis (33%), acute fetal distress (42%) or as an incidental prenatal ultrasound finding (25%). Underlying maternal conditions, which included chronic conditions (hypertension and diabetes mellitus), acute conditions (pyelonephritis and preeclampsia) and thrombophilia, were present in 58% of the patients [43].

Hypertension

In newborns, a thromboembolism caused by umbilical artery catheters most often leads to hypertension [44,45] and it has been advocated as the most common cause of hypertension in the post-natal period [13,46]. Renal arterial stenosis from RAT accounts for 10% - 24% of cases of infantile hypertension [17].

Acute and Chronic Renal Failure

RAT and RVT can result in renal failure if they are bilateral conditions or even if they occur in a solitary kidney [47,48]. Acute renal failure associated with severe hypertension was described in newborns and young children with a solitary kidney or after massive thromboembolisms [49-51]. However, a reduced glomerular filtration rate at follow up was described in 2 out of 4 infants with bilateral RVT [52]. Finally, in a retrospective study of 53 newborns, the main clinical presentations of RVT included renal failure in 56%, thrombocytopenia, anemia, or both in 51%, and renal mass in 49% [11].

Other Clinical Features

Median presentation of symptoms in 23 newborns was on day 1; 83% of these had pre- or peri-natal problems, including fetal distress, intrauterine growth retardation or other pre-identified renal abnormalities [23]. One newborn (gestational age of 37 weeks) with bilateral RVT showed a severe macrohematuria within 24 hours after birth [53]. Preterm infants of diabetic mothers presented with intestinal obstruction secondary to extrinsic compression by the mass effect of the enlarged hemorrhagic adrenal and thrombosed kidney on the left hemicolon [54].

Children

Symptoms manifest rapidly in some patients while others have no symptoms at all. The onset of acute RVT at any age may cause pain in the lower back and sides of the abdomen, fever, blood in the urine, decreased urine output and sometimes kidney failure. On examination, the child's abdomen may disclose kidney enlargement. If RVT is present, when placing the stethoscope over the child's abdomen, one may hear an abnormal "whooshing" sound as blood tries to flow through the blocked vessel. Another symptom is high blood pressure.

Children with RVT may suffer acute renal failure along with oliguria and increased nitrogen and creatinine levels, hypertension, gross or microscopic hematuria, thrombocytopenia and enlarged kidneys [25,49,55,56]. A 13-day-old infant presented with acute renal failure secondary to a large thrombus formation involving the umbilical aorta and both renal arteries. The initial clinical manifestations were hematuria, followed by anuria, severe dehydration, grunting while breathing and cyanosis of the feet [57]. Duncan et al, who studied 11 children with RVT, reported that some of them developed pulmonary emboli associated with thrombosis of the inferior vena cava. After RVT many children develop a consumptive coagulopathy [58].

No significant differences were detected among 44 unselected patients with nephrotic syndrome between plasma fibrinogen, serum cholesterol, β-lipoprotein, triglycerides and phospholipid concentrations in those diagnosed with RVT and those who were not [59]. However, 48 patients with various degrees of nephrotic syndrome, hypoalbuminemia, hypercholesterolemia and edema were associated with the loss of coagulation factors, which led to thrombophilic states [26]. Moreover, Uthman et al, in a review of the medical literature between 1968 and 2005, concluded that a-PL could be greatly involved in cases of renal artery stenosis, hypertension and unexplained deterioration of renal function [60].

Clinical Evaluation

Evaluation of RVT and RAT includes laboratory analyses and at least an ultrasonography of the kidneys, which can reveal renal enlargement with disruption of the normal echo pattern, followed by computed tomography and renal isotope scanning [25]. Although there are many imaging techniques to choose from, ultrasound is the technique most commonly used in the evaluation of newborn infants with suspected RVT.

Laboratory Investigation

Laboratory tests in cases of suspect thrombosis are blood cell count, especially of platelets, PT, aPTT and fibrinogen. D-Dimer in newborns has low specificity; it is used to exclude rather than confirm thrombosis. Therefore, a low platelet count is the most sensible indicator of thrombosis (sepsis). Again, reduced numbers of platelets and low fibrinogen indicate a suspicion of thrombosis [61]. Other diagnostic tests are to check antithrombin activity and to assess protein C and S, genetic tests such as factor V of Leiden (prevalence 2-4%), prothrombin mutation 20210 (prevalence 1-3%) in association or not with hyperhomocistinemia, and lipoprotein (a), since their increased levels in newborns are associated with an increased risk of thrombosis. Antiphospholipid antibodies (lupus anticoagulant, anti cardiolipin and anti-β2-glycoprotein) should be assessed in newborns of mothers affected by lupus or antiphospholipid syndrome [62]. Increased levels of factors VII, VIII, IX, XI and a deficiency of factor XII are associated with increased risk of thromboembolism [63]. Hereditary thrombophilia must be recognized in a newborn with significant and spontaneous thromboembolism associating purpura. Asymptomatic newborns do not need to be examined if they have no history of familial fulminant purpura.

In conclusion, coagulative screening and thrombophilias in neonatal thrombosis must include a blood cell count (platelets), PT, aPTT, fibrinogen, antithrombin activity, protein C and S, lupus anticoagulant (mother) and antiphospholipid antibodies (mother).

Ultrasound

In the post-natal period, renal ultrasound is helpful in making a differential diagnosis among renal diseases [64]. However, the assessment of a peculiar neonatal ultrasound pattern (enlarged kidney, distinct clumps of echoes randomly scattered throughout the kidney, sometimes surrounding echo-free spaces) and clinical features (hematuria, proteinuria and right flank masses) allow a diagnosis of RVT without the need for invasive vascular studies [65]. Schlengel et al reported their experience in three cases of RVT, one of which was a child. Sonograms and computed radionuclide urograms used to detect conditions sustaining RAT or RVT are both non-invasive and safe methods with no adverse effects in the presence of azotemia or even anuria [66].

Prenatal Ultrasound

In a case report, prenatal ultrasound was able to detect fetal renal abnormalities described as suspected neoplasm and subsequently confirmed as prenatal thrombosis [67]. However, another case report described prenatal calcifications of the inferior vena cava and renal veins as a rare condition with unclear etiology and prognosis. It was a case of RVT in utero and was associated with congenital anomalies and abnormal prenatal hemodynamic status [68]. In 42% of 11 cases of prenatal thrombosis of the inferior vena cava and renal veins, a prenatal ultrasound revealed an enlarged and hyper-echogenic affected kidney [43]. In one case report, postnatal ultrasonography confirmed the prenatal diagnosis of RVT. Both gray-scale and Doppler techniques were used to follow the resolution of the thrombosis and the fate of the kidney [67].

Hyperecogenic Kidney

A review of 1600 abdominal ultrasound results revealed 103 newborn infants (56 females and 47 males, with birth weight between 560 and 3,700 grams and gestational age between 25 and 42 weeks) whose kidneys showed increased echogenicity. Prenatal ultrasound hyperechogenicity of the kidney identified RVT in 2 of the 103 newborns.

Ultrasound appearances depend on the fetal stage at which the scan is performed and the extention of the thrombus. Initially, the interlobular and interlobar thrombi appear as highly echogenic streaks [69]. Ultrasonic follow-up of 3 cases of RVT showed that initially the kidneys were enlarged and echogenic, with echogenic streaking having vascular or perivascular distribution. These streaks commenced in a peripheral, focal segment of the involved kidney and only persisted for a few days [70]. In one newborn, perivascular streaks were first seen by ultrasound at 3 days of age with a diffusely enlarged and echogenic right kidney. Echolucency gradually appeared over the medulla area with shrinking renal size [71]. In a case of bilateral RVT, sonography of the kidneys showed a dense cortical parenchyma with loss of cortico-medullary differentiation [53]. Grey-scale ultrasound readily showed a thrombus in the renal vein in two infants with RVT. Adrenal hemorrhage may be an acknowledged association identified ultrasonically. In the first week, the affected kidney swelled and became echogenic with prominent echo-poor medullary pyramids. However, the apex of the renal papilla became hypo-echoic and a ring of reduced echogenicity around the affected pyramids may have appeared 1-2 weeks after the acute phase [72]. Ultimately, the swelling increased in an 8-month-old infant, whose kidney became heterogenous with loss of cortico-medullary differentiation or atrophy [19].

Color Doppler

Vascular ultrasound is a non-invasive method that examines blood circulation to detect blood clots. Vascular ultrasound may confirm RVT in asymptomatic newborns. Argyropoulou et al reported a newborn whose initial ultrasonographic image of RAT appeared normal or revealed minor abnormalities, whereas a renal scan showed little or no blood flow. Furthermore, very high arterial resistance with reversed diastolic flow was observed in the main renal artery and its intraparenchymal branches [73]. In the early stages of RVT, color Doppler may identify the absence of intrarenal and renal venous flow. In a report on three cases, Lalmand et al showed that, over time, the ultrasonographic image of RVT may show an enlarged, swollen kidney, and the renal scan typically shows decreased blood flow. Color Doppler can show a thrombus within the renal vein or the inferior vena cava [74]. In a case of bilateral RVT in a newborn twin, a negative diastolic flow in both renal arteries and veins were diagnostic [53]. To rule out RVT, careful Doppler studies of the renal vasculature are advisable in any patient with persistently positive a-PL that develops sudden heavy proteinuria [29].

Renal Calcification

Detection of renal calcification may indicate a previous RVT and has a virtually diagnostic lace-like radiological pattern on a prenatal ultrasound performed at 37 weeks of gestation [75].

Selective Renal Venography

Renal venography, or renal angiography or phlebography, is an X-ray examination of the renal veins used to diagnose RVT. A catheter is inserted into the femoral vein and threaded first into the right kidney vein and then into the vein of the left kidney. The contrast material is injected through the catheter into each vein and X-rays are taken. This test may be performed to locate the narrowing or blockage in the renal vein. Renal venography may delineate a clot in the main renal veins or indicate areas of reduced blood flow due to thromboses in intrarenal venules [34]. This method has been widely accepted for an evaluation of the renal venous bed in patients with suspected RVT or hematuria of unknown etiology [76].

In 10 out of 44 patients, aged 12–65 years, with nephrotic syndrome, RVT was confirmed by selective renal venography. Extension of the thrombus from the renal veins into the inferior vena cava was seen in 3 patients, 2 of which died. Evidence of thrombo-embolism elsewhere in the body has been seen in the form of thrombophlebitis in the lower extremities, pulmonary embolism and myocardial infarction [59]. Anuria of acute onset was evaluated in 6 patients, aged 11–67 years, by renal scan and arteriogram to detect those patients with proximal renal artery occlusion in preparation for revascularization [77]. Aortography confirmed the occlusion of the left renal artery and developing renovascular hypertension in a 16-year-old boy with primary antiphospholipid syndrome [78].

Renal Scintigraphic Scan

Radionuclides are frequently used in the estimation of renal function. A newborn with RVT showed a rim sign on renal scan with Technetium DTPA. The rim sign on renal scan was differentiated from severe hydronephrosis or multicystic kidney since both of them may have a peripheral thin cortex, whose functions appear late on the renal scan [79]. In a rare case of simultaneous RVT and bilateral adrenal hemorrhage, DMSA scintigraphy was able to assess renal function. The characteristic appearances were suprarenal tracer-free areas encircled by peripheral radioactive rims over the inferiorly displaced kidneys on a Tc-99m DTPA renal scan [80]. Finally, concomitant loss of renal function was demonstrated by DMSA scan at the age of 1 year in a case of neonatal RVT [71].

Magnetic Resonance Imaging and Computed Tomography Scans, Angio-MRI

Magnetic resonance imaging (MRI) and computed tomography scans (CT scans) aid the physician in making an accurate diagnosis of RVT or RAT. A CT scan proved to be informative for recurrent episodes of venous or arterial thrombosis in 32 patients out of 751 with primary antiphospholipid syndrome, 1 of which patient had hepatic, portal and renal vein involvement [81]. However, emergency abdominal CT scans revealed left RAT in a 13-year-old Japanese boy with an 11-month history of systemic lupus erithematosus; a renal scintigraphy revealed reduced blood flow in the left kidney [32]. Moreover, MRI showed low signal intensity of the renal pyramids on T1- and T2-weighted images, suggesting acute hemorrhage in the case of a newborn infant with hereditary thrombophilia [73].

Treatment

One of the major goals of treatment for RVT is to prevent pulmonary embolism which can have serious complications. Thus, the serious sequelae of thromboembolism (mortality, and short- and long-term morbidity) require careful therapeutic intervention.

In a retrospective cohort study of 43 newborns with RVT, interventions included anti-coagulants and thrombolytic agents: subcutaneous low-molecular weight heparin (LMWH, 40%), systemic heparin (16%), t-PA (7%) and warfarin (2%) in 28 patients, antihypertensive medication in 9 patients (21%), peritoneal dialysis in 2 patients (5%), and nephrectomy in 2 patients (5%) [11]. A 15-year retrospective study showed that 50% of the newborn infants with RVT (13 cases out of 271) were treated with supportive therapy. Of those patients who received anticoagulation therapy, unfractioned heparin or LMWH alone were given in 21.6% and 20.7% of cases, respectively. Fibrinolytic treatment alone was used in 11.2% of the patients. Only a minority of patients were treated with antithrombin (1.7%), warfarin alone (0.9%) or underwent surgery (0.3%) [8]. Prospective controlled trials are still lacking, and to date there are no evidence-based guidelines available for the treatment of newborn babies with RVT [8].

Supportive Care

The initial treatment of RVT is supportive. Supportive therapy is necessary in all cases to correct dehydration and sepsis. In particular, thromboembolism with associated pyrexia, dehydration, anemia, coagulative defects and piastrinopenia (<50.000/µl) must be corrected [82,83]. Different approaches should be used and different outcomes expected for patients with RVT secondary to congenital absence of coagulation factors and for those with severely altered blood flow secondary to sepsis and shock. Severe dehydration requires medical treatment with intravenous fluids and may require hospitalization. Bedrest or limited activity may be recommended for brief periods.

Hypertension

Blood pressure medication may be prescribed to treat high blood pressure from RVT, something that is often difficult to treat. In a prospective trial, intravenous nicardipine was reported as the first-line antihypertensive drug in 17 newborns out of 20 with RVT: the initial nicardipine dosage was 0.5 µg/kg/min. The mean nicardipine dosage was 0.74±0.41 µg/kg/min (range 0.5-2.0 µg/kg/min). The duration of treatment was 14.6±11.6 days [84]. In a 2-day-old newborn with unilateral RVT, because hypertension remained sustained despite aggressive antihypertensive therapy including hydralazine (0.7 mg/kg per dose every 4 hours) and enalaprilat (highest dose: 10 µg/kg per dose twice daily), on day 4 of life he developed clinical signs of hypertensive encephalopathy and significant cardiac dysfunction [85].

Anticoagulant and Thrombolytic Therapy

In newborns, therapy for RVT should be aimed at limiting the extension of the clot by removal of the umbilical arterial catheter; then anticoagulant or fibrinolytic therapy can be considered, particularly if the clot is large [15,16,86,87]. Thrombolytic agents and anticoagulants are often used in combination. Treatment with heparin, recombinant t-PA and fibrinogenolytic agents gave partially satisfactory results in patients suffering from Familial Mediterranean Fever with nephrotic syndrome. Thus, the authors suggested prompt renal phlebography when renal function began to fall, followed by anticoagulant treatment to prevent further thromboembolic complications [34]. Multiple single centers have reported or described the successful use of heparin, streptokinase and recombinant t-PA in preterm infants, children and older people [5,88-91]. In a neonatal case of acute renal failure due to bilateral RVT, reperfusion of the left kidney was achieved by treatment with urokinase (4,400 U/kg/hour for 5 days) and heparin (760 U/kg/day for 10 days), infused simultaneously. Prophylactic oral anticoagulation (INR $\approx$ 2.3) was used for 21 days after the heparin was stopped [92]. In a 3-day-old infant with acute renal failure secondary to a large thrombus formation involving the umbilical aorta and both renal arteries, heparinization and fibrinolytic therapies gave unsuccessful results in dissolving the clot. However, the aortic clot recanalized spontaneously a few weeks later, but the renal arteries remained permanently occluded [57].

Ellis et al reported a newborn with RVT who underwent dialysis and received general supportive care, together with concurrent anticoagulation therapy (continuous infusion of heparin with INR $\approx$ 2) and continuous aggressive intrathrombic instillation with urokinase (single dose of 16,000 U, followed by continuous infusion of urokinase at a rate of 4,400 - 6,600 U/kg/hour). Adjustments of the therapy were based on sequential plasma fibrinogen measurements which ranged from 100-200 mg/dl [18]. Moreover, a retrospective study showed that 15 out of 35 cases of RVT occurred in premature babies. For 8 babies the therapeutic approaches were mainly supportive. Low dose heparin was used in 14 patients (from 4 to 10 U/kg/hour not aimed at prolonging the aPTT], full heparinization in 9 (from 12 to 50 U/kg/hour) and thrombolytic therapy in 2 patients with recombinant t-PA or streptokinase [9]. However, the Montreal experience reported long-term renal function impairment in 100% of those who did not receive heparin, and in 33% of those who did receive heparin. In particular, 12 patients (52%) received either intravenous heparin or subcutaneous enoxaparin. Of these, 5 patients received heparin alone, 5 patients received enoxaparin alone, and 2 patients received heparin followed by enoxaparin [89]. Whereas some authors reported successful recovery of renal function, others noted a significant incidence of bleeding complications and significant renal atrophy on long-term follow-up. Prelog et al reported a retrospective outcome study of 28 newborns with RVT, of which 10 babies received either unfractioned or low molecular weight heparin (LMWH) for 3 days and 7 months. Three infants with unilateral RVT treated with heparin alone did not seem to benefit from such therapy. Seven newborns were treated with fibrinolytics and unfractioned heparin (4 infants with unilateral RVT and 3 with bilateral RVT). Treatment with fibrinolytics did not restore renal function in the 4 infants with unilateral RVT, but it was associated with restoration of quite normal renal function in the 2 newborns with bilateral

RVT who received fibrinolytics immediately after the diagnosis of RVT. Two newborns treated with fibrinolytics suffered bleeding complications at the area of adrenal hemorrhage. Finally, two newborns (not treated for RVT) died because of underlying disease [53].

Thrombolytic Drugs

Recombinant t-PA is the treatment of choice in newborns because of its low half-live (5 minutes). In newborns with local or systemic thrombosis, the recommended doses of recombinant t-PA ranged between 0.1 and 0.5 mg/kg, with a starting dose of 0.06 mg/kg/hour [93]. Simultaneous infusion of intravenous heparin at 10 U/kg/hour may sometimes be advisable. In cases of fibrinogenemia <100 mg/dl, it is advisable to reduce the dose by 50% or to do an infusion of fibrinogen or fresh frozen plasma and to maintain the platelets at levels of >50,000/μl. Counter-indications for thrombolytic therapy in newborns are previous bleeding and surgical intervention (10 days before), asphyxia (7 days before), convulsions (3 days before), preterm delivery under 32 weeks of gestation, severe asphyxia, active bleeding, platelets persistently <50,000-100,00/μl or fibrinogen <100 mg/dl. Moreover, during treatment it is essential to monitor the chemicals to avoid intramuscular injections and arterial invasive procedures. Success of the treatment can be clinically and radiologically assessed. Table 2 shows the thrombolytic scheme recommended for newborn infants [94,95].

Table 2. Thrombolysis with urokinase or recombinant t-PA in neonatal age. The mornitoring of thrombolysis must include imaging, fibrinogen (minimum 100 mg/dl), platelet (minimum 50-100,000/μl) coagulative tests, plasminogen and D-dimer

	Urokinase	Recombinant t-PA
Dose attack	4,400 UI/kg in 5 minutes	Only if increased risk 0.1-0.2 mg/kg
Maintenance dosages	4,400 U/kg/hour for 72 hours	0.1-0.3 mg/kg/hour for 6 hour, 0.03-0.06 mg/kg/hour for 12-96 hours
Associations	Heparin 15-20 UI/kg/hour, LMWH 1.5 mg/kg	Heparin 15-20 UI/kg/hour, LMWH 1.5 mg/kg

Research has shown that clot-busting medications are most effective when given within 2 hours of the onset of symptoms. Molteni et al reported a case in which a continuous intrathrombic urokinase infusion induced complete clot lysis and reperfusion of the right kidney in an at-term infant with aortic and renal artery thrombosis in whom the right kidney experienced complete ischemia for 5 days [96]. Rosembaum et al reported a 15-year-old boy with thromboses of the inferior vena cava, the femoral, inguinal and renal veins of unknown origin. Although the thrombosis was 2 weeks old, thrombolytic therapy with recombinant t-PA (maximum dosage: 0.4 mg/kg/hour) was started as this appeared to be the only change to re-establish normal kidney function. After 1 week, the treatment was discontinued because of generalized bleeding [97].

Anticoagulants

The aim of anticoagulant therapy is to avoid worsening of the thrombus. The drug of choice for anticoagulation is heparin. Optimal duration of anticoagulant treatment in the newborn is generally a rather brief period (15-30 days) with strict mornitoring of the thrombus [83,98]. Rarely is secondary prophylaxis necessary for a long time, mainly because of the low risk of relapse and the peculiar hemostatic system in newborns.

Anticoagulant or antiaggregant medication, including heparin or warfarin and low-dose aspirin, can be prescribed to prevent existing blood clots from getting larger and to prevent the formation of new clots. There have been controversial reports regarding anticoagulant therapy in children with RVT [25]. The use of aspirin in children is controversial because of the risk of Reye's syndrome. Unfractioned heparin has shown the following disadvantages: age-dependent unpredictable pharmacokinetics, the need for intravenous access for therapy and monitoring, delays in achieving therapeutic ranges, risk of bleeding, the risk of heparin-induced thrombocytopenia, and osteoporosis after long-term use. Oral anticoagulants, in addition to some of the above-mentioned disadvantages, show considerable variations in anticoagulation depending on diet (especially if there is a change from breast to bottle-feeding), concomitant medication and intercurrent illness. In two newborns with severe cardiac disease and RAT, neither patient recovered renal function in the affected kidney despite systemic anticoagulation [12]. Nuss et al reported treatment for RVT, bilateral in 3 out of 6 newborns, with standard heparin infusion rates between 8 and 40 U/kg/hour for 7-14 days. Two infants developed hemorrhages; one suffered disseminated intravascular coagulation but did not hemorrhage until heparin reached toxic levels, and the other was well until an umbilical catheter was removed while he was on heparin [88].

RVT requires mornitoring of extension when no treatment is in progress or for anticoagulation with standard heparin or LMWH for unilateral thrombosis without renal failure or in absence of extension in vena cava. Anticoagulation therapy with standard heparin or LMWH may be advisable for 6 weeks to 3 months if extension occurs in the inferior vena cava. The reported dosages of standard heparin must be adjusted for the gestational age of the newborns. In particular, in newborns <28 weeks of gestational age, begin with 25 U/Kg and then with 15 U/Kg/hour; in infants born between 28 and 37 weeks, begin with 50 U/kg and then with 15 U/Kg/hour; and in newborns born after 37 weeks, begin with 100 U/Kg and then with 28 U/kg/hour. The dose for unfractioned heparin is 10 U/kg/hour in continuous infusion. Anticoagulation with standard heparin for 6 weeks - 3 months and thrombolysis are advisable if it is a case of bilateral thrombosis with renal failure. The therapeutic dose for bolus is 100 U/kg in 10 minutes maintaining 28 U/kg/hour, adjusted for a therapeutic level of anti-FXa activity of 0.35-0.7 U/ml or aPTT range 60-85 seconds. Since newborns show an increased clearance of the drug from reduced levels of antithrombin, it is necessary to use a plasma infusion or an antithrombin or to increase the heparin dosages [99].

Sutor et al, who studied 728 children with thromboembolic complications, reported the following advantages of LMWH over unfractioned heparin: minimal monitoring, easy administration (subcutaneous), and possibly equal efficacy and safety. Dosages were calculated according to body weight: infants <3 months (or <5 kg) need approximately 50% less LMWH than older children or adults to reach prophylactic or therapeutic anti-factor Xa levels [100]. In cases of renal failure, LMWH must not be used because it is cleared through the kidneys. Different LMWHs (Table 3) with different molecular weights and anti-factor Xa activity are available [101]. For neonatal ages, the main experience regards enoxaparine

[102]. Guidelines for the treatment of newborns with standard heparin according to gestational age have been published [103]. The initial recommended dose is 1.6-1.7 mg/kg subcutaneously every 12 hours for at-term newborns, and 2.1 mg/kg subcutaneously every 12 hours in preterm infants (<37 weeks of gestational age) if there is no risk of bleeding, with increments of 0.125 mg/kg/dose adjusting for the anti-factor Xa therapeutic range [104]. The main side effects of LMWH are bleeding and thrombocytopenia. The treatment of choice for bleeding from heparin is protamine and free frozen plasma. For example, to neutralize 100U (1 mg) enoxaparine, infused 3-4 hours before, it is necessary to use 1 mg protamine; if infused 8 hours previously, it is necessary to use 0.5 mg of protamine; and if infused 12 hours before, no protamine is necessary.

Possibly, anticoagulation medication prevents existing thromboses from progressing to uninvolved parenchyma or to the other kidney; however, there are no controlled, multicenter studies to determine the effectiveness of heparin, aspirin and other anticoagulants in children with RVT or RAT.

Table 3. Therapeutic doses of LMWH in the newborn. The mornitoting of LMWH therapy is based on anti FXa (therapeuric range 0.5-1.0 U/ml)

	Therapy	Prophylaxis
Enoxaparine	1.7-1.5 mg/kg/12 hours	0.75 mg/kg/12 hours
Dalteparine	130-160 UI/kg/24 hours	92 IU/kg/24 hours
Nodraparine	100-225 IU/kg/12 hours	50-110 IU/kg/12 hours
Tinzaparine	280 IU/kg/24 hours	-
Reviparine	150 IU/kg/12 hours	50 IU/kg/12 hours

New Drugs

New oral or parenteral drugs for anticoagulation are currently under investigation [105].

Surgery

Normally, a surgical approach is not advisable in cases of thromboembolic complications due to the high risk of mortality and bleeding [83,98]. Indeed, surgical intervention is not indicated in the acute phase of RVT except in the rare instance of bilateral disease.

Angiography

Angiography is a non-operative method, an alternative to surgery, for intervening on renal arteries that are partially or completely obstructed. A catheter inserted into a vein or artery may be slowly directed to the blocked blood vessel using X-ray guidance (angiography). A specialized balloon tip or other device at the end of the catheter can be used to open the blocked or narrowed vessel. The balloon is rapidly inflated and deflated to open or widen the area. In some patients, a stent (metal mesh tube) can be placed to act as a scaffold to hold the area open. Intra-arterial thrombolysis involves threading a catheter with clot-busting medication through a large blood vessel in the groin up to the site of the clot.

Grützmacher et al described the transluminal angioplasty technique they used to obtain renal artery revascularization in 16 consecutive patients with 17 complete main renal artery occlusions and high operative risk [106]. In the case of a 13-year-old Japanese boy with systemic lupus erithematosus, the prompt use of intravenous anticoagulants was not effective in controlling the infarction-reduced renal arterial blood supply. Moreover, the patient developed stupor due to central nervous system lupus a week after the occurrence of the hypertensive episode. Finally, a percutaneous transluminal angioplasty successfully relieved the occlusion of the left renal artery at its origin [32].

Thrombectomy

A thrombectomy may be attempted when bilateral non-visualization on urography is associated with a positive venacavogram [58]. In a renal thrombectomy (endarterectomy), a vascular surgeon removes the blockage from the inner lining of the renal artery. Bypass surgery re-routes the blood flow around the narrowed or blocked sections of the renal artery. Endarterectomy and surgical bypass are two surgical treatment options, but they are not common in children. However, when venous thrombosis involves the entire venous system, a thrombectomy is rarely indicated or possible. Surgical thrombectomy is advisable only in cases of immediate risk of life or organ loss (for instance, complex thrombosis involving the heart, or occlusive septic thrombosis). Since there is a high risk of re-occlusion, it is advisable to associate concomitant or further anticoagulant treatment.

Nephrectomy

It is rare, but when there is complete blockage of the renal vein in infants, the kidney must be surgically removed. Patients with thrombosis of the inferior vena cava may require surgical nephrectomy- especially children who develop severe hypertension refractory to antihypertensive medication. Therefore, a period of treatment with drugs should be attempted before opting for unilateral nephrectomy. The literature describes a newborn infant with RAT and embolism from an umbilical artery catheter, in which the hypertension was transient and kidney function returned to normal [45]. Evans et al described a newborn with persistent hypokalemia and hyper-reninemia in the presence of a small left kidney and normal right kidney which led to the decision to perform a left nephrectomy [107]. The syndrome of neonatal renal arterial embolism, discussed in eight cases recorded in the literature and in one case report, presumably from the ductus arteriosum, resulted in congestive heart failure, respiratory distress and increased renin secretion, which could result in malignant hypertension. A nephrectomy promptly brought the blood pressure into the normal range [108]. Of 320 children who underwent a nephrectomy between 1991 and 2001, 22 underwent sugery to manage hypertension and one had renal artery thrombosis [109]. In one case of unilateral RVT, a renal angiography showed complete, likely thrombotic occlusion of the right renal artery. Renal MAG3 imaging showed minimal function of the affected kidney, and a nephrectomy secondary to medically uncontrollable hypertension and worsening cardiac dysfunction was performed [85].

Follow-up

When a child has been diagnosed with RVT, it is important a closely monitor the patient's condition. If an anticoagulant medication has been prescribed, it is essential to keep all scheduled laboratory appointments so that the effectiveness of the medication can be checked. If the child has developed any new symptoms, the patient should be re-assessed.

Differential Diagnosis

Increased echogenicity of the kidneys in newborns has many causes, some of which reflect serious renal disease. A differential diagnosis of bilateral RVT includes other causes of bilateral renal enlargement, such as autosomal recessive polycystic kidney disease, multicystic dysplasia, hydronephrosis and Wilms tumor [110].

A patient with bilateral RVT may be difficult to distinguish from those with hemolytic-uremic syndrome. Both disorders can be preceeded by a gastrointestinal disorder associated with dehydration, pallor, and evidence of microangiopathic hemolytic anemia, thrombocytopenia and acute renal failure. Market renal enlargement and absence of renal vein flow by renal Doppler ultrasonography is consistent with RVT. Acute renal failure is an uncommon but alarming complication of idiopathic nephrotic syndrome. The renal failure could be secondary to causes evident from the history and evaluation, such as severe intravascular volume depletion, acute tubular necrosis, allergic interstitial nephritis, bilateral renal vein thrombosis, acute pyelonephritis or rapid progression of the original glomerular disease [111].

Intrinsic acute renal failure includes a variety of disorders characterized by renal parenchymal damage, including sustained hypoperfusion/ischemia. A variety of conditions including prerenal conditions, such as dehydration, sepsis, etc, and intrinsic renal conditions, such as hemolytic-uremic syndrome, glomerulonephritis and postrenal conditions, may be involved. Laboratory test abnormalities may include anemia and thrombocytopenia (as in SLE and RVT). The prognosis for recovery of renal function is unusual when acute renal failure results from bilateral RVT. Management with drugs may be necessary for a prolonged period to treat the sequel of acute renal failure.

In newborns, cortical necrosis is most commonly associated with hypoxic/ischemic insults caused by perinatal asphyxia, placental abruption, and twin-twin or fetal-maternal transfusion. Other causes include renal vascular thrombosis and congenital heart disease. After the neonatal period, cortical necrosis is most commonly seen in children with septic shock or hemolytic-uremic syndrome as well as in adolescents with pregnancy-related acute renal failure. The involved portion of the renal cortex shows infarction, with congestion of the glomeruli, thrombosis of the arterioles, and necrosis of the tubules. Cortical necrosis develops when endothelial cell injury occurs in conjunction with diminished renal cortical blood flow. Toxins or other mediators that presumably develop during shock, hemolytic-uremic syndrome or sepsis may injure the endothelial cells and initiate intrarenal coagulation, leading to thrombosis and cortical necrosis.

PROGNOSIS

In a retrospective survey of forty-three patients with neonatal RVT, the median age at follow-up was 3.7 years (range, 0.5-20.2 years). Thirteen patients (34%) had hypertension and 11 patients (29%) had renal failure. End-stage renal disease developed in 3 patients who underwent live-related renal transplants. Twelve out of 28 patients (43%) examined had prothrombotic abnormalities [11]. Long-term follow-up of newborns disclosed abnormalities in 28 out of 34 (82%) affected kidneys. The mean glomerular filtration rate was 93.6 versus 70.2 ml/min/1.73 m2 in unilateral versus bilateral RVT (difference 23.4; 95% confidence interval 6.4 to 40.4; p = 0.01). Twenty-three patients with neonatal RVT showed no correlation between procoagulant tendencies and outcome, but renal length had a significant negative correlation. The mean fall in an estimated single kidney glomerular filtration rate was 3 ml/min/1.73 m2 (95% confidence interval 3.7 to -2.2; p = 0.001) per 1 mm increase, and kidneys larger than 6 cm at presentation never had a normal outcome [23].

Nephrectomy

A nephrectomy may be necessary because of hypertension, persistent infection and scarring [58]. RAT frequently required a nephrectomy (83%) [112]. Vigorous thrombolytic therapy with urokinase followed by t-PA dissolved the thrombus in the inferior vena cava and restored perfusion of both kidneys in a newborn with bilateral RVT and adrenal hemorrhage. However, a hemorrhagic rupture of the right kidney occurred, requiring emergency nephrectomy followed by adrenal insufficiency and dialysis dependent faction [41].

Renal Failure

Late sequelae of RVT included impairment of renal function, shrunken hypoplastic kidney, arterial hypertension and tubular defects [25]. In a newborn with bilateral RAT from severe dehydration, renal function recovery began 11 days after the onset of anuria. Despite ischemic atrophy of the left kidney, renal function and blood pressure were normal on follow-up [18]. Most cases of RVT resolve over time without permanent injury to the kidneys, which highlights the role of revascularization in the recovery of significant renal function [77]. Anuria resulting from obstruction of the renal arteries in both kidneys or in a solitary kidney is unusual. Bilateral fetal RVT is quite uncommon, and postnatal recovery of a kidney severely affected by RVT is very rare [113].

Compensating Collateralization

The tolerance of a kidney to ischemia is largely dependent on the presence of collaterals, stimulated by pre-existing arterial disease. In a case of nephrotic syndrome, decreased flow with congestion, a large kidney with parenchymal thickening, pelvocalyceal thinning, good function, and no obstruction in the proper clinical settings indicated the diagnosis of a chronic form of RVT with compensating collateralization [114]. In an infant with thrombosis of a renal artery treated with anticoagulants and fibrinolytic therapy, the kidneys showed bilateral blood flow, probably by reperfusing the kidneys through collateral circulation [57]. Renal arterial and venous Doppler signals in pediatric RVT showed that 7 out of 8 native kidneys had atrophied in the months following the acute event. Perirenal collateral vessels were shown with color Doppler US in one baby [115].

Death

Death from RVT is rare; a death is often caused by the blood clot detaching and lodging in the heart or lungs.

Renal Athrophy

The outcome in 6 newborns with RVT (3 had bilateral) at 3 months to 6 years disclosed hypertension in one baby, atrophic kidneys in two and both hypertension and an atrophic kidney in one [88]. At follow-up after a median time of 11.5 months, renal atrophy was present in 26 out of 39 affected kidneys [9]. In a retrospective study, the majority (70.6%) of the involved kidneys in newborns became atrophic despite anticoagulant and/or antithrombotic intervention. A total of 9 infants in a 13-case series died from non-RVT-related conditions during the study period [8].

Restoration

The presence of branching calcification at US and normal renal size probably indicated a good prognosis for renal function in two newborns with RVT and may have indicated prenatal thrombosis. The kidneys remained normal in size, and uptake of 99mTc-labelled dimercaptosuccinic acid (99mTc-DMSA) was normal at a follow-up examination [116].

References

[1] Saxonhouse, MA; Manco-Johnson, MJ. The evaluation and management of neonatal coagulation disorders. *Semin Perinatol,* 2009 33, 52-65.

[2] Monagle, P; Barnes, C; Ignjatovic, V; Furmedge, J; Newall, F; Chan, A; De Rosa, L; Hamilton, S; Ragg, P; Robinson, S; Auldist, A; Crock, C; Roy, N; Rowlands, S. Developmental haemostasis. Impact for clinical haemostasis laboratories. *Thromb Haemost,* 2006 95, 362-372.

[3] Andrew, M; Paes, B; Milner, R; Johnston, M; Mitchell, L; Tollefsen, DM; Powers, P. Development of the human coagulation system in the full-term infant. *Blood,* 1987 70, 165-172.
[4] Nowak-Göttl, U; von Kries, R; Göbel, U. Neonatal symptomatic thromboembolism in Germany: two year survey. *Arch Dis Child Fetal Neonatal Ed,* 1997 76, F163-167.
[5] Schmidt, B; Andrew, M. Neonatal thrombosis: report of a prospective Canadian and international registry. *Pediatrics,* 1995 96, 939-943.
[6] Chalmers, EA. Neonatal thrombosis. *J Clin Pathol,* 2000 53, 419-423.
[7] Andrew, M; Brooker, LA. Hemostatic complications in renal disorders of the young. *Pediatr Nephrol,* 1996 10, 88-99.
[8] Lau, KK; Stoffman, JM; Williams, S; McCusker, P; Brandao, L; Patel, S; Chan, AK. Neonatal renal vein thrombosis: review of the English-language literature between 1992 and 2006. *Pediatrics,* 2007 120, 1278-1284.
[9] Bökenkamp, A; von Kries, R; Nowak-Göttl, U; Göbel, U; Hoyer, PF. Neonatal renal venous thrombosis in Germany between 1992 and 1994: epidemiology, treatment and outcome. *Eur J Pediatr,* 2000 159, 44-48.
[10] Kuhle, S; Massicotte, P; Chan, A; Mitchell, L. A case series of 72 neonates with renal vein thrombosis. Data from the 1-800-NO-CLOTS Registry. *Thromb Haemost,* 2004 92, 729-733.
[11] Marks, SD; Massicotte, MP; Steele, BT; Matsell, DG; Filler, G; Shah, PS; Perlman, M; Rosenblum, ND; Shah, VS. Neonatal renal venous thrombosis: clinical outcomes and prevalence of prothrombotic disorders. *J Pediatr,* 2005 146, 811-816.
[12] Kavaler, E; Hensle, TW. Renal artery thrombosis in the newborn infant. *Urology,* 1997 50, 282-284.
[13] Lam, HS; Chu, WC; Lee, CH; Wong, W; Ng, PC. Renal artery thrombosis and ischaemia presenting as severe neonatal hypertension. *Arch Dis Child Fetal Neonatal,* 2007 92, F264.
[14] Zaffanello, M; Franchini, M. Thromboembolism in childhood nephrotic syndrome: a rare but serious complication. *Hematology,* 2007 12, 69-73.
[15] Ellis, D. Recurrent renal vein thrombosis and renal failure associated with antithrombin-III deficiency. *Pediatr Nephrol,* 1992 6, 131-134.
[16] Payne, RM; Martin, TC; Bower, RJ; Canter, CE. Management and follow-up of arterial thrombosis in the neonatal period. *J Pediatr,* 1989 114, 853-858.
[17] Kasaragod, AB; Lucia, MS; Lum, GM; Caldwell, S; Stork, L; Stenmark, KR. Solitary renal myofibromatosis: an unusual cause of infantile hypertension. *Pediatrics,* 1999 103, e66.
[18] Ellis, D; Kaye, RD; Bontempo, FA. Aortic and renal artery thrombosis in a neonate: recovery with thrombolytic therapy. *Pediatr Nephrol,* 1997 11, 641-644.
[19] Hibbert, J; Howlett, DC; Greenwood, KL; MacDonald, LM; Saunders, AJ. The ultrasound appearances of neonatal renal vein thrombosis. *Br J Radiol,* 1997 70, 1191-1194.
[20] Alexander, F; Campbell, WA. Congenital nephrotic syndrome and renal vein thrombosis in infancy. *J Clin Pathol,* 1971 24, 27-40.

[21] Lewy, PR; Jao, W. Nephrotic syndrome in association with renal vein thrombosis in infancy. *J Pediatr,* 1974 85, 359-365.

[22] Messinger, Y; Sheaffer, JW; Mrozek, J; Smith, CM; Sinaiko, AR. Renal outcome of neonatal renal venous thrombosis: review of 28 patients and effectiveness of fibrinolytics and heparin in 10 patients. *Pediatrics,* 2006 118, e1478-1484.

[23] Winyard, PJ; Bharucha, T; De Bruyn, R; Dillon, MJ; van't Hoff, W; Trompeter, RS; Liesner, R; Wade, A; Rees, L. Perinatal renal venous thrombosis: presenting renal length predicts outcome. *Arch Dis Child Fetal Neonatal,* 2006 91, F273-278.

[24] Murphy, A. Proceedings: Renal venous thrombosis in hypertonic dehydration. *Arch Dis Child,* 1974 49, 823-824.

[25] Reimold, EW; Wittel, RA. Renal venous thrombosis in children: changes in management. *South Med J,* 1983 76, 1277-1284.

[26] Kauffmann, RH; Veltkamp, JJ; Van Tilburg, NH; Van Es, LA. Acquired antithrombin III deficiency and thrombosis in the nephrotic syndrome. *Am J Med,* 1978 65, 607-613.

[27] Moore, HL; Katz, R; McIntosh, R; Smith, F; Michael, AF; Vernier, RL. Unilateral renal vein thrombosis and the nephrotic syndrome. *Pediatrics,* 1972 50, 598-608.

[28] Lai, NS; Lan, JL. Renal vein thrombosis in Chinese patients with systemic lupus erythematosus. *Ann Rheum Dis,* 1997 56, 562-564.

[29] D'Cruz, DP. Renal manifestations of the antiphospholipid syndrome. *Lupus,* 2005 14, 45-48.

[30] Louis, CU; Morgenstern, BZ; Butani, L. Thrombotic complications in childhood-onset idiopathic membranous nephropathy. *Pediatr Nephrol,* 2003 18 1298-1300.

[31] Bradley, WG Jr; Jacobs, RP; Trew, PA; Biava, CG; Hopper, J Jr. Renal vein thrombosis: occurrence in membranous glomerulonephropathy and lupus nephritis. *Radiology,* 1981 139, 571-576.

[32] Tsugawa, K; Tanaka, H; Kudo, M; Nakahata, T; Ito, E. Renal artery thrombosis in a pediatric case of systemic lupus erythematosus without antiphospholipid antibodies. *Pediatr Nephrol,* 2005 20, 1648-1650.

[33] Beard, ME; Taylor, DJ. Renal vein thrombosis in cases of polyarteritis nodosa and of the Henoch-Schoenlein syndrome. *J Clin Pathol,* 1969 22, 396-400.

[34] Reuben, A; Hirsch, M; Berlyne, GM. Renal vein thrombosis as the major cause of renal failure in familial Mediterranean fever. *Q J Med,* 1977 46, 243-258.

[35] Barth, RA. Fibromuscular dysplasia with clotted renal artery aneurysm. *Pediatr Radiol,* 1993 23, 296-297.

[36] Münchow, N; Kosch, A; Schobess, R; Junker, R; Auberger, K; Nowak-Göttl, U. Role of genetic prothrombotic risk factors in childhood caval vein thrombosis. *Eur J Pediatr,* 1999 158 Suppl 3, S109-112.

[37] Sutor, AH; Uhl, M. Diagnosis of thromboembolic disease during infancy and childhood. *Semin Thromb Hemost,* 1997 23, 237-246.

[38] Schobess, R; Junker, R; Auberger, K; Münchow, N; Burdach, S; Nowak-Göttl, U. Factor V G1691A and prothrombin G20210A in childhood spontaneous venous thrombosis-evidence of an age-dependent thrombotic onset in carriers of factor V G1691A and prothrombin G20210A mutation. *Eur J Pediatr,* 1999 158 Suppl 3, S105-108.

[39] Llach, F. Hypercoagulability, renal vein thrombosis, and other thrombotic complications of nephrotic syndrome. *Kidney Int,* 1985 28, 429-439.

[40] Llach, F; Papper, S; Massry, SG. The clinical spectrum of renal vein thrombosis: acute and chronic. *Am J Med,* 1980 69, 819-827.

[41] Haffner, D; Wühl, E; Zieger, B; Grulich-Henn, J; Mehls, O; Schaefer, F. Bilateral renal venous thrombosis in a neonate associated with resistance to activated protein C. *Pediatr Nephrol,* 1996 10, 737-739.

[42] Magid, D; Fishman, EK; Charache, S; Siegelman, SS. Abdominal pain in sickle cell disease: the role of CT. *Radiology* 1987 163, 325-328.

[43] Smorgick, N; Herman, A; Wiener, Y; Halperin, R; Sherman, D. Prenatal thrombosis of the inferior vena cava and the renal veins. *Prenat Diagn,* 2007 27, 603-607.

[44] Plumer, LB; Kaplan, GW; Mendoza, SA. Hypertension in infants--a complication of umbilical arterial catheterization. *J Pediatr,* 1976 89, 802-805.

[45] Siegler, RL. Conservative management of neonatal renal artery embolism. *Urology,* 1976 8, 484-487.

[46] Arar, MY; Hogg, RJ; Arant, BS Jr; Seikaly, MG. Etiology of sustained hypertension in children in the southwestern United States. *Pediatr Nephrol,* 1994 8, 186-189.

[47] Andreoli, SP. Acute renal failure in the newborn. *Semin Perinatol,* 2004 28, 112-123.

[48] Bellini, C; Campone, F. A neonate with acute renal failure. Renal vein thrombosis (RVT). *Pediatr Nephrol,* 2008 23, 49-53.

[49] Stewart, CL; Barnett, R.Acute renal failure in infants, children and adults. *Crit Care Clin,* 1997 13, 575-590.

[50] Bauer, SB; Feldman, SM; Gellis, SS; Retik, AB. Neonatal hypertension. A complication of umbilical-artery catheterization. *N Engl J Med,* 1975 293, 1032-1033.

[51] Adelman, RD. The hypertensive neonate. *Clin Perinatol,* 1988 15, 567-585.

[52] Rasoulpour, M; McLean, RH. Renal venous thrombosis in neonates. Initial and follow-up abnormalities. *Am J Dis Child,* 1980 134, 276-279.

[53] Prelog, M; Fischer, H; Gassner, I; Tzankov, A; Glatz-Krieger, K; Mihatsch, M; Zimmerhackl, LB. Bilateral renal vein thrombosis in a twin newborn without known risk factors. *Clin Nephrol,* 2006 66, 135-139.

[54] Levine, C. Intestinal obstruction in a neonate with adrenal hemorrhage and renal vein thrombosis. *Pediatr Radiol,* 1989 19, 477-478.

[55] Keidan, I; Lotan, D; Gazit, G; Boichis, H; Reichman, B; Linder, N. Early neonatal renal venous thrombosis: long-term outcome. *Acta Paediatr,* 1994 83, 1225-1227.

[56] Pinto, E; Guignard, JP.Renal masses in the neonate. *Biol Neonate,* 1995 68, 175-184.

[57] Muñoz-Arizpe, R; Walsh, RF; Edge, W. Obstructive aortic and renal thrombosis in the newborn--spontaneous recovery. *Pediatr Nephrol,* 1992 6, 190-191.

[58] Duncan, RE; Evans, AT; Martin, LW. Natural history and treatment of renal vein thrombosis in children. *J Pediatr Surg,* 1977 12, 639-645.

[59] Chugh, KS; Malik, N; Uberoi, HS; Gupta, VK; Aggarwal, ML; Singhal, PC; Suri, S; Jain, SK. Renal vein thrombosis in nephrotic syndrome--a prospective study and review. *Postgrad Med J,* 1981 57, 566-570.

[60] Uthman, I; Khamashta, M. Antiphospholipid syndrome and the kidneys. *Semin Arthritis Rheum,* 2006 35, 360-367.

[61] Manco-Johnson, MJ; Grabowski, EF; Hellgreen, M; Kemahli, AS; Massicotte, MP; Muntean, W; Peters, M; Schlegel, N; Wang, M; Nowak-Göttl, U. Recommendations for tPA thrombolysis in children. On behalf of the Scientific Subcommittee on Perinatal and Pediatric Thrombosis of the Scientific and Standardization Committee of the International Society of Thrombosis and Haemostasis. *Thromb Haemost,* 2002 88, 157-158.

[62] Roach, ES; Golomb, MR; Adams, R; Biller, J; Daniels, S; Deveber, G; Ferriero, D; Jones, BV; Kirkham, FJ; Scott, RM; Smith, ER; American Heart Association Stroke Council; Council on Cardiovascular Disease in the Young. Management of stroke in infants and children: a scientific statement from a Special Writing Group of the American Heart Association Stroke Council and the Council on Cardiovascular Disease in the Young. *Stroke,* 2008 39, 2644-2691.

[63] Simioni, P. Thrombophilia and gestational VTE. *Thromb Res,* 2009 123 Suppl 2, S41-44.

[64] McInnis, AN; Felman, AH; Kaude, JV; Walker, RD. Renal ultrasound in the neonatal period. *Pediatr Radiol,* 1982 12, 15-20.

[65] Rosenberg, ER; Trought, WS; Kirks, DR; Sumner, TE; Grossman, H. Ultrasonic diagnosis of renal vein thrombosis in neonates. *AJR Am J Roentgenol,* 1980 134, 35-38.

[66] Schlegel, JU; Lang, EK. Computed radionuclide urogram for assessing acute renal failure. *AJR Am J Roentgenol,* 1980 134, 1029-1034.

[67] Fishman, JE; Joseph, RC. Renal vein thrombosis in utero: duplex sonography in diagnosis and follow-up. *Pediatr Radiol,* 1994 24, 135-136.

[68] Ranch, D; Aigbe, MO; Gorospe, EC. Prenatal calcification of the inferior vena cava and renal veins in a normal neonate. *ScientificWorldJournal,* 2006 6, 734-736.

[69] Chiara, A; Chirico, G; Comelli, L; De Vecchi, E; Rondini, G. Increased renal echogenicity in the neonate. *Early Hum Dev,* 1990 22, 29-37.

[70] Cremin, BJ; Davey, H; Oleszczuk-Raszke, K. Neonatal renal venous thrombosis: sequential ultrasonic appearances. *Clin Radiol,* 1991 44, 52-55.

[71] Lin, GJ; Yang, PH; Wang, ML. Neonatal renal venous thrombosis--a case report describing serial sonographic changes. *Pediatr Nephrol,* 1994 8, 589-591.

[72] Wright, NB; Blanch, G; Walkinshaw, S; Pilling, DW. Antenatal and neonatal renal vein thrombosis: new ultrasonic features with high frequency transducers. *Pediatr Radiol,* 1996 26, 686-689.

[73] Argyropoulou, MI; Giapros, VI; Papadopoulou, F; Drougia, AA; Nikolopoulos, P; Vartholomatos GA, Andronikou S. Renal venous thrombosis in an infant with predisposing thrombotic factors: color Doppler ultrasound and MR evaluation. *Eur Radiol,* 2003 13, 2027-2030.

[74] Lalmand, B; Avni, EF; Nasr, A; Ketelbant, P; Struyven, J. Perinatal renal vein thrombosis. Sonographic demonstration. *J Ultrasound Med,* 1990 9, 437-442.

[75] Sanders, LD; Jequier, S. Ultrasound demonstration of prenatal renal vein thrombosis. *Pediatr Radiol,* 1989 19, 133-135.

[76] Beckmann, CF; Abrams, HL. Renal venography: anatomy, technique, applications, analysis of 132 venograms, and a review of the literature. *Cardiovasc Intervent Radiol,* 1980 3, 45-70.

[77] Flye, MW; Anderson, RW; Fish, JC; Silver, D. Successful surgical treatment of anuria caused by renal artery occlusion. *Ann Surg,* 1982 195, 346-353.
[78] Riccialdelli, L; Arnaldi, G; Giacchetti, G; Pantanetti, P; Mantero, F.Hypertension due to renal artery occlusion in a patient with antiphospholipid syndrome. *Am J Hypertens,* 2001 14, 62-65.
[79] Howman-Giles, R; Gett, M; Roy, P. Renal subcapsular rim sign. Radionuclide pattern. *Clin Nucl Med,* 1986 11, 285-286.
[80] Suga, K; Hara, A; Motoyama, K; Ishikawa, Y; Kume, N; Matsunaga, N. Coexisting renal vein thrombosis and bilateral adrenal hemorrhage: renoscintigraphic demonstration. *Clin Nucl Med,* 2000 25, 263-267.
[81] Kim, JH; Ha, HK; Yoon, KH; Lee, YS; Park, KB; Lee, IJ; Kim, PN; Lee, MG; Auh, YH. CT features of abdominal manifestations of primary antiphospholipid syndrome. *J Comput Assist Tomogr,* 1999 23, 678-683.
[82] Veldman, A; Nold, MF; Michel-Behnke, I. Thrombosis in the critically ill neonate: incidence, diagnosis, and management. *Vasc Health Risk Manag,* 2008 4, 1337-1348.
[83] Monagle, P; Chalmers, E; Chan, A; DeVeber, G; Kirkham, F; Massicotte, P; Michelson, AD; American College of Chest Physicians. Antithrombotic therapy in neonates and children: American College of Chest Physicians Evidence-Based Clinical Practice Guidelines (8th Edition). *Chest,* 2008 133 Suppl 6, 887S-968S.
[84] Milou, C; Debuche-Benouachkou, V; Semama, DS; Germain, JF; Gouyon, JB. Intravenous nicardipine as a first-line antihypertensive drug in neonates. *Intensive Care Med,* 2000 26, 956-958.
[85] Kiessling, SG; Wadhwa, N; Kriss, VM; Iocono, J; Desai, NS. An unusual case of severe therapy-resistant hypertension in a newborn. *Pediatrics,* 2007 119, e301-304.
[86] Chevalier, RL. What treatment do you advise for bilateral or unilateral renal thrombosis in the newborn, with or without thrombosis of the inferior vena cava? *Pediatr Nephrol,* 1991 5, 679.
[87] Mocan, H; Beattie, TJ; Murphy, AV. Renal venous thrombosis in infancy: long-term follow-up. *Pediatr Nephrol,* 1991 5, 45-49.
[88] Nuss, R; Hays, T; Manco-Johnson, M. Efficacy and safety of heparin anticoagulation for neonatal renal vein thrombosis. *Am J Pediatr Hematol Oncol,* 1994 16, 127-131.
[89] Zigman, A; Yazbeck, S; Emil, S; Nguyen, L. Renal vein thrombosis: a 10-year review. *J Pediatr Surg,* 2000 35, 1540-1542.
[90] Weinschenk, N; Pelidis, M; Fiascone, J. Combination thrombolytic and anticoagulant therapy for bilateral renal vein thrombosis in a premature infant. *Am J Perinatol,* 2001 18, 293-297.
[91] Markowitz, GS; Brignol, F; Burns, ER; Koenigsberg, M; Folkert, VW. Renal vein thrombosis treated with thrombolytic therapy: case report and brief review. *Am J Kidney Dis,* 1995 25, 801-806.
[92] Pohl, M; Zimmerhackl, LB; Hausser, I; Ludwig, H; Hildebrandt, F; Gordjani, N; Sutor, AH; Anton-Lamprecht, I; Brandis, M. Acute bilateral renal vein thrombosis complicating Netherton syndrome. *Eur J Pediatr,* 1998 157, 157-160.
[93] Wang, M; Hays, T; Balasa, V; Bagatell, R; Gruppo, R; Grabowski, EF; Valentino, LA; Tsao-Wu, G; Manco-Johnson, MJ; Pediatric Coagulation Consortium. Low-dose tissue

plasminogen activator thrombolysis in children. *J Pediatr Hematol Oncol,* 2003 25, 379-386.
[94] Thornburg, C; Pipe, S. Neonatal thromboembolic emergencies. *Semin Fetal Neonatal Med,* 2006 11, 198-206.
[95] Saxonhouse, MA; Manco-Johnson, MJ. The evaluation and management of neonatal coagulation disorders. *Semin Perinatol,* 2009 33, 52-65.
[96] Molteni, KH; George, J; Messersmith, R; Puppala, BL; Mangurten, HH; Kallen, RJ. Intrathrombic urokinase reverses neonatal renal artery thrombosis. *Pediatr Nephrol,* 1993 7, 413-415.
[97] Rosenbaum, T; Rammos, S; Kniemeyer, HW; Göbel, U. Extended deep vein and inferior vena cava thrombosis in a 15-year-old boy: successful lysis with recombinant tissue-type plasminogen activator 2 weeks after onset of symptoms. *Eur J Pediatr,* 1993 152, 978-980.
[98] Veldman, A; Nold, MF; Michel-Behnke I. Thrombosis in the critically ill neonate: incidence, diagnosis, and management. *Vasc Health Risk Manag,* 2008 4, 1337-1348.
[99] Newall, F; Johnston, L; Ignjatovic, V; Monagle, P. Unfractionated heparin therapy in infants and children. *Pediatrics,* 2009 123, e510-518.
[100] Sutor, AH; Chan, AK; Massicotte, P. Low-molecular-weight heparin in pediatric patients. *Semin Thromb Hemost,* 2004 30 Suppl 1, 31-39.
[101] van Ommen, CH; van den Dool, EJ; Peters, M. Nadroparin therapy in pediatric patients with venous thromboembolic disease. *J Pediatr Hematol Oncol,* 2008 30, 230-234.
[102] Malowany, JI; Monagle, P; Knoppert, DC; Lee, DS; Wu, J; McCusker, P; Massicotte, MP; Williams, S; Chan, AK; Canadian Paediatric Thrombosis And Hemostasis Network. Enoxaparin for neonatal thrombosis: a call for a higher dose for neonates. *Thromb Res,* 2008 122, 826-830.
[103] Manco-Johnson, MJ. How I treat venous thrombosis in children. *Blood,* 2006 107, 21-29.
[104] Ramasethu, J. Complications of vascular catheters in the neonatal intensive care unit. *Clin Perinatol,* 2008 35, 199-222.
[105] Young, G. New anticoagulants in children. *Hematology Am Soc Hematol Educ Program,* 2008, 245-250.
[106] Grützmacher, P; Bussmann, WD; Meyer, TH; Starck, E; Kollath, J; Baum, RP; Fassbinder, W; Schoeppe, W. Non-operative revascularisation of renal artery occlusion by transluminal angioplasty. *Nephrol Dial Transplant,* 1988 3, 130-137.
[107] Evans, DJ; Silverman, M; Bowley, NB. Congenital hypertension due to unilateral renal vein thrombosis. *Arch Dis Child,* 1981 56, 306-308.
[108] Durante, D; Jones, D; Spitzer, R. Neonatal renal arterial embolism syndrome. *J Pediatr,* 1976 89, 978-981.
[109] Báez-Trinidad, LG; Lendvay, TS; Broecker, BH; Smith, EA; Warshaw, BL; Hymes, L; Kirsch, AJ. Efficacy of nephrectomy for the treatment of nephrogenic hypertension in a pediatric population. *J Urol,* 2003 170, 1655-1657.
[110] Slovis, TL; Bernstein, J; Gruskin, A. Hyperechoic kidneys in the newborn and young infant. *Pediatr Nephrol,* 1993 7, 294-302.

[111] Agarwal, N; Phadke, KD; Garg, I; Alexander, P. Acute renal failure in children with idiopathic nephrotic syndrome. *Pediatr Nephrol,* 2003 18, 1289-1292.

[112] Hansen, KJ; Deitch, JS; Oskin, TC; Ligush, J Jr; Craven, TE; Dean, RH. Renal artery repair: consequence of operative failures. *Ann Surg,* 1998 227, 678-689.

[113] Lau, KK; Fernandez y Garcia, E; Kwan, WY; Albrecht, L; Stein-Wexler, R. Bilateral renal venous thrombosis and adrenal hemorrhage: sequential prenatal US with postnatal recovery. *Pediatr Radiol,* 2007 37, 912-915.

[114] Sfakianakis, GN; Zilleruelo, G; Thompson, T; Al-Sheikh, W; Strauss, J. Tc-99m glucoheptonate scintigraphy in a case of renal vein thrombosis. *Clin Nucl Med,* 1985 10, 75-79.

[115] Laplante, S; Patriquin, HB; Robitaille, P; Filiatrault, D; Grignon, A; Décarie, JC.Renal vein thrombosis in children: evidence of early flow recovery with Doppler US. *Radiology,* 1993 189, 37-42.

[116] Wilkinson, AG; Murphy, AV; Stewart, G. Renal venous thrombosis with calcification and preservation of renal function. *Pediatr Radiol,* 2001 31, 140-143.

In: Thrombosis: Causes, Treatment and Prevention ISBN 978-1-61668-696-3
Editor: D. G. Macri and L. D. Procaccini, pp. 119-130

Chapter IV

FACTORS AFFECTING THROMBOSIS IN WOMEN

G. Murtagh and Vincent Maher
Adelaide, Meath and National Childrens' Hospital, Tallaght, Dublin, Ireland

Thrombosis in women is subject to many hormonal influences. Menstruation and pregnancy can be associated with accelerated presentation of either coagulopathies or inherited thrombophilia. There is also a rise in the incidence of arterial thrombosis at the onset of menopause, which had been thought to represent a loss of the protective effects of oestrogen. Not only are there alterations in native hormone levels as women age, but women may also opt to use exogenous hormones, in the form of the oral contraceptive pill, or in later years, hormone replacement therapy.

Thus at certain times in a woman's life, the interplay between the various hormone systems may result in an increased risk of thrombosis due to either physiological factors, or exogenous hormone intake. Underlying conditions such as diabetes, renal failure and smoking may also alter thrombotic tendencies. Thus, it may be advisable to tailor both preventative and treatment options in terms of diet, lifestyle and antiplatelet or anticoagulant therapies in order to incorporate these hormonal variations. Female patients may require somewhat different strategies than their male counterparts. We present a discussion of the mechanisms underlying these processes, and review recent evidence in order to optimize clinicians' awareness of these risks.

CHILDHOOD TO TEENAGE YEARS

Venous thromboembolism is more likely to occur than arterial until the age of 40 years. Central venous catheters contribute to cases of thrombosis in young patients, although as patients enter young adulthood, other factors come into play - particularly in female patients. The normal menstrual cycle involves cyclical variations in the level of several coagulation factors. During ovulation, factor VIII levels peak [1,2]. Activated factor VII levels tend to drop from the follicular into the luteal phase [3]. Both fibrinogen and van Willebrand factor rise in the luteal phase, while D-dimer levels drop simultaneously [4].

The inherited thrombophilias are one of the other main causes of thromboembolism in both sexes in younger age groups, comprising Factor V Leiden (the most prevelant), Protein C and S deficiencies and Dysfibrinogenaemias. Factor V Leiden, for example, involves an inherited genetic mutation. Factor V is usually activated by protein C to Factor Va, which acts as a cofactor in the conversion of prothrombin to thrombin. In this mutation, arginine at position 506 being replaced by glutamine. This gene product is inactivated more slowly since it is less susceptible to cleavage. Patients are particularly susceptible to VTE and atherothrombosis.

Diagnosis and Treatment

Contrast venography is considered the gold standard in diagnosis of VTE in young patients, however difficulty with venous access means the ultrasound is often frequently used. Treatment falls along the same general lines as in adults, with initial use of unfractionated heparin or low molecular weight heparin, followed by a period of oral anticoagulant therapy [5].

Conditions such as the inherited thrombophilias become more relevant in women towards adulthood, when reproductive and contraceptive issues arise.

Adulthood OCP VTE

The oral contraceptive pill has been on the market since the early 1960s. The use of oral contraceptives (OC) has been associated with both venous and arterial thrombosis, even when lower doses of oestrogen are used, as is more common nowadays [6,7]. It is the progestogen that suppresses ovulation by antagonising luteinising hormone, thus proventing pregnancy. The oestrogen is used so that breakthrough bleeding does not occur.

The first studies that alerted clinicians to these risks were published in the late 1960s. The RCGP case control study reported a 3-fold higher risk of VTE in those taking the OCP compared to those who did not [8]. This was followed by further data in the subsequent years that consolidated this evidence [9-11]. Smoking and obesity probably also contribute to the thromboembolic risk [12]. Although hormone doses have been reduced, the risk remains significant with the use of third generation OCPs [13]. The first doses used were in the region of 100 to 150 mcg, whereas newer products usually contain 30 mcg oestrogen, or even less. Despite this, the pooled analysis by Douketis et al revealed that the risk ratio for VTE in first and second generation OCPs was 3 in case-control studies, 4.8 in retrospective cohort studies and 2.4 in prospective cohort studies [14].

Progestogens were once thought to be less dangerous in terms of thrombotic risk. However, even in 2009, evidence published by van Hylckama et al reported that users of desogestrel have over 7 times the risk of VTE than non-users of the OCP, with the risk increasing 6.8-fold in the case of cyproterone acetate. Overall, the pooled risk ratio for all currently available OCPs was reported as 5 [15].

Concerns relating to progestogens were initially raised in the mid 1990s, when several trials were published that suggested that Desogestrel and Gestodene were not without risk, [16], a fact consolidated by a statement by the World Health Organisation [17]. One large case control study suggested that desogestrel or gestodene combined with low-dose ethinyl estradiol versus no use results in an odds ratio of 4.8 for a venous thromboembolic event [18]. The most likely underlying mechanism relates to acquired resistance to activated protein C [19,20]. In the case of those heterozygous for Factor V Leiden, the use of combined oral contraceptives increases the risk of VTE by a factor of approximately 6, but this may be as high as 40 fold or even 50 fold in homozygotes using third generation agents [21,22].

Progesin-only methods seem to have less effect on coagulation pathways, though data is limited. [23]. Based on these findings, it would seem that in general, the combination with the least risk is levonorgestrel or norethisterone with as low a dose of oestrogen as is possible.

Other Contraceptives

Newer forms of combined contraceptive include the transdermal patch and vaginal ring. There is little evidence relating to these, however one randomized clinical trial with 24 women published in 2008 reported declines in protein S, antithrombin while fibrinogen increased. Transdermal patch patients had a more significant decline in protein S levels [24]. Another study published by Kluft and Meijer demonstrated that both oral and transdermal contraceptives increases levels of prothrombin fragment 1+2 levels and D-Dimers. Again, there was a greater decline in protein S levels with the patch. Authors concluded that overall, both methods increased procoagulant processes to a similar degree [25]. Meanwhile, data from 120 women who switched from oral to either transdermal patch or contraceptive ring showed that those who switched to the ring exhibited higher protein S and overall less procoagulant tendencies [26]. There is little conclusive data relating to the thrombotic risk of the IUCD, however it appears to invoke less resistance to activated protein C, with several studies suggesting that this effect makes it less risky in terms of VTE [27].

Diagnosis and Treatment

Current guidelines recommend compression ultrasonography for the diagnosis of suspected deep vein thrombosis, and CT pulmonary angiography for suspected pulmonary embolus. Contrast venography can be considered for other extremity thrombosis, or in cases where ultrasound is not feasible. Treatment should be with unfractionated heparin or low molecular weight heparin initially, followed by at least three months of oral anticoagulation, with a longer duration if the cause will remain a factor or several events have occurred [28].

Atherothrombosis

An increased rate of myocardial infarction was observed in the RCGP study amongst women who were over the age of 35 who smoked while using the OCP [29]. Several other studies have since been published that coroborate this finding, including a WHO collaborative study that resulted in a statement warning of such risks [30]. Ischaemic stroke rates are also higher in this population, as demonstrated in a prospective cohort study by Mant et al [31]. The mechanism behind this increased risk is still being eludcidated, though increased fibrinogen levels and fibrinogen deposition, along with an increase in monocyte procoagulant tissue factor B15 expression [32,33] have been discovered in such patients. It should be borne in mind, however, that since atherothrombotic events remain rare overall in this age group, the risk is still very low.

Diagnosis and Treatment

This follows conventional lines, with diagnosis based on biomarkers and electrocardiography followed by either CT coronary angiography, or conventional coronary angiography if an infarct is definite or intervention is likely [34].

Pregnancy VTE

As adulthood progresses, a powerful hormonal process comes to the fore, as many women become pregnant. A large population-based cohort study from Rochester, Minnesota, provided an insight into the incidence of VTE. It was estimated that the risk ranges from 4 to 50 times higher in pregnant versus non-pregnant women, with an absolute incidence rate of 1 in 500 to 2000 pregnancies [35].

Meanwhile in the UK, a retrospective cohort and case-control study on 395,335 women with pregnancies reaching 24 weeks of gestation were followed [36]. The incidence of VTE was 85 per 100,000 maternities, the majority of which occurred in the postpartum period, with those who had a premature delivery, c-section or history of cardiac disease being at particular risk.

Pregnancy naturally promotes all three components of Virchow's triad.

Venous Stasis

This occurs as the uterus enlarges. Compression of the inferior vena cava was reported on extensively in the 1950s and 60s [37,38]. Reports more recently concentrated on the demonstration of venous dilatation earlier in pregnancy [39,40].

Changes in the Vessel Wall

At the time of delivery, there can be disruption at the uteroplacental surface, local inflammation and endothelial damage. This is more prevalent in those who have had forceps, vacuum or caesarean section [41].

Changes within the Composition of the Blood

Pregnancy generally induced a rise in several procoagulant factors such as factor I, II, VII, VIII, IX, and X, along with a decline in the level of protein S. There is increased fibrin production along with decreased fibrinolysis [42]. This is beneficial in terms of reduced haemorrhagic complications during and after labour. However, for many women it leads to venous thromboembolic events.

Inherited Thrombophilias

Inherited thrombophilias and the antiphospholipid syndrome increase the risk for venous thromboembolism both during pregnancy and within the period after delivery [43]. In fact, studies suggest that retrospective analysis of women who have had a venous thromboembolic event during pregnancy reveals that over 50% test positive for an inherited thrombophilia [44]. It should be borne in mind that testing can be inaccurate during pregnancy or VTE treatment, but after this period the results become more reliable.

Diagnosis and Treatment

This is a controversial area. Although consideration should be given to minimising the dose of radiation the foetus is exposed to, ultrasound, ventilation perfusion lung scanning and CT pulmonary angiography are all acceptable when VTE is suspected in pregnancy. Low-molecular-weight heparin (LMWH) seems to be the safest treatment option, and has been shown to reduce mortality [45]. Those felt to be at particularly high risk for bleeding can be started on unfractionated heparin as it is amenable to rapid reversal with protamine. Neuraxial anaesthesia should be avoided in anticoagulated patients due to the risk of spinal haematoma. Those diagnosed with an inherited thrombophilia, or who have had a VTE event in the past, can be started on prophylaxis if deemed suitable, and this can be continued into the postpartum period. Oral anticoagulation can be started postpartum, though it is advisable to wait until breastfeeding is not an issue. Duration of therapy is decided upon based upon conventional guidelines as above.

Pregnancy Arterial Thrombosis

In a large study from the United States published in 2006, an incidence of 6.2 myocardial infarcts in 100,000 pregnancies was reported. It was estimated that there is a 3 -4 fold risk of MI in pregnancy, with anterior wall infarcts being the most common. Diabetic women, hypertensives and those in an older age bracket were more commonly affected. However as discussed above, pregnancy does induce a procoagulant state, and those with a history of thrombophilia were found to have an odds ratio 25.6, indicating that physicians must seek expert help if they find themselves caring for such a patient [46].

In terms of cerebral infarction, rates tend to be low during pregnancy, but increase in the six week period after delivery. A comprehensive study published by Kittner et al demonstrated the relative risk during this time to be 8.7 [47]. Again, those women with a history of thromboembolic disorders or inherited thrombophilia are at risk, but pre-eclampsia and eclampsia play a major causative role also.

Diagnosis and Treatment

Generally, diagnosis and treatment follow the usual guidelines [48], but maternal deterioration is an indication for urgent delivery. Percutaneous coronary intervention and even coronary artery bypass grafting have been successfully performed and are indicated in the appropriate circumstances. However, thrombolysis remains relatively contraindicated in pregnancy. Angiotensin converting enzyme inhibitors are, of course, contraindicated in pregnancy, and although nitrates and beta blockers are not contraindicated, care must be taken to avoid hypotension. Labetolol remains the first line agent for beta blockade in the pregnant woman [49].

Infertility Treatment

For those women who wish to become pregnant but have difficulty in conceiving, treatments include exogenous gonadotrophins. One complication includes Ovarian hyperstimulation syndrome (OHSS), which can be associated with venous thromboembolism [50].

Hormone Replacement Therapy VTE

After the reproductive phase of a woman's life, hormonal influences still exert a huge influence on the risk of VTE and arterial thromboses. The majority of women progress to the menopause, or ovarian failure, around the age of 51 years. This can be associated with several undesirable symptoms, such as hot flushes, mood swings and vaginal dryness. Many women were commenced on HRT prior to 2002 in order to alleviate these symptoms. The menopause was also thought to involve a loss of cardiovascular protection when oestrogen levels dropped, and HRT was considered beneficial in terms of cardiovascular risk.

However, the findings of the Women's Health Initiative, published in 2002 [51], refuted this. The WH Initiative sought to determine the true effects of hormone replacement therapy on the female population in terms of cardiovascular risk. The WHI consisted of a set of clinical trials and an observational study. In total it involved over 160,000 generally healthy postmenopausal women, and it's findings have become pivotal in terms of known risks associated with HRT. In terms of VTE, those taking combined oestrogen and progestin agents were twice as likely as those on placebo to suffer a venous thromboembolic event, and the risk was further increased if the patient was obese or in an older age group. It is possible that Activated Protein C resistance is the culprit for this [52]. The inherited thrombophilia Factor V Leiden was also associated with a higher rate of VTE (HR 6.9). In terms of risk reduction, transdermal HRT would seem to be associated with a lower risk of VTE [53,54], but there has been no randomised control trial to confirm this to date. Selective oestrogen receptor modulators were designed to overcome some of the side effects of conventional HRT. However, they have also been associated with an increased risk of VTE [55].

Diagnosis and Treatment

Again, conventional guidelines, as above, apply. Future use of similar hormonal agents is discouraged.

HRT Arterial Thrombosis

Oestrogen has several beneficial cardiovascular effects. It has been shown to improve lipid profiles by lowering LDL and raising HDL levels by around 8 - 15% [56,57], though triglyceride levels rose in some trials. It seems to improve endothelial function in healthy women. However it also seems to activate procoagulant pathways and increase levels of inflammatory markers such as C-reactive protein [58]. As with VTE, this may be less pronounced in the case of transdermal delivery systems [59].

Progestins, on the other hand, seem to reverse some of the beneficial effects oestrogens do have, and have been noted to reduce HDL [60].

The net effect of these observations was studied as part of the WHI, described above, and the HERS trial. Although it had been thought in earlier decades that HRT was cardioprotective, one arm of the WHI was discontinued early due to higher rates of coronary disease and stroke than were expected on combined oestrogen - progestin therapy, with a hazard ratio for coronary disease development reported as being 1.24, and an increased stroke risk in the order of 31%. The oestrogen alone arm was also discontinued early due to higher stroke rates than predicted [61].

This was supported by findings from the HERS trial (RR fatal stroke 1.61), with over 2.700 women enrolled. However, there was no associated increase in risk for nonfatal stroke or transient ischaemic attack, and authors overall concluded that combined HRT did not significantly increase the stroke risk [62]. The data for stroke risk remain conflicting and based on current evidence, most physicians would still prescribe HRT for healthy women, and discontinue only if a stroke occurs.

Diagnosis and Treatment

There are no special considerations in this case, only that hormonal agents should be discouraged if an atherothrombotic event occurs while the patient was taking one of these medications.

Breast Cancer Treatment – Tamoxifen

With increasing age comes an increased risk of malignancy, including breast cancer. One of the more successful treatments for those whose tumours are oestrogen receptor positive is Tamoxifen [59]. Not only is malignancy itself a risk factor for VTE, but Tamoxifen magnifies this risk [60,61].Thus many hormonal processes influence the risk of thrombosis throughout a woman's life. Recognition of the potential for such an event is the responsibility of every clinician.

References

[1] Kadir, RA, Economides, DL et al. Variations in coagulation factors in women: effects of age, ethnicity, menstrual cycle and combined oral contraceptive, *Thromb Haemost* 1999; 82:1456–1461.

[2] Mandalaki T, Louizou C, et al. Variations in factor VIII during the menstrual cycle in normal women, *N Engl J Med* 1980; 302:1093–1094.

[3] Kapiotis S, Jilma B, et al. Plasma levels of activated factor VII decrease during the menstrual cycle, *Thromb Haemost* 1998; 80:588–591.

[4] Giardina EG, Chen HJ, et al. Dynamic variability of hemostatic and fibrinolytic factors in young women, *J Clin Endocrinol Metab* 2004, 89:6179–6184.

[5] Monagle, P, Chalmers, E, et al. Antithrombotic therapy in neonates and children: *American College of Chest Physicians Evidence-Based Clinical Practice Guidelines (Eighth Edition)*. Chest 2008; 133:887S.

[6] Vandenbroucke JP, Rosing J et al. Oral contraceptives and the risk of venous thrombosis. *N Engl J Med* 2001;344(20):1527 35.

[7] Poulter, Meirik et al. Cardiovascular disease and use of oral and injectable progestagen-only contraceptives and combined injectable contraceptives. Results of an international, multicenter, case-control study. World Health Organization Collaborative Study of Cardiovascular Disease and Steroid Hormone Contraception. *Contraception* 1998; 57(5):315 24.

[8] Records Unit and Research Advisory Service of the Royal College of General Practitioners. Oral contraception and thrombo-embolic disease. *J R Coll Gen Pract.* 1967;13:267–279.
[9] Vessey MP, Doll R. Investigation of relation between use of oral contraceptives and thromboembolic disease. *BMJ.* 1968;1:199–205.
[10] Vessey MP, Doll R. Investigation of relation between use of oral contraceptives and thromboembolic disease: a further report. *BMJ.* 1969;2:651–657.
[11] Boston Collaborative Drug Surveillance Program. Oral contraceptives and venous thromboembolic disease, surgically confirmed gall bladder disease and breast tumours. *Lancet.* 1973;1:1399–1404.
[12] Farmer RD, Lawrenson RA, et al. A comparison of the risks of venous thromboembolic disease in association with different combined oral contraceptives. *Br J Clin Pharmacol* 2000;49(6):580 90.
[13] Kemmeren JM, Algra A, et al. Third generation oral contraceptives and risk of venous thrombosis: metaanalysis.*Br Med J* 2001;323:131 4.
[14] Douketis, JD, Ginsberg, JS, et al. A reevaluation of the risk for venous thromboembolism with the use of oral contraceptives and hormone replacement therapy. *Arch Intern Med* 1997; 157:1522.
[15] The venous thrombotic risk of oral contraceptives, effects of oestrogen dose and progestogen type: results of the MEGA case-control study. van Hylckama Vlieg A, Helmerhorst FM, et al, *BMJ.* 2009 Aug 13;339:b2921.
[16] Bloemenkamp KWM, Rosendaal FR, et al. Enhancement by factor V Leiden mutation of risk of deep-vein thrombosis associated with oral contraceptives containing a third-generation progestagen. *Lancet.* 1995;346:1593–1596.
[17] World Health Organization. Effect of different progestagens in low oestrogen oral contraceptives on venous thromboembolic disease. World Health Organization Collaborative Study of Cardiovascular Disease and Steroid Hormone Contraception. *Lancet.* 1995;346:1582–1588.
[18] Spitzer, WO, Lewis, MA, et al. Third generation oral contraceptives and risk of venous thromboembolic disorders: An international case-control study. *BMJ* 1996; 312:83.
[19] Tans G, Curvers J, et al. A randomized cross-over study on the effects of levonorgestreland desogestrel-containing oral contraceptives on the anticoagulant pathways. *Thromb Haemost* 2000;84(1): 15 21.
[20] Rosing J, Middeldorp S, et al. Low-dose oral contraceptives and acquired resistance to activated protein C: a randomised cross-over study. *Lancet* 1999; 354:2036 40.
[21] Vandenbroucke, JP, Koster, T, et al. Increased risk of venous thrombosis in oral-contraceptive users who are carriers of factor V Leiden mutation. *Lancet* 1994; 344:1453.
[22] Bloemenkamp, KWM, Rosendaal, FR, et al. Enhancement by factor V Leiden of risk of deep vein thrombosis associated with oral contraceptives containing a third-generation prostagen. *Lancet* 1995; 346:1593.
[23] Creinin, MD, Lisman, R, et al. Screening for factor V Leiden mutation before prescribing combination oral contraceptives. *Fertil Steril* 1999; 72:646.

[24] Johnson, JV, Lowell, J, et al. Effects of Oral and Transdermal Hormonal Contraception on Vascular Risk Markers: A Randomized Controlled Trial. *Obstet Gynecol* 2008; 111:278.

[25] Kluft, C, Meijer, P, et al. Comparison of a transdermal contraceptive patch vs. oral contraceptives on hemostasis variables. *Contraception* 2008; 77:77.

[26] Fleischer, K, van Vliet, HA, et al. Effects of the contraceptive patch, the vaginal ring and an oral contraceptive on APC resistance and SHBG: A cross-over study. *Thromb Res* 2009; 123:429.

[27] The effect of the levonorgestrel-releasing intrauterine system on the resistance to activated protein C (APC). van Vliet HA, Tchaikovski SN, et al. *Thromb Haemost.* 2009 Apr;101(4):691-5.

[28] Kearon, C, Kahn, SR, et al. Antithrombotic therapy for venous thromboembolic disease: American College of Chest Physicians Evidence-Based Clinical Practice Guidelines (8th Edition). *Chest* 2008; 133:454S

[29] Croft, P, Hannaford, PC. Risk factors for acute myocardial infarction in women: Evidence from the Royal College of General Practitioners' Oral Contraception Study. *BMJ* 1989; 298:165.

[30] Acute myocardial infarction and combined oral contraceptives: results of an international multicentre case-control study. WHO Collaborative Study of Cardiovascular Disease and Steroid Hormone Contraception. *Lancet* 1997; 349:1202.

[31] Risk of myocardial infarction, angina and stroke in users of oral contraceptives: an updated analysis of a cohort study.Mant J, Painter R, Vessey M.*Br J Obstet Gynaecol.* 1998 Aug;105(8):890-6.

[32] Increased monocyte tissue factor activity in women following cerebral venous thrombosis. Hölschermann H, Haberbosch W, et al. *J Neurol.* 2003 May;250(5):631-2.

[33] Scarabin, PY, Vissac, AM, et al. Elevated plasma fibrinogen and increased fibrin turnover among healthy women who both smoke and use low-dose oral contraceptives--a preliminary report. *Thromb Haemost* 1999; 82:1112.

[34] Antman, EM, Hand, M, et al. 2007 focused update of the ACC/AHA 2004 Guidelines for the Management of Patients With ST-Elevation Myocardial Infarction: a report of the American College of Cardiology/American Heart Association Task Force on Practice Guidelines (Writing Group to Review New Evidence and Update the ACC/AHA 2004 Guidelines for the Management of Patients With ST-Elevation Myocardial Infarction*). J Am Coll Cardiol* 2008; 51

[35] Heit, JA, Kobbervig, CE, et al. Trends in the incidence of venous thromboembolism during pregnancy or postpartum: a 30-year population-based study. *Ann Intern Med* 2005; 143:697.

[36] Simpson, EL, Lawrenson, RA, et al. Venous thromboembolism in pregnancy and the puerperium: incidence and additional risk factors from a London perinatal database. *BJOG* 2001; 108:56.

[37] Goodrich, S, Wood, JE. Peripheral venous distensibility and velocity of venous blood flow during pregnancy or during oral contraceptive therapy. *Am J Obstet Gynecol* 1964; 90:740.

[38] Wright, H, Osborn, S, et al. Changes in the rate of flow of venous blood in the leg during pregnancy, measured with radioactive sodium. *Surg Gynecol Obstet* 1950; 90:481.

[39] Macklon NS, Greer IA. The deep venous system in the puerperium: an ultrasound study. *Br J Obstet Gynaecol* 1997;104:198-200.

[40] Macklon NS, Greer IA. Venous thromboembolic disease in obstetrics and gynaecology: the Scottish experience. *Scott Med J* 1996;41:83-86.

[41] Marik, PE, Plante, LA. Venous thromboembolic disease and pregnancy. *N Engl J Med* 2008; 359:2025

[42] American College of Obstetricians and Gynecologists. Thromboembolism in pregnancy. ACOG Practice Bulletin 19. *ACOG 2000*; Washington, DC.

[43] James AH, Jamison MG, et al. Venous thromboembolism during pregnancy and the postpartum period: incidence, risk factors, and mortality. *Am J Obstet Gynecol* 2006;194:1311-1315.

[44] Greer IA. Thrombosis in pregnancy: maternal and fetal issues. Lancet 1999;353:1258-1265. Rosendaal FR. Venous thrombosis: a multicausal disease. *Lancet* 1999;353:1167-1173.

[45] van Dongen, CJ, van den Belt, AG et al. Fixed dose subcutaneous low molecular weight heparins versus adjusted dose unfractionated heparin for venous thromboembolism. *Cochrane Database Syst Rev* 2004; :CD001100.

[46] James, AH, Jamison, MG, et al. Acute myocardial infarction in pregnancy: a United States population-based study. *Circulation* 2006; 113:1564.

[47] Kittner, SJ, Stern, BJ, et al. Pregnancy and the risk of stroke. *N Engl J Med* 1996; 335:768.

[48] *Cardiac Problems in Pregnancy*, 3rd ed, Elkayam, U, Gleicher, N (Eds), Wiley-Liss, New York 1998.

[49] Rubin, PC. Current concepts: beta-blockers in pregnancy. *N Engl J Med* 1981; 305:1323.

[50] Diagnosis, prevention and management of ovarian hyperstimulation syndrome. Brinsden PR, Wada I, et al. *Br J Obstet Gynaecol.* 1995 Oct;102(10):767-72.

[51] Rossouw, JE, Anderson, GL, et al. Risks and benefits of estrogen plus progestin in healthy postmenopausal women: principal results From the Women's Health Initiative randomized controlled trial. *JAMA* 2002; 288:321.

[52] Post, MS, Rosing, J, et al. Increased resistance to activated protein C after short-term oral hormone replacement therapy in healthy post-menopausal women. *Br J Haematol* 2002; 119:1017

[53] Canonico, M, Oger, E, et al. Hormone therapy and venous thromboembolism among postmenopausal women: impact of the route of estrogen administration and progestogens: the ESTHER study. *Circulation* 2007; 115:840.

[54] Canonico, M, Plu-Bureau, G, et al. Hormone replacement therapy and risk of venous thromboembolism in postmenopausal women: systematic review and meta-analysis. *BMJ* 2008; 336:1227.

[55] Grady, D, Ettinger, B, et al. Safety and adverse effects associated with raloxifene: multiple outcomes of raloxifene evaluation. *Obstet Gynecol* 2004; 104:837.

[56] Darling, GM, Johns, JA, et al. Estrogen and progestin compared with simvastatin for hypercholesterolemia in postmenopausal women. *N Engl J Med* 1997; 337:595.

[57] [57] Binder, EF, Williams, DB, et al. Effects of hormone replacement therapy on serum lipids in elderly women. A randomized, placebo-controlled trial. *Ann Intern Med* 2001; 134:754.

[58] Sumino, H, Ichikawa, S, et al. Different effects of oral conjugated estrogen and transdermal estradiol on arterial stiffness and vascular inflammatory markers in postmenopausal women. *Atherosclerosis* 2006; 189:436.

[59] Brosnan, JF, Sheppard, BL, et al. Haemostatic activation in post-menopausal women taking low-dose hormone therapy: Less effect with transdermal administration?. *Thromb Haemost* 2007; 97:558.

[60] Ottosson, UB, Johansson, BG, et al. Subfractions of high-density lipoprotein cholesterol during estrogen replacement therapy: A comparison between progestogens and natural progesterone. *Am J Obstet Gynecol* 1985; 151:746.

[61] Rossouw,JE, Anderson, GL, et al. Risks and benefits of estrogen plus progestin in healthy postmenopausal women: principal results From the Women's Health Initiative randomized controlled trial. *JAMA* 2002; 288:321.

[62] Simon, JA, Hsia, J, et al. Postmenopausal hormone therapy and risk of stroke: The Heart and Estrogen-progestin Replacement Study (HERS). *Circulation* 2001; 103:638.

[63] Effects of chemotherapy and hormonal therapy for early breast cancer on recurrence and 15-year survival: an overview of the randomised trials. *Lancet* 2005; 365:1687.

[64] Pritchard, KI, Paterson, AH, et al. Increased thromboembolic complications with concurrent tamoxifen and chemotherapy in a randomized trial of adjuvant therapy for women with breast cancer. National Cancer Institute of Canada Clinical Trials Group Breast Cancer Site Group. *J Clin Oncol* 1996; 14:2731.

[65] McDonald, CC, Alexander, FE, et al. Cardiac and vascular morbidity in women receiving adjuvant tamoxifen for breast cancer in a randomised trial. The Scottish Cancer Trials Breast Group. *BMJ* 1995; 311:977.

In: Thrombosis: Causes, Treatment and Prevention ISBN 978-1-61668-696-3
Editor: D. G. Macri and L. D. Procaccini, pp. 131-153

Chapter V

PATHOPHYSIOLOGY DIAGNOSIS AND MANAGEMENT OF PORTAL VEIN THROMBOSIS

Francesca R. Ponziani*, Maria A. Zocco and Antonio Gasbarrini
Catholic University of Rome, Italy.

ABSTRACT

Portal vein thrombosis (PVT) is considered a rare event in general population, more common in patients with an advanced liver disease and hepatocellular carcinoma. Local and systemic factors - or a combination of them - may contribute to PVT development, making often difficult to identify certainly its original cause. However, thanks to innovations in non-invasive imaging, the diagnosis of PVT is now possible in the most part of suggestive cases. Clinical experience has also a pivotal role in PVT early diagnosis, even if, sometimes, patients may be completely asymptomatic or may present only few symptoms. In particular, it depends on the modality of PVT onset (acute or chronic) and on the extension of the thrombosis since, sometimes, PVT may progress to intestinal ischemia or cause a massive gastrointestinal bleeding. These extreme consequences are the manifestation of a complex alteration in liver and splanchnic hemodynamic, resulting in portal hypertension, hyperdinamic circulation and impairment in liver function. Thus, a prompt therapeutic management is essential to avoid complications, preserving patients' health and, sometimes, life.

Keywords: thrombosis, portal vein, thrombophilia, liver cirrhosis, anticoagulants.

* Correspondence concerning this article should be addressed to: Francesca R. Ponziani, Largo A. Gemelli 8, Catholic University of Rome, 00168 Rome. Tel. 06/30156018; E-mail francesca.ponziani@yahoo.it.

INTRODUCTION

The term portal vein thrombosis (PVT) is used to describe a complete or partial obstruction of the portal vein, due to the presence of a thrombus in the vasal lumen, with a consequent impairment in splanchnic blood circulation [1]. The presence of a thrombosis within portal vein can be recognized in 5-10% of the overall cases of portal hypertension; it is less frequent among subjects without an overt liver disease, more common in cirrhotic patients, with a prevalence of 4.4-15% [2]. PVT etiology is heterogeneous, frequently resulting by the interaction of both local and systemic risk factors. Furthermore, PVT clinical presentation depends by the modality of onset and the activation of compensatory mechanisms. Intestinal congestion and ischemia, associated with abdominal pain, diarrhea, rectal bleeding, abdominal distention, nausea, vomiting, anorexia, progressing to lactacidosis and sepsis are possible consequences of acute PVT, while patients with chronic PVT are, often, completely asymptomatic, or present splenomegaly, pancytopenia, varices, and, rarely, ascites. PVT has always to be suspected in apparently healthy subjects with portal hypertension, and in cirrhotic patients when clinical conditions worsen and there are signs of alteration in splanchnic hemodynamic [2,3]. Clinical suspicion may lead to an early diagnosis and an appropriate management of complications and original causes, preserving patients' health and, sometimes, life. Therapeutic options may be more or less invasive, but their risks and benefits have still to be clearly assessed and their feasibility should be considered for case by case.

EPIDEMIOLOGY

The first case of PVT was described by Balfour and Stewart more than a hundred years ago; at present, a large study reported that PVT can be incidentally found in 1% of the autopsies, in the general population [4]. Even if, in patients without an overt liver disease, PVT is a relatively rare finding, about 0.6 to 16% of cirrhotics present an obstruction of the portal vein. In specimen, PVT is more frequent in patients with a primary or metastatic liver cancer or with an advanced liver disease. Indeed, PVT prevalence ranges from 1%, at the earlier stages, to 30% in candidates for liver transplantation [5,6], and in patients affected by hepatocellular carcinoma the reported PVT incidence is of about 6.5% [7], with a prevalence of 10-40% [8]. By the way, PVT incidence in the general population has been increasing in the past years for the advance in diagnostic techniques, and it is responsible for about 5 to 10% of overall cases of portal hypertension, 40% in developing countries [3,7,9,10].

ETIOLOGY

Several causes are usually involved in PVT development, frequently combined. The most common local and systemic factors are shown in tables 1 and 2.

Table 1. Local risk factors for PVT (70%)

Cancer
- Any abdominal organ
Focal inflammatory lesions
- Neonatal omphalitis, ombilical vein catheterization
- Diverticulitis, Appendicitis
- Pancreatitis
- Duodenal ulcer
- Cholecystitis
- Tuberculous lymphadenitis
- Crohn's disease, Ulcerative colitis
- Cytomegalovirus hepatitis
Injury to the portal venous system
- Splenectomy
- Colectomy, Gastrectomy
- Cholecystectomy
- Liver transplantation
- Abdominal trauma
- Surgical portosystemic shunting, TIPS,
- Iatrogenic (fine needle aspiration of abdominal masses etc.)
Cirrhosis
- Preserved liver function with precipitating factors (splenectomy, surgical portosystemic shunting, TIPS dysfunction, thrombophilia)
- Advanced disease in the absence of obvious precipitating factors

Table 2. Systemic risk factors for PVT (30%)

Inherited:
- Factor V Leiden mutation
- Factor II (prothrombin) mutation
- Protein C deficiency
- Protein S deficiency
- Antithrombin deficiency
Acquired:
- Myeloproliferative disorder
- Antiphospholipid syndrome
- Paroxysmal nocturnal hemoglobinuria
- Oral contraceptives
- Pregnancy or puerperium
- Hyperhomocysteinemia
- Malignancy

Inflammatory abdominal diseases, liver cirrhosis and tumors, represent the most common local thrombotic triggers [4,5]. About 20% of portal vein occlusions are imputable to malignancies, most of them hepatic or pancreatic [11,12]. The mechanism is, in part, unknown; indeed, even if the thrombosis may result from vascular compression or invasion by the tumor, the role of a hypercoagulable state or hormonal alterations is less clear [7,13,14]. PVT incidence in cirrhotic patients has still been discussed in this chapter; however, it is important to remember that it is strictly connected to the severity of liver disease and to the presence of hepatocellular carcinoma. Adenopaties, systemic inflammatory response syndrome, surgical traumas to the portal venous system (i.e. portosystemic shunting, splenectomy, liver transplantation, ablative therapy for HCC and fine needle aspiration of abdominal masses) are less common local causes of PVT [1].

A systemic risk factor is present in about 30% of PVT and are mainly represented by myeloproliferative neoplasms (MPN) and prothrombotic conditions (Table 3) [5,15].

Table 3. Prevalence of thrombotic risk factors in adult patients with non tumorous and non cirrhotic, acute or chronic, PVT

RISK FACTOR	PVT PATIENTS
Myeloproliferative disorders - atypical - classical	30-40% 14% 17%
Antithrombin deficiency	0-26%
Protein C deficiency	0-26%
Protein S deficiency	2-30%
Factor V Leiden mutation	6-32%
Prothrombine mutation	14-40%
TT677 Methylene Tetrahydrofolate Reductase (MTHFR) genotype	11-50%
Antiphospholipid syndrome	6-19%
Hyperomocisteinemia	12-22%
Recent pregnancy	6-40%
Recent oral contraceptive use	12%

Factor V Leiden and protein C deficiency are the most frequent inherited prothrombotic conditions associated to PVT [16-18]. Prothrombin G20210A gene mutation is generally considered a weak prothrombotic condition, and its role in PVT development, in absence of an overt liver disease, is not clear. By the way, among cirrhotic patients with PVT, prothrombin G20210A gene mutation and MTHFR C677-T genotype seem to be a common finding [2,19-22]. Moreover, it is interesting to note that a transient positivity of anticardiolipin antibodies is frequent, but often resulting from liver damage or intercurrent infections, thus it has to be carefully evaluated in clinical practice [23-26].

However, the difficulty in assessing cirrhotic patients' haemocoagulative state is well known. In this condition, both of pro- and anticoagulative factors are reduced, revealing a complex alteration of the whole haemostatic system which may mask the presence of inherited coagulative disorders [27]. Basing on this considerations, the major part of clinicians is usually prone to refer the alterations of haemostatic system to the impaired liver function, omitting to search for inherited coagulative disorders [28]. Familial screening is useful to confirm the nature of this alterations, but it is sometimes not applicable in clinical practice. Although, recently, some authors proposed other tools to overcome the problem, such as the ratio of PS or PC or AT to [(factor II + factor X)/2], their reliability needs to be validated [1].

Finally, a myeloproliferative neoplasm (MPN) could manifest with the thrombosis of the portal venous system as the first symptom and is reported to be responsible of 22–48% of cases of PVT. Even if, sometimes, clinical manifestations may be lacking, a latent MPN may successively emerge in 51% of patients [2,13,29,30]. A simple method to investigate a latent MPN in PVT patients, especially when diagnosis is difficult to be assessed or unclear, is the screening of V617F point mutation in the gene encoding tyrosine-protein kinase JAK2 [31-36]. Recently, it has been reported the presence of the JAK2 V617F gene mutation in about 17-35% of PVT patients without a known underlying disease [37,38] but, at present, its prevalence among cirrhotics is unknown.

The diagnosis of idiopathic PVT may be established when no original cause could be recognized. Nowadays, PVT is rarely labeled as idiopathic, thanks to the advance in diagnostic techniques and to clinicians' better awareness of this pathologic entity [4]. As a consequence, the new practice in PVT management includes a detailed investigation of its possible original cause, since an inherited predisposition, associated to sporadic local or systemic triggers, may realize a complex interaction, resulting, finally, in PVT development [1,39].

PATHOPHYSIOLOGY

On the cessation of portal blood flow, both systemic and splanchnic hemodynamic change and liver loses about two thirds of its blood supply [40]. However, the activation of support systems makes possible to keep safe, in some limits, liver function. Two mechanisms are principally involved. The first one, is a vascular reflex called "arterial vasodilation", typical of those organs with a "portal" vascular system, which means the presence of both an arterial and a venous circulation. While arterial vasodilation occurs early after PVT occurrence, the second mechanism starts within 3-5 weeks after portal vein obstruction; it is called "venous rescue" and consists in the development of new collateral vessels which bypass the obstruction [41,42]. The result will be the fibrosis of the original portal vein, replaced by a net of newborn vessels called "cavernoma" (Figure 1) [5,8]. However, as reported by several studies performed in animal models, the reduction of portal venous flow causes a damage of the liver tissue in the less perfused lobe, increasing the mithotic activity in the normal perfused one [43]. The presence of a slightly impaired liver function in patients with an advanced chronic PVT may confirm this evidence [11]. Furthermore, at this stage, a hyperkinetic circulation, with low systemic vascular resistance and high cardiac output, is a common finding [3].

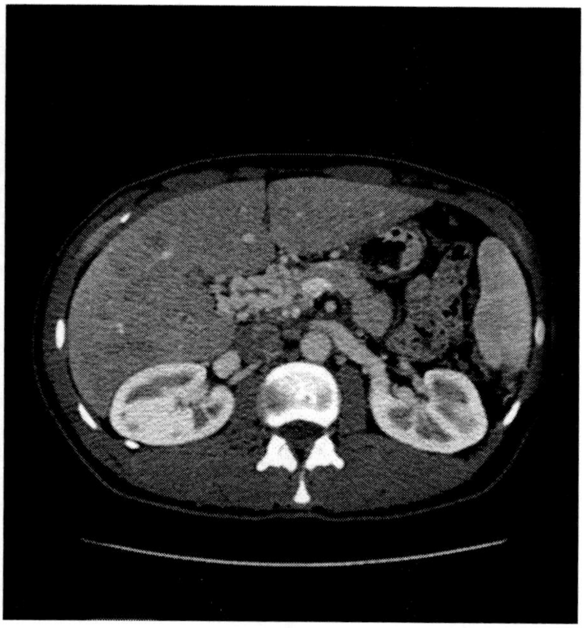

Figura 1. Portal cavernoma (CT scan).

Classification

Anatomical classification of PVT is based on its extension; four cathegories can be recognized: (1) thrombosis confined to the portal vein beyond the confluence of the splenic vein; (2) thrombosis extended to the superior mesenteric vein, but with patent mesenteric vessels; (3) thrombosis extended to the whole splanchnic venous system, but with large collaterals or (4) with only fine collaterals [45]. This classification may help to simply assess patients' clinical outcome, since, the more extended is the thrombosis, the higher will be the risk of bowel ischemia or infarction [46].

Basing on clinical presentation, PVT may develop in acute or chronic manner. Even if it is an arbitrary distinction, it is widely accepted that, in acute-onset PVT, symptoms develop within sixty days before hospital admission [47,48].

Clinical Presentation

PVT clinical presentation may be acute or chronic, depending on the extension of the vascular obstruction and on the presence of collaterals [49]. Acute PVT is characterized by intestinal congestion and ischemia, sometimes associated to abdominal pain or distention, diarrhea, rectal bleeding, nausea, vomiting, anorexia, fever, lactacidosis, splenomegaly and sepsis [50,51]. Progression to intestinal perforation leading to peritonitis, shock, and death is certain if portal venous circulation is not restored [5]. Physical examination do not shows typical features and signs of peritoneal irritation are unusual, before the onset of intestinal infarction or perforation [15]. Splenomegaly is a common finding, in contrast to ascites, which is mainly due to venous congestion, differently to what happens in cirrhotic patients [50,51,30]. Similarly, in the most cases of chronic PVT ascites is absent; it may transiently develop, similarly to encephalopathy, associated to renal failure or sepsis in older patients or after an episode of gastrointestinal bleeding [5,51]. Indeed, esophageal varices are a common feature of chronic PVT, differently to the acute onset, and an episode of gastrointestinal bleeding is frequently the first presenting symptom [8]. The risk of bleeding is higher in cirrhotic patients but the outcome is more favorable than in subjects without an overt liver disease [52,53]. It is therefore reasonable to investigate the presence of varices at the time of PVT diagnosis [50]. Varices are not the sole manifestation of the portal hypertension characterizing chronic PVT. Cutaneous collaterals and hypersplenism with pancytopenia are present in various degrees, depending by the partial or complete obstruction of the portal vein [1,49]. Moreover, the extrahepatic biliary tree can be indirectly affected in more than 80% of patients, because of compression (by choledochal or periportal varices or by the cavernoma), pericholedochal fibrosis and ischemic stricturing [54-57]. Physical examination and biochemical markers are usually normal and cholangitis, choledocholithiasis, cholecystitis rare, as liver injury [57]; retrograde cholangiopancreatography may reveal the so called "pseudocholangiocarcinoma sign" [1,6,44], representing the displacement, stricturing or thumprinting of the biliary ducts by neo-formed vessels. Differential diagnosis between this "portal biliopathy" and local tumors has always to be considered [58-,60]. Overall, it is to remember that the typical feature of chronically developed PVT is the presence of few symptoms, especially in subjects without an overt liver disease; often patients don't remember any trigger event and diagnosis is frequently delayed [15,50,51].

DIAGNOSIS

Nowadays, PVT is usually recognized at an early stage demonstrating the presence of solid material in the vasal lumen [15]. Ultrasonography (US) is the most employed diagnostic tool, capable to discover hyperechoic material into an enlarged portal vein or its tributaries, the presence of collateral vessels or a cavernoma, with a sensitivity and specificity between 60% and 100%(Figures 2, 3) [6,11,15,61]. Doppler imaging enhances the diagnosis if blood flow within the portal vein is not detectable, and confirms the presence a cavernomatous transformation [15]. In spite of some limits, related to the impossibility to visualize the distal superior mesenteric vein and the intrahepatic portion of the portal vein [62], the endoscopic use of ultrasound (EUS) was demonstrated to be 81% sensitive and 93% specific in PVT diagnosis [62]. EUS is more reliable than other imaging in detecting small and non-occluding thrombi and the invasion of the portal vein by tumors [63,64]. By the way, the assessment of thrombosis extension through the mesenteric system is difficult to obtained with ultrasonography [30] and the use of CT scan and magnetic resonance imaging (MRI) is preferable. CT scan may detect with accuracy hyperattenuating material in the portal vein lumen, surrounded by contrast enhancement, or the stop of the contrast medium in the proximal part of the vein in case of complete thrombosis. Hypoperfused areas are easily recognizable, appearing highlighted during the arterial phase and darker in the portal phase after contrast injection. Moreover, CT scan and MRI are the gold standard to investigate intestinal ischemia and other PVT complications, such as the impairment of other abdominal organs, and the original cause of the thrombosis [15]. The presence of isointense material within the portal vein lumen on T1-weighted RMI sequences, which become hyperintense on T2 images, is highly suggestive of PVT; gradient echo MRI may resolve any uncertainty [65], while contrast-enhanced MR angiography may give additional and more detailed informations about portal flow direction, cavernoma, varices, and surgical shunts functionality [66,67]. Moreover, MRI is the best choice in patients' follow-up before and after liver transplantation since, using particular techniques of imaging procession (i.e. fast imaging with steady state precession, *true FISP*), can obtain good results in patients with difficult venous access and when the images are degraded by respiratory motion [67-71].

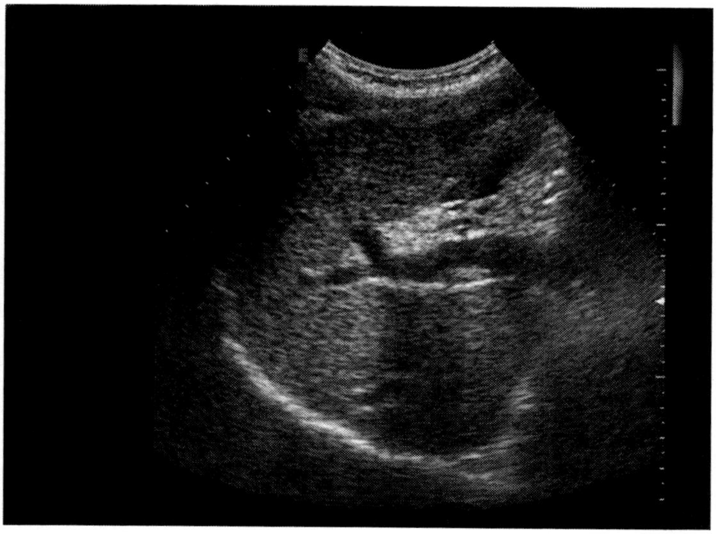

Figure 2. Partial portal vein thrombosis (ultrasonography).

PVT diagnosis is completed by laboratory investigations, useful to recognize predisposing conditions and to monitor liver function. Hepatic synthetic and metabolic functionality is typically conserved in PVT patients, unless the coexistence of an underling liver disease. Sometimes, prothrombin and other coagulation factors plasmatic levels could be decreased, in contrast to the increase of D-dimer [5,15].

However, the first step in the management of any common or rare disease is to recognize and treat its original cause, then the second step is resolving or preventing eventual complications. The identification of PVT etiology is based on the exclusion of the most common local causes, such as cirrhosis, primary or metastatic malignancies, pylephlebitis, liver cysts, vascular abnormalities (webs or aneurysms) and pancreatitis. Imaging (US+Doppler, MRI or CT scan) [15] and needle biopsy of the obstructed portal vein may be helpful [72]. In absence of a manifest predisposing local cause, trombophilic disorders have to be investigated and, if excluded, PVT is considered idiopathic. By the way, in about 72% of idiopathic PVT, some authors reported the evidence a subclinical prothrombotic condition [73-75].

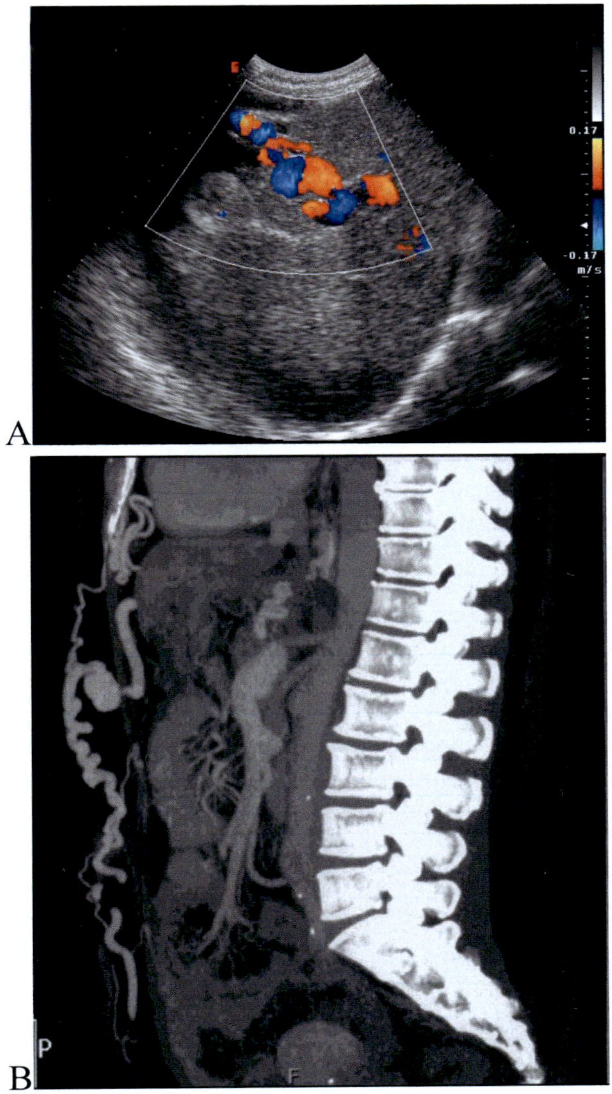

Figure 3. Collateral circulation. A: recanalization of paraumbilical vein (ultrasonography + doppler); B: recanalization of paraumbilical vein (CT scan).

PVT complications are strictly related to the degree of the obstruction (complete or partial, limited or extensive). Partial thrombosis is associated with few symptoms, in contrast to a rapid and complete obstruction; if mesenteric venous arches are not involved, the result will be only intestinal congestion, otherwise, intestinal infarction will occur. Intestinal congestion does not imply impairment in liver function or other organs' failure probably for the increased hepatic arterial blood and the developing of collateral circulation and is reversible. Intestinal infarction, instead, is a point of no return, often life threatening for patients.

It is a common belief in medical practice that to prevent is better than to treat a morbid condition after its onset, especially in case of PVT, an event so frequent in patients with liver cirrhosis to be defined "**a milestone**" in the natural course of the disease. To prevent means to avoid the occurrence of serious complications too, reducing morbidity and mortality [76]. Several studies tried to identify the most reliable factors predicting PVT development. Male sex, previous surgery or interventional treatment for portal hypertension, previous variceal bleeding, low platelet count and advanced liver failure have been associated with an increased risk of PVT development [2,19,70,77]. In a recent study, Zocco et al. [78] demonstrated that portal flow velocity is strongly predictive of PVT development, confirming the importance of Virchow triad in its pathogenesis. In this study, 47.8% of patients with a portal flow velocity lower than 15 cm/sec at Doppler Ultrasound developed PVT, in contrast to only 2% of those with a measured velocity above 15 cm/sec. Probably, the reduced removal of thrombin due to blood stagnation, together with reduced levels of circulating anticoagulants, may produce the local conditions predisposing to PVT. This study opens new interesting perspectives, considering also that evaluation of portal flow velocity needs only a Doppler Ultrasound measurement, in clinical practice. However, further studies are necessary to confirm these data and to identify other factors helpful to recognize patients at high risk of PVT development [79].

Prognosis

PVT prognosis is good in non-cirrhotic and non-neoplastic patients and also in acute onset, before the occurrence of intestinal infarction [46,52,80-85]. In case of bowel ischemia and multiorgan dysfunction or failure, patients in-hospital mortality rate is approximately of 20-50% [46].

In PVT chronic onset, mortality is less than 10% [11,86], except for patients with malignancy or cirrhosis – about 26% [50]. In addition to liver cirrhosis, advanced age, malignancy, mesenteric vein thrombosis, absence of abdominal inflammation, serum levels of aminotransferase and albumin are associated with reduced survival [1,4,15,30,52]. Systemic risk factors seems not to affect short term survival [87].

PVT and Liver Transplantation

The thrombosis of the portal vein represented a source of technical difficulties and surgical complications during the course of orthotopic liver transplantation (OLT) [88]. Shaw et al. in 1985 reported the first successful liver transplant in a patient with a thrombosed portal vein [89]. Thanks to recent innovations in surgery, medical care and radiological interventions, it is now possible to consider PVT by itself as an indication for liver transplantation [44,51]. Surgical thrombectomy, thromboendovenectomy with venous reconstruction, interposition of vein graft, porto-caval hemitransposition and radiological endovascular interventions are the principal procedures used to resolve the portal vein obstruction in liver transplant recipients [90-95]. To choose the correct procedure, PVT intra-operatory grading (i.e. **Yerdel's** grading) [6] is absolutely necessary: terminal to terminal portal vein anastomosis with or without thrombectomy is the common choice in low grade

PVT (less than 50% occlusion of the portal vein), while porto-caval hemitransposition is mandatory in grade 4 (complete thrombosis of portal vein and proximal and distal superior mesenteric vein) [70,96].

The outcome of liver transplantation in recipients with or without PVT is similar, with the same survival after 1 and 5 years of follow-up [96-99]. On the contrary, other studies reported a more complex surgical procedure, an increased risk of complications (such as primary non function or dysfunction, thrombosis of the hepatic artery, re-laparotomy, postoperative pancreatitis, sepsis, and renal failure), a poorer survival and a higher mortality, especially in those patients with an extended thrombosis [70,90,96-98]. On the whole, for low grade PVT survival appears better and, almost, as equal as non-PVT transplanted patients, but these data has to be confirmed [70,100]. In cirrhotics with PVT, post transplantation outcome is the same of those without, even if some authors reported more difficulties and complications (re-thrombosis or re-intervention) [96,98]. By the way, the rate of thrombosis recurrence after OLT is about 9-42%, especially in male patients with an advanced liver disease, often alcohol-related, and who underwent previous local treatments [70,90,91,97,99,101-103].

The development of a new thrombosis after liver transplantation has been reported in 1-2% of recipients, as always in the early postoperative period and at the anastomotic site [45,104,105]. Technical complications, a small diameter of the portal vein, pediatric recipients, history of PVT or surgical shunting pre–OLT, and splenectomy are the principal predisposing factors [105]. Immediate retransplantation must be quickly attempted in case of severe worsening of liver function, since acute liver failure, bleeding from esophageal varices, and massive ascites could rapidly occur [105,106].

For all these reasons and the good results reported in literature, nowadays portal vein thrombosis has no longer to be considered a contraindication but only a disadvantage and, rather, sometimes may represent by itself a possible indication to liver transplantation [97,99].

Treatment

To treat portal vein thrombosis is essential to prevent the occurrence of possible complications, since, according to literature, a spontaneous resolution is a rare event [83,84]. Thus, on one hand, to correct the original cause is the first step to achieve portal vein recanalization or, at least, to prevent its extension; on the other hand, a specific treatment of the thrombosis is required. Anticoagulant therapy is the best choice to obtain a complete recanalization, even if a consensus on its application does not exist; other modalities of treatment should be adopted only in case of partial or absent PVT resolution [4,107].

There are no randomized controlled trials regarding the use of anticoagulants in acute PVT [107]. Recanalization is reported in about half of patients after 6 months of therapy, even in case of extension to the mesenteric vein and with a low incidence of complications. In addition, anticoagulants administered previous to laparotomy for intestinal infarction seem to have a consistent benefit on survival [108-110]. By the way, about 10% of PVTs are resistant to anticoagulants [80-85].

According to the general opinion, the sooner the treatment is given the better is the outcome for acute PVT; anticoagulant treatment, if instituted within the first week after PVT onset, can achieve recanalization is about 69% of patients, decreasing to 25% if instituted after the second week [8,48,111].

In contrast, the management of chronic PVT has not been universally codified yet. Only 30% of patients receive the medical treatment, since clinicians are scared to administer anticoagulants in the presence of gastro-esophageal varices, low platelet counts and coagulation dysfunctions [30]. However, anticoagulant therapy seems not to increase the number of bleeding episodes and the mortality, and can prevent the occurrence of new thrombotic events [53,107]. By the way, a pragmatic approach, such as the endoscopic eradication of varices prior to begin anticoagulation, should be reasonable [30].

Anticoagulation should be administered for 3-6 months in patients with a recent PVT with no thrombophilic condition, since sometimes a complete recanalization could be delayed [30,82,83,112-114]. Recently, a panel of expert recommended the prosecution of anticoagulant therapy only in PVT patients with a proved thrombophilic disorder or familial history of venous thrombosis [114,115], with a considerable benefit on survival and a reduced risk of gastrointestinal bleeding [116,117]. However, regarding cirrhotic patients, the ubiquitary and long-term use of anticoagulants is not considered a correct practice, until their safety and efficacy will be completely tested [47]. Anticoagulants should be administered to cirrhotics only in case of intestinal ischemia or infarction or an underlying thrombophilic condition, and only after an adequate prophylaxis for variceal bleeding [2,107]. In candidates for liver transplantation with a high risk PVT (obstruction of more than 50% of the portal vein), anticoagulation should be recommended, even if a scheduled prophylactic treatment has not yet been assessed [51,70,91,100].

Apart from the anticoagulant treatment, thrombolytic treatment, surgical thrombectomy, transjugular intrahepatic porto-systemic shunt (TIPS) placement and shunt surgery represent other available therapeutic options. Thrombolytic treatment, given into the systemic venous circulation, or the superior mesenteric artery or the portal vein via a transjugular or transhepatic route, is effective to provide recanalization of acute PVT, especially when anticoagulant therapy fails [118-123]. However, it has a lower efficacy and a higher mortality and it is not clear in which conditions it should be preferred to anticoagulation [48,118124,125]. Surgical thrombectomy is routinely not recommended, for the reported morbidity and mortality; percutaneous transhepatic mechanical thrombectomy may also be effective in recent thrombosis, but vascular traumas are frequent and may stimulate re-thrombosis [126]. TIPS placement is reserved for patients developing PVT before or after liver transplantation, or in alternative to thrombolysis when anticoagulation fails [127,128]. It seems to be effective in resolving portal biliophathy, ascites and portal hypertension, but it is not feasible if portal vein is not catheterizable or a cavernomatous vein cannot be dilated [129-131]. Finally, shunt surgery (distal spleno-renal shunt or Rex shunt, in children) might be applied as the last choice, but its use has been abandoned in clinical practice [132].

CONCLUSION

PVT is a rare event in healthy subjects, while it is comparable to a "milestone" in the natural evolution of liver cirrhosis. Local or systemic factors, or a combination of them, may contribute to PVT onset, with peculiar features for each patient. As a result, splanchnic and hepatic hemodynamic is profoundly altered and bowel ischemia and infarction, vascular neo-formation and gastrointestinal bleeding are possible complications of PVT development. Liver function is usually conserved, in absence of an underlying liver disease, while it may worsen considerably in cirrhotic patients with PVT. Even if, in the past, PVT diagnosis presented some technical difficulties, thanks to the recent advance in imaging and laboratory investigations the early identification of the obstruction and its original cause is now possible. PVT treatment has been notably improved too, since different less invasive and better-tolerated options, as well as more effective, are now available. However, the future target of PVT management will be to improve the safety of the treatment and to realize a scheduled, preemptive, therapeutic approach to the patient, to stop the development of PVT complications before their occurrence, especially in cirrhotic patients.

REFERENCES

[1] Bayraktar Y, Harmanci O. Etiology and consequences of thrombosis in abdominal vessels *World J Gastroenterol.* 2006; 12(8):1165-74. PMID: 16771946.

[2] Amitrano L, Guardascione MA, Brancaccio V, Margaglione M, Manguso F, Iannaccone L, Grandone E, Balzano A. Risk factors and clinical presentation of portal vein thrombosis in patients with liver cirrhosis *J Hepatol.* 2004; 40(5):736-41. doi:10.1016/j.jhep.2004.01.001 PMID:15094219.

[3] Wang JT, Zhao HY, Liu YL. Portal vein thrombosis. *Hepatobiliary Pancreat Dis Int.* 2005; 4(4):515-8. PMID: 16286254.

[4] Ogren M, Bergqvist D, Björck M, Acosta S, Eriksson H, Sternby NH. Portal vein thrombosis: Prevalence, patient characteristics and lifetime risk: A population study based on 23796 consecutive autopsies *World J Gastroenterol.* 2006; 12(13):2115-9. PMID: 16610067.

[5] Condat B, Valla D. Nonmalignant portal vein thrombosis in adults *Nat Clin Pract Gastroenterol Hepatol.* 2006; 3(9):505-15. doi:10.1038/ncpgasthep0577 PMID: 16951667.

[6] Chawla Y, Duseja A, Dhiman RK. Review article: Modern management of portal vein thrombosis. *Aliment Pharmacol Ther.* 2009 12. doi: 10.1111/j.1365-2036.2009.04116.x PMID: 19678814.

[7] Pirisi M, Avellini C, Fabris C, Scott C, Bardus P, Soardo G, Beltrami CA, Bartoli E. Portal vein thrombosis in hepatocellular carcinoma: age and sex distribution in an autopsy study *J J Cancer Res Clin Oncol.* 1998; 124(7):397-400. doi:10.1007/s004320050189 PMID: 9719503.

[8] Hoekstra J, Janssen HL. Vascular liver disorders (II): portal vein thrombosis. *Neth J Med.* 2009; 67(2):46-53. PMID: 19299846.

[9] Alpern MB, Rubin JM, Williams DM, Capek P. Porta hepatis: duplex Doppler US with angiographic correlation. Radiology 1987; 162:53–56. PMID: 3538152.

[10] Bradbury MS, Kavanagh PV, Bechtold RE, Chen MY, Ott DJ, Regan JD, Weber TM. Mesenteric venous thrombosis: diagnosis and noninvasive imaging. *Radiographics* 2002; 22:527–541. PMID: 12006685.

[11] Cohen J, Edelman RR, Chopra S. Portal vein thrombosis: A review. *Am J Med.* 1992; 92(2):173-82. doi:10.1016/0002-9343(92)90109-O PMID: 1543202.

[12] Witte CL, Brewer ML, Witte MH, Pond GB. Protean manifestations of the pylethrombosis. A review of thirty-four patients. *Ann Surg.* 1985; 202(2):191-202. PMID: 3874612.

[13] Valla DC, Condat B. Portal vein thrombosis in adults: Pathophysiology, pathogenesis and management. A review. *J Hepatol* 2000; 32:865–71. doi:10.1016/S0168-8278(00)80259-7 PMid:10845677.

[14] Bick RL. Coagulation abnormalities in malignancy. *Semin Thromb Hemost* 1992; 18:353–72. doi:10.1055/s-2007-1002575 PMID:1470924.

[15] Kocher G, Himmelmann A. Portal vein thrombosis (PVT): a study of 20 non-cirrhotic cases. *Swiss Med Wkly.* 2005 25; 135(25-26):372-6. doi: 2005/25/smw-11035 PMID: 16106327.

[16] Janssen HL, Meinardi JR, Vleggaar FP, van Uum SH, Haagsma EB, van Der Meer FJ, van Hattum J, Chamuleau RA, Adang RP, Vandenbroucke JP, van Hoek B, Rosendaal FR. Factor V Leiden mutation, prothrombin gene mutation, and deficiencies in coagulation inhibitors associated with Budd-Chiari syndrome and portal vein thrombosis: results of a case-control study. *Blood* 2000; 96: 2364-2368. PMID: 11001884.

[17] Mohanty D, Shetty S, Ghosh K, Pawar A, Abraham P. Hereditary thrombophilia as a cause of Budd-Chiari syndrome: a study from Western India. *Hepatology* 2001; 34:666-670. doi:10.1053/jhep.2001.27948 PMID:11584361.

[18] Bhattacharyya M, Makharia G, Kannan M, Ahmed RP, Gupta PK, Saxena R. Inherited prothrombotic defects in Budd-Chiari syndrome and portal vein thrombosis: a study from North India. *Am J Clin Pathol* 2004; 121:844-847. doi:10.1309/F2U1XBV4RXYUAYG0 PMID:15198356.

[19] Amitrano L, Brancaccio V, Guardascione MA, Margaglione M, Sacco M, Martino R, De Nucci C, Mosca S, Iannaccone L, Ames PR, Romano L, Balzano A. Portal vein thrombosis after variceal endoscopic sclerotherapy in cirrhotic patients: role of genetic thrombophilia. *Endoscopy* 2002; 34:535–538. doi:10.1055/s-2002-33210 PMID:12170404.

[20] Erkan O, Bozdayi AM, Disibeyaz S, Oguz D, Ozcan M, Bahar K, Karayalcin S, Ozden A, Bozkaya H, Yurdaydin C, Uzunalimoglu O. Thrombophilic gene mutations in cirrhotic patients with portal vein thrombosis. *Eur J Gastroenterol Hepatol* 2005; 17:339–343. PMID: 15716659.

[21] Guyatt G. Determining prognosis and creating clinical decision rules. In: Haynes B, Sackett DL, Guyatt G, Tulliez M, editors.*Clinical epidemiology*. Lippincott Williams & Wilkins; 2006. p. 323–355.

[22] Walker AP. Portal vein thrombosis: what is the role of genetics? *Eur J Gastroenterol Hepatol* 2005; 17:705–707. doi:10.1097/01.meg.0000170927.60979.1d PMID: 15947546.

[23] Mangia A, Margaglione M, Cascavilla I, Gentile R, Cappucci G, Facciorusso D, Grandone E, Di Minno G, Rizzetto M, Andriulli A. Anticardiolipin antibodies in patients with liver disease. *Am J Gastroenterol.* 1999; 94(10):2983-7. doi:10.1111/j.1572-0241.1999.01447.x PMID:10520856.

[24] Wahl DG, Guillemin F, de Maistre E, Perret-Guillaume C, Lecompte T, Thibaut G. Meta-analysis of the risk of venous thrombosis in individuals with antiphospholipid antibodies without underlying autoimmune disease or previous thrombosis. *Lupus.* 1998; 7(1):15-22. doi:10.1191/096120398678919688 PMID:9493144.

[25] Liappis AP, Roberts AD, Schwartz AM, Simon GL. Thrombosis and infection: a case of transient anti-cardiolipin antibody associated with pylephlebitis. *Am J Med Sci.* 2003; 325(6):365-8. doi:10.1097/00000441-200306000-00008 PMID:12811233.

[26] Gervais A, Czernichow B, Grunebaum L, Wiesel ML, Auperin A, Rivalland D, Gabanyi J, Goldstein L, Cazenave JP, Doffoël M. Serum cardiolipin antibodies in patients with alcohol cirrhosis. *Gastroenterol Clin Biol.* 1996; 20(10):736-42. PMID: 8991142.

[27] Ponziani FR, De Stefano V, Gasbarrini A. Viral cirrhosis: an overview of haemostatic alterations and clinical consequences. *Med J Hemat in press.*

[28] Fisher NC, Wilde JT, Roper J, Elias E. Deficiency of natural anticoagulant proteins C, S, and antithrombin in portal vein thrombosis: a secondary phenomenon? *Gut* 2000; 46:534-539. doi:10.1136/gut.46.4.534 PMID:10716684.

[29] Valla D, Casadevall N, Huisse MG, Tulliez M, Grange JD, Muller O, Binda T, Varet B, Rueff B, Benhamou JP. Etiology of portal vein thrombosis in adults. A prospective evaluation of primary myeloproliferative disorders. *Gastroenterology* 1998; 94:1063-9. PMID: 3345875.

[30] Webster GJ, Burroughs AK, Riordan SM. Review article: portal vein thrombosis – new insights into aetiology and management. *Aliment Pharmacol Ther.* 2005; 21(1):1-9. doi:10.1111/j.1365-2036.2004.02301.x PMID: 15644039.

[31] Lamy T, Devillers A, Bernard M, Moisan A, Grulois I, Drenou B, Amiot L, Fauchet R, Le Prise PY. Inapparent polycythemia vera: an unrecognized diagnosis. *Am J Med* 1997; 102:14–20. PMID: 9209196.

[32] Baxter EJ, Scott LM, Campbell PJ, East C, Fourouclas N, Swanton S, Vassiliou GS, Bench AJ, Boyd EM, Curtin N, Scott MA, Erber WN, Green AR. Acquired mutation of the tyrosine kinase JAK2 in human myeloproliferative disorders. *Lancet.* 2005; 365(9464):1054-61. doi:10.1016/S0140-6736(05)71142-9 PMID: 15781101.

[33] James C, Ugo V, Le Couedic JP, Staerk J, Delhommeau F, Lacout C, Garcon L, Raslova H, Berger R, Bennaceur-Griscelli A, Villeval JL, Constantinescu SN, Casadevall N, Vainchenker W. A unique clonal JAK2 mutation leading to constitutive signalling causes polycythaemia vera. *Nature* 2005; 434:1144-1148. doi:10.1038/nature03546 PMID:15793561.

[34] Kralovics R, Passamonti F, Buser AS, Teo SS, Tiedt R, Passweg JR, Tichelli A, Cazzola M, Skoda RC. A gain-of-function mutation of JAK2 in myeloproliferative

disorders. *N Engl J Med.* 2005; 352(17):1779-90. doi:10.1056/NEJMoa051113 PMID:15858187.

[35] Xavier SG, Gadelha T, Pimenta G, Eugenio AM, Ribeiro DD, Gomes FM, Bonamino M, Zalcberg IR, Spector N. JAK2V617F Mutation in Patients with Splanchnic Vein Thrombosis. *Dig Dis Sci.* 2009; 19. doi:10.1007/s10620-009-0933-y PMID: 19690956.

[36] Levine RL, Wadleigh M, Cools J, Ebert BL, Wernig G, Huntly BJ, Boggon TJ, Wlodarska I, Clark JJ, Moore S, Adelsperger J, Koo S, Lee JC, Gabriel S, Mercher T, D'Andrea A, Fröhling S, Döhner K, Marynen P, Vandenberghe P, Mesa RA, Tefferi A, Griffin JD, Eck MJ, Sellers WR, Meyerson M, Golub TR, Lee SJ, Gilliland DG. Activating mutation in the tyrosine kinase JAK2 in polycythemia vera, essential thrombocythemia, and myeloid metaplasia with myelofibrosis. *Cancer Cell.* 2005; 7(4):387-97. doi:10.1016/j.ccr.2005.03.023 PMID: 15837627.

[37] Colaizzo D, Amitrano L, Tiscia GL, Scenna G, Grandone E, Guardascione MA, Brancaccio V, Margaglione M. The JAK2 V617F mutation frequently occurs in patients with portal and mesenteric venous thrombosis. *J Thromb Haemost* 2007; 5:55-61. doi:10.1111/j.1538-7836.2006.02277.x PMID: 17059429.

[38] Primignani M, Barosi G, Bergamaschi G, Gianelli U, Fabris F, Reati R, Dell'Era A, Bucciarelli P, Mannucci PM. Role of the JAK2 mutation in the diagnosis of chronic myeloproliferative disorders in splanchnic vein thrombosis. *Hepatology* 2006; 44:1528-1534. doi:10.1002/hep.21435 PMID: 17133457.

[39] Denninger MH, Chait Y, Casadevall N, Hillaire S, Guillin MC, Bezeaud A, et al. Cause of portal or hepatic venous thrombosis in adults: the role of multiple concurrent factors. *Hepatology* 2000; 31:587–591. doi: 10.1002/hep.510310307 PMID: 10706547.

[40] Lebrec D, Bataille C, Bercoff E, et al. Hemodynamic changes in patients with portal venous obstruction. *Hepatology* 1983; 3:550. PMID: 6862366.

[41] Ohnishi K, Okuda K, Ohtsuki T, Nakayama T, Hiyama Y, Iwama S, Goto N, Nakajima Y, Musha N, Nakashima T. Formation of hilar collaterals or cavernous transformation after portal vein obstruction by hepatocellular carcinoma. Observations in ten patients. *Gastroenterology* 1984; 87:1150-1153. PMID: 6090259.

[42] De Gaetano AM, Lafortune M, Patriquin H, De Franco A, Aubin B, Paradis K. Cavernous transformation of the portal vein: patterns of intrahepatic and splanchnic collateral circulation detected with Doppler sonography. *AJR Am J Roentgenol* 1995; 165: 1151-1155. PMID 7572494.

[43] Ogren M, Bergqvist D, Wahlander K, Eriksson H, Sternby NH. Trousseau's syndrome-what is the evidence? A population based autopsy study. *Thromb Haemost* 2006; 95:541-545. doi:10.1267/THRO06030541 PMID: 16525584.

[44] Harmanci O, Bayraktar Y. Portal hypertension due to portal venous thrombosis: etiology, clinical outcomes. *World J Gastroenterol.* 2007;13(18):2535-40. PMID: 17552000.

[45] Jamieson NV. Changing perspectives in portal vein thrombosis and liver transplantation. *Transplantation* 2000; 69:1772–4. doi:10.1097/00007890-200005150-00006 PMID:10830208.

[46] Kumar S, Sarr MG, Kamath PS. Mesenteric venous thrombosis. *N Engl J Med* 2001; 345:1683–8. PMID: 11759648.

[47] Gertsch P, Matthews J, Lerut J, Luder P, Blumgart LH. Acute thrombosis of the splanchnic veins. *Arch Surg* 1993; 128: 341–5. PMID: 8442693.

[48] Malkowski P, Pawlak J, Michalowicz B, Szczerban J, Wroblewski T, Leowska E, Krawczyk M. Thrombolytic treatment of portal thrombosis. *Hepatogastroenterology*. 2003; 50(54):2098-100. PMID: 14696472.

[49] Northup PG, Sundaram V, Fallon MB, Reddy KR, Balogun RA, Sanyal AJ, Anstee QM, Hoffman MR, Ikura Y, Caldwell SH. Hypercoagulation and thrombophilia in liver disease. *J Thromb Haemost*. 2008; 6(1):2-9. doi:10.1111/j.1538-7836.2007.02772.x PMID: 17892532.

[50] Sogaard KK, Astrup LB, Vilstrup H, Gronbaek H. Portal vein thrombosis: risk factors, clinical presentation and treatment. *BMC Gastroenterol*. 2007;7:34. doi:10.1186/1471-230X-7-34 PMID:17697371.

[51] Sobhonslidsuk A, Reddy KR. Portal vein thrombosis: a concise review. *Am J Gastroenterol*. 2002; 97(3):535-41. doi:10.1111/j.1572-0241.2002.05527.x PMID:11922544.

[52] Janssen HL, Wijnhoud A, Haagsma EB, Van Uum SH, Van Nieuwkerk CM, Adang RP, Chamuleau RA, Van Hattum J, Vleggaar FP, Hansen BE, Rosendaal FR, Van Hoek B. Extrahepatic portal vein thrombosis: aetiology and determinants of survival. *Gut*. 2001; 49(5):720-4. doi:10.1136/gut.49.5.720 PMID:11600478.

[53] Condat B, Pessione F, Hillaire S, Denninger MH, Guillin MC, Poliquin M, Hadengue A, Erlinger S, Valla D. Current outcome of portal vein thrombosis in adults: risk and benefit of anticoagulant therapy. *Gastroenterol*. 2001; 120(2):490-7. doi:10.1053/gast.2001.21209 PMID:11159889.

[54] Perlemuter G, Béjanin H, Fritsch J, Prat F, Gaudric M, Chaussade S, Buffet C. Biliary obstruction caused by portal cavernoma: a study of 8 cases. *J Hepatol*. 1996; 25(1):58-63. PMID: 8836902.

[55] Dhiman RK, Puri P, Chawla Y, Minz M, Bapuraj JR, Gupta S, Nagi B, Suri S. Biliary changes in extrahepatic portal venous obstruction: compression by collaterals or ischemic? *Gastrointest Endosc*. 1999; 50(5):646-52. doi:10.1016/S0016-5107(99)80013-3 PMID:10536320.

[56] Colle I, Van Vlierberghe H, Pattyn P, Troisi R, Vogelaers D, de Hemptinne B, De Vos M. Cholestasis as presenting symptom of portal cavernoma. *Hepatol Res*. 2003; 25(1):32-37. doi:10.1016/S1386-6346(02)00172-9 PMID:12644036.

[57] Chandra R, Kapoor D, Tharakan A, Chaudhary A, Sarin SK. Portal biliopathy. *J Gastroenterol Hepatol*. 2001; 16(10):1086-92. doi:10.1046/j.1440-1746.2001.02562.x PMID:11686833.

[58] Sarin SK, Agarwal SR. Extrahepatic portal vein obstruction. *Semin Liver Dis*. 2002; 22(1):43-58. doi:10.1055/s-2002-23206 PMID: 11928078.

[59] Bayraktar Y, Balkanci F, Kayhan B, Ozenç A, Arslan S, Telatar H. Bile duct varices or "pseudo-cholangiocarcinoma sign" in portal hypertension due to cavernous transformation of the portal vein. *Am J Gastroenterol*. 1992; 87(12):1801-6. PMID: 1449145.

[60] Bayraktar Y, Balkanci F, Ozenc A, Arslan S, Koseoglu T, Ozdemir A, Uzunalimoglu B, Telatar H, Gurakar A, Van Thiel DH, et al. The "pseudo-cholangiocarcinoma sign"

in patients with cavernous transformation of the portal vein and its effect on the serum alkaline phosphatase and bilirubin levels. *Am J Gastroenterol.* 1995; 90(11):2015-9. PMID: 7485013.

[61] Belli L, Puttini M, Marni A. Extrahepatic portal obstruction— clinical experience and surgical treatment in 105 patients. *J Cardiovasc Surg.* 1980; 21(4):439-48. PMID: 7191422.

[62] Lai L, Brugge WR. Endoscopic ultrasound is a sensitive and specific test to diagnose portal venous system thrombosis (PVST). *Am J Gastroenterol.* 2004; 99(1):40-4. doi:10.1046/j.1572-0241.2003.04020.x PMID:14687139.

[63] Sugiyama M, Hagi H, Atomi Y, Saito M. Diagnosis of portal venous invasion by pancreatobiliary carcinoma: Value of endoscopic ultrasonography. *Abdom Imaging.* 1997; 22(4):434-8. doi:10.1007/s002619900227 PMID:9157867.

[64] Brugge WR, Lee MJ, Kelsey PB, Schapiro RH, Warshaw AL. The use of EUS to diagnose ,malignant portal venous system invasion by pancreatic cancer. *Gastrointest Endosc.* 1996; 43(6):561-7. doi:10.1016/S0016-5107(96)70191-8 PMID:8781933.

[65] Ueno N, Sasaki A, Tomiyama T, Tano S, Kimura K. Color doppler ultrasonography in the diagnosis of cavernous transformation of the portal vein. *J Clin Ultrasound.* 1997; 25(5):227-33. doi:10.1002/(SICI)1097-0096(199706)25:5<227::AID-JCU2>3.0.CO;2-F PMID:9314103.

[66] Haddad MC, Clark DC, Sharif HS, Al Shahed M, Aideyan O, Sammak BM. MR, CT, and ultrasonography of splanchnic venous thrombosis. *Gastrointest Radiol.* 1992; 17(1):34-40. doi:10.1007/BF01888505 PMID:1544556.

[67] Ito K, Siegelman ES, Stolpen AH, Mitchell DG. MR imaging of the complications after liver transplantation. *Am J Roentgenol* 2000; 175:1145–9. PMID: 11000180.

[68] Okumura A, Watanabe Y, Dohke M, Ishimori T, Amoh Y, Oda K, Dodo Y. Contrast-enhanced three-dimensional MR portography. *Radiographics.* 1999; 19(4):973-87. PMID: 10464804.

[69] Glockner JF, Forauer AR, Solomon H, Varma CR, Perman WH. Three-dimensional gadolinium-enhanced MR angiography of vascular complications after liver transplantation. *AJR Am J Roentgenol.* 2000; 174(5):1447-53. PMID: 10789810.

[70] Yerdel MA, Gunson B, Mirza D, Karayalçin K, Olliff S, Buckels J, Mayer D, McMaster P, Pirenne J. Portal vein thrombosis in adults undergoing liver transplantation. Risk factors, screening, management and outcome. *Transplantation.* 2000 15; 69(9):1873-81. PMID: 10830225.

[71] Smith CS, Sheehy N, McEniff N, Keogan MT. Magnetic resonance portal venography: use of fast-acquisition true FISP imaging in the detection of portal vein thrombosis. *Clin Radiol.* 2007; 62:1180-8. doi:10.1016/j.crad.2007.06.007 PMID: 17981166.

[72] De Sio I, Castellano L, Calandra M, Romano M, Persico M, Del Vecchio-Blanco C. Ultrasound-guided fine needle aspiration biopsy of portal vein thrombosis in liver cirrhosis: results in 15 patients. *J Gastroenterol Hepatol.* 1995; 10(6):662-5. doi:10.1111/j.1440-1746.1995.tb01367.x PMID:8580410.

[73] Plemmons RM, Dooley DP, Longfield RN. Septic thrombophlebitis of the portal vein (pylephlebitis): diagnosis and management in the modern era. *Clin Infect Dis.* 1995; 21(5):1114-20. PMID: 8589130.

[74] Tsujikawa T, Ihara T, Sasaki M, Inoue H, Fujiyama Y, Bamba T. Effectiveness of combined anticoagulant therapy for extending portal vein thrombosis in Crohn's disease. *Dis Colon Rectum*. 1996; 39(7):823-5. doi:10.1007/BF02054451 PMID: 8674378.

[75] Hassn AM, Al-Fallouji MA, Ouf TI, Saad R. Portal vein thrombosis following splenectomy. Br J Surg. 2000; 87(3):362-73. doi:10.1046/j.1365-2168.2000.01383-16.x PMID:10718950.

[76] Garcia-Pagan JC, Valla DC. Portal vein thrombosis: A predictable milestone in cirrhosis? *J Hepatol*. 2009. doi:10.1016/j.jhep.2009.06.009 PMID: 19660824.

[77] Francoz C, Belghiti J, Vilgrain V, Sommacale D, Paradis V, Condat B, Denninger MH, Sauvanet A, Valla D, Durand F. Splanchnic vein thrombosis in candidates for liver transplantation: usefulness of screening and anticoagulation. *Gut* 2005; 54:691–697. doi:10.1136/gut.2004.042796 PMID: 15831918.

[78] Zocco MA, Stasio ED, Cristofaro RD, Novi M, Ainora ME, Ponziani F, Riccardi L, Lancellotti S, Santoliquido A, Flore R, Pompili M, Rapaccini GL, Tondi P, Gasbarrini GB, Landolfi R, Gasbarrini A. Thrombotic risk factors in patients with liver cirrhosis: Correlation with MELD scoring system and portal vein thrombosis development. *J Hepatol* 2009; 51: 682-9.

[79] Garcia-Pagan JC, Salmeron JM, Feu F, Luca A, Ginés P, Pizcueta P, Claria J, Piera C, Arroyo V, Bosch J. Effects of low-sodium diet and spironolactone on portal pressure in patients with compensated cirrhosis. *Hepatology* 1994; 19: 1095–1099.

[80] Plessier A, Murad SD, Hernandez-Guerra M, et al. A prospective multicentric follow-up study on 105 patients with acute portal vein thrombosis (PVT): Results from the european network for vascular disorders of the liver (en-vie). *Hepatology*. 2007; 46:310a-a.

[81] Amitrano L, Guardascione MA, Scaglione M, Pezzullo L, Sangiuliano N, Armellino MF, Manguso F, Margaglione M, Ames PR, Iannaccone L, Grandone E, Romano L, Balzano A. Prognostic factors in noncirrhotic patients with splanchnic vein thromboses. *Am J Gastroenterol*. 2007; 102:2464-70. doi:10.1111/j.1572-0241.2007.01477.x PMID: 17958760.

[82] Sheen CL, Lamparelli H, Milne A, Green I, Ramage JK. Clinical features, diagnosis and outcome of acute portal vein thrombosis. *Q J Med* 93:531–534. PMID: 10924535.

[83] Condat B, Pessione F, Denninger MH, Hillaire S, Valla D. Recent portal or mesenteric venous thrombosis: increased recognition and frequent recanalization on anticoagulant therapy. *Hepatology* 2000; 32:466–470. doi:10.1053/jhep.2000.16597 PMID:10960436.

[84] Baril N, Wren S, Radin R, Ralls P, Stain S. The role of anticoagulation in pylephlebitis. *Am J Surg* 1996; 172:449–452. doi:10.1016/S0002-9610(96)00220-6 PMID: 8942542.

[85] Lagasse JP, Bahallah ML, Salem N, Debillon G, Labarrière D, Serve MP, Advenier V, Causse X, Legoux JL. Acute thrombosis of the portal system. Treatment with alteplase and heparin or with heparin alone in 10 patients. *Gastroenterol Clin Biol* 1997; 21:919–923. PMID: 9587554.

[86] Voorhees AB, Price JB. Extrahepatic portal hypertension. A retrospective analysis of 127 cases and associated clinical implications. *Arch Surg* 1974; 108:338–41. PMID: 4544312.

[87] Kiladjian JJ, Cervantes F, Leebeek FWG, et al. Role of JAK 2 mutation detection in budd-chiari syndrome (BCS) and portal vein thrombosis (PVT) associated to MPD. *Blood.* 2006;108:116a-a.

[88] Van Thiel DH, Schade RR, Starzl TE, Iwatsuki S, Shaw BW Jr, Gavaler JS, Dugas M. Liver transplantation in adults. *Hepatology* 1982; 2:637–40. PMID: 6749636.

[89] Shaw BW Jr, Iwatsuki S, Bron K, Starzl TE. Portal vein grafts in hepatic transplantation. *Surg Gynecol Obstet* 1985; 161:66–8. PMID: 3892734.

[90] Manzanet G, Sanjuan F, Orbis P, Lopez R, Moya A, Juan M, Vila J, Asensi J, Sendra P, Ruiz J, Prieto M, Mir J. Liver transplantation in patients with portal vein thrombosis. *Liver Transpl* 2001; 7:125-131. doi:10.1053/jlts.2001.21295 PMID: 11172396.

[91] Dumortier J, Czyglik O, Poncet G, Blanchet MC, Boucaud C, Henry L, Boillot O. Eversion thrombectomy for portal vein thrombosis during liver transplantation. *Am J Transplant* 2002; 2:934-938. PMID: 12482145.

[92] Gerunda GE, Merenda R, Neri D, Angeli P, Barbazza F, Valmasoni M, Feltracco P, Zangrandi F, Gangemi A, Miotto D, Gagliesi A, Faccioli AM. Cavoportal hemitransposition: a successful way to overcome the problem of total portosplenomesenteric thrombosis in liver transplantation. *Liver Transpl* 2002; 8:72-75. doi:10.1053/jlts.2002.30404 PMID: 11799489.

[93] Egawa H, Tanaka K, Kasahara M, Takada Y, Oike F, Ogawa K, Sakamoto S, Kozaki K, Taira K, Ito T. Single center experience of 39 patients with preoperative portal vein thrombosis among 404 adult living donor liver transplantations. *Liver Transpl* 2006; 12:1512-1518. doi:10.1002/lt.20777 PMID: 17004256.

[94] Selvaggi G, Weppler D, Nishida S, Moon J, Levi D, Kato T, Tzakis AG. Ten-year experience in porto-caval hemitransposition for liver transplantation in the presence of portal vein thrombosis. *Am J Transplant* 2007; 7:454-460. doi:10.1111/j.1600-6143.2006.01649.x PMID:17229075.

[95] Gomez-Gutierrez M, Quintela J, Marini M, Gala B, Suarez F, Cao I, Selles CC, Aguirrezabalaga J, Otero A, Mosteiro S. Portal vein thrombosis in patients undergoing orthotopic liver transplantation: intraoperative endovascular radiological procedures. *Transplant Proc* 2005; 37:3906-3908. doi:10.1016/j.transproceed.2005.10.063 PMID: 16386580.

[96] Lladó L, Fabregat J, Castellote J, Ramos E, Torras J, Jorba R, Garcia-Borobia F, Busquets J, Figueras J, Rafecas A. Management of portal vein thrombosis in liver transplantation: influence on morbidity and mortality. *Clin Transplant.* 2007; 21(6):716-21. doi:10.1111/j.1399-0012.2007.00728.x PMID: 17988264.

[97] Gimeno FA, Calvo J, Loinaz C, Meneu JC, Pérez B, Gomez R, Jiménez C, Abradelo M, Moreno A, Sesma A, García I, Moreno E. Comparative analysis of the results of orthotopic liver transplantation in patients with and without portal vein thrombosis. *Transplant Proc.* 2005; 37(9):3899-903. doi:10.1016/j.transproceed.2005.10.085 PMID: 16386578.

[98] Lendoire J, Raffin G, Cejas N, Duek F, Barros Schelotto P, Trigo P, Quarin C, Garay V, Imventarza O. Liver transplantation in adult patients with portal vein thrombosis: risk factors management and outcome. *HPB (Oxford).* 2007; 9(5):352-6. doi:10.1080/13651820701599033 PMID: 18345318.

[99] Arcadipane A, Nadalin S, Gruttadauria S, Panarello G, Burgio G, Vizzini G, Luca A, Gridelli B. The recipient with portal thrombosis and/or previous surgery. *Transplant Proc.* 2008; 40(4):1183-6. doi:10.1016/j.transproceed.2008.03.073 PMID: 18555144.

[100] Seu P, Shackleton CR, Shaked A, Imagawa DK, Olthoff KM, Rudich SR, et al. Improved results of liver transplantation in patients with portal vein thrombosis. *Arch Surg* 1996;131:840-4. PMID: 8712907.

[101] Stieber AC, Zetti G, Todo S et al. The spectrum of portal vein thrombosis in liver transplantation. *Ann Surg* 1991; 213:199. PMID: 1998400.

[102] Davidson B, Gibson M, Dick R, Burroughs A, Rolles K. Incidence, risk factors, management, and outcome of portal vein abnomalities at orthotopic liver transplantation. *Transplantation* 1994; 57:1174. doi:10.1097/00007890-199404270-00006 PMID:8178342.

[103] Robles R, Fernandez JA, Hernández Q, Marín C, Ramírez P, Sánchez-Bueno F, Luján JA, Rodríguez JM, Acosta F, Parrilla P. Eversion thromboendovenectomy in organized portal vein thrombosis during liver transplantation. *Clin Transplant* 2004: 18:79. PMID: 15108774.

[104] Langnas AN, Marujo W, Stratta RJ, Wood RP, Shaw BW Jr. Vascular complications after orthotopic liver transplantation. *Am J Surg* 1991; 161:76–83. PMID: 1987861.

[105] Lerut J, Tzakis AG, Bron K, Gordon RD, Iwatsuki S, Esquivel CO, Makowka L, Todo S, Starzl TE. Complications of venous reconstruction in human orthotopic liver transplantation. *Ann Surg* 1987; 205:404–14. PMID: 3551857.

[106] Duffy JP, Hong JC, Farmer DG, Ghobrial RM, Yersiz H, Hiatt JR, Busuttil RW. Vascular complications of orthotopic liver transplantation: experience in more than 4,200 patients. *J Am Coll Surg.* 2009; 208(5):896-903; discussion 903-5. doi:10.1016/j.jamcollsurg.2008.12.032 PMID: 19476857.

[107] De Leve LD, Valla DC, Garcia-Tsao G. Vascular disorders of the liver. *Hepatology.* 2009; 49(5):1729-64. doi:10.1002/hep.22772 PMID:19399912.

[108] Clavien PA. Diagnosis and management of mesenteric infarction. *Br J Surg* 1990; 77:601-603. doi:10.1002/bjs.1800770602 PMID:2200547.

[109] Brunaud L, Antunes L, Collinet-Adler S, Marchal F, Ayav A, Bresler L, Boissel P. Acute mesenteric venous thrombosis: case for nonoperative management. *J Vasc Surg* 2001; 34:673-679. doi:10.1067/mva.2001.117331 PMID: 11668323.

[110] Abdu RA, Zakhour BJ, Dallis DJ. Mesenteric venous thrombosis–1911 to 1984. *Surgery* 1987; 101:383-388. PMID: 3563882.

[111] Turnes J, García-Pagán JC, González M, Aracil C, Calleja JL, Ripoll C, Abraldes JG, Bañares R, Villanueva C, Albillos A, Ayuso JR, Gilabert R, Bosch J. Portal hypertension-related complications after acute portal vein thrombosis: impact of early anticoagulation. *Clin Gastroenterol Hepatol.* 2008; 6:1412-7. doi:10.1016/j.cgh.2008.07.031 PMID: 19081529.

[112] Rahmouni A, Mathieu D, Golli M, Douek P, Anglade MC, Caillet H, Vasile N. Value of CT and sonography in the conservative management of acute splenoportal and superior mesenteric venous thrombosis. *Gastrointest Radiol* 1992; 17:135-140. PMID: 1551509.

[113] Sarin SK, Sollano JD, Chawla YK, Amarapurkar D, Hamid S, Hashizume M, Jafri W, Kumar A, Kudo M, Lesmana LA, Sharma BC, Shiha G, Janaka de Silva H. Consensus on extra-hepatic portal vein obstruction. *Liver Int.* 2006; 26:512-9. doi:10.1111/j.1478-3231.2006.01269.x PMID: 16761994.

[114] De Franchis R. Evolving consensus in portal hypertension. Report of the Baveno IV consensus workshop on methodology of diagnosis and therapy in portal hypertension. *J Hepatol.* 2005; 43:167-76. doi:10.1016/j.jhep.2005.05.009 PMID:15925423.

[115] Garcia-Pagan JC, Hernandez-Guerra M, Bosch J. Extrahepatic portal vein thrombosis. *Seminars in Liver diseases* 2008; 28:282-92. doi:10.1055/s-0028-1085096 PMID: 18814081.

[116] Orr DW, Harrison PM, Devlin J, Karani JB, Kane PA, Heaton ND, O'Grady JG, Heneghan MA. Chronic mesenteric venous thrombosis: evaluation and determinants of survival during long-term follow-up. *Clin Gastroenterol Hepatol.* 2007; 5(1):80-6. doi:10.1016/j.cgh.2006.09.030 PMID: 17142105.

[117] Kitchens CS, Weidner MH, Lottenberg R. Chronic oral anticoagulant therapy for extrahepatic visceral thrombosis is safe. *J Thromb Thrombolysis* 2007; 23:223-228. doi:10.1007/s11239-006-9017-4 PMID:17221331.

[118] Schafer C, Zundler J, Bode JC. Thrombolytic therapy in patients with portal vein thrombosis: case report and review of the literature. *Eur J Gastroenterol Hepatol* 2000; 12:1141–5. PMID: 11057461.

[119] Henao EA, Bohannon WT, Silva MB Jr. Treatment of portal venous thrombosis with selective superior mesenteric artery infusion of recombinant tissue plasminogen activator. *J Vasc Surg* 2003; 38:1411–5. doi:10.1016/S0741-5214(03)01052-8 PMID:14681650.

[120] Tateishi A, Mitsui H, Oki T, Morishita J, Maekawa H, Yahagi N, Maruyama T, Ichinose M, Ohnishi S, Shiratori Y, Minami M, Koutetsu S, Hori N, Watanabe T, Nagawa H, Omata M. Extensive mesenteric vein and portal vein thrombosis successfully treated by thrombolysis and anticoagulation. *J Gastroenterol Hepatol* 2001; 16:1429–33. PMID: 11851847.

[121] Aytekin C, Boyvat F, Kurt A, Yologlu Z, Coskun M. Catheterdirected thrombolysis with transjugular access in portal vein thrombosis secondary to pancreatitis. *Eur J Radiol* 2001; 39:80–2. doi:10.1016/S0720-048X(01)00289-3 PMID:11522414.

[122] Lopera JE, Correa G, Brazzini A, Ustunsoz B, Patel S, Janchai A, Castaneda-Zuniga W. Percutaneous transhepatic treatment of symptomatic mesenteric venous thrombosis. *J Vasc Surg* 2002; 36:1058–61. PMID: 12422118.

[123] Kercher KW, Sing RF, Watson KW, Matthews BD, LeQuire MH, Heniford BT. Transhepatic thrombolysis in acute portal vein thrombosis after laparoscopic splenectomy. Surg Laparosc *Endosc Percutan Tech* 2002; 12:131–6. doi:10.1097/00129689-200204000-00013 PMID: 11948303.

[124] Hollingshead M, Burke CT, Mauro MA, Weeks SM, Dixon RG, Jaques PF. Transcatheter thrombolytic therapy for acute mesenteric and portal vein thrombosis. *J Vasc Interv Radiol* 2005; 16:651-661. doi:10.1097/01.RVI.0000156265.79960.86 PMID: 15872320.
[125] Grisham A, Lohr J, Guenther JM, Engel AM. Deciphering mesenteric venous thrombosis: imaging and treatment. *Vasc Endovascular Surg* 2005; 39:473-479. doi:10.1177/153857440503900603 PMID:16382268.
[126] Rosendaal FR. Venous thrombosis: a multicausal disease. *Lancet.* 1999; 353:1167-73.
[127] Ciccarelli O, Goffette P, Laterre PF, Danse E, Wittebolle X, Lerut J. Transjugular intrahepatic portosystemic shunt approach and local thrombolysis for treatment of early posttransplant portal vein thrombosis. *Transplantation* 2001; 72:159–61. PMID: 11468552.
[128] Liatsos C, Vlachogiannakos J, Patch D, Tibballs J, Watkinson A, Davidson B, Rolles K, Burroughs AK. Successful recanalization of portal vein thrombosis before liver transplantation using transjugular intrahepatic portosystemic shunt. *Liver Transpl* 2001; 7:453–60. doi:10.1053/jlts.2001.23914 PMID: 11349268.
[129] Senzolo M, Tibbals J, Cholongitas E, Burroughs AK. Transjugular intrahepatic portosystemic shunt for portal vein thrombosis with and without cavernous transformation. *Aliment Pharmacol Ther.* 2006; 23:767-75. doi:10.1111/j.1365-2036.2006.02820.x PMID: 16556179.
[130] Bilbao JI, Elorz M, Vivas I, Martínez-Cuesta A, Bastarrika G, Benito A. Transjugular intrahepatic portosystemic shunt (TIPS) in the treatment of venous symptomatic chronic portal thrombosis in non-cirrhotic patients. *Cardiovasc Intervent Radiol.* 2004; 27:474-80. doi:10.1007/s00270-004-0241-z PMID: 15383850.
[131] Van Ha TG, Hodge J, Funaki B, Lorenz J, Rosenblum J, Straus C, Leef J. Transjugular intrahepatic portosystemic shunt placement in patients with cirrhosis and concomitant portal vein thrombosis. *Cardiovasc Intervent Radiol.* 2006;29:785-90. doi:10.1007/s00270-005-0090-4 PMID:16850140.
[132] Wolff M, Hirner A. Current state of portosystemic shunt surgery. *Langenbecks Arch Surg.* 2003; 388:141-9. doi:10.1007/s00423-003-0367-5 PMID: 12942328.
[133] Ponziani FR, Zocco MA, Campanale C, Rinninella E, Tortora A, Di Maurizio L, Bombardieri G, De Cristofaro R, De Gaetano AM, Landolfi R, Gasbarrini A. Portal vein thrombosis: insight into physiopathology, diagnosis and treatment. *World J Gastroenterol. 2010;16:143-155* doi:10.3748/wjg.v16.i2.143 PMID:20066733.

In: Thrombosis: Causes, Treatment and Prevention ISBN 978-1-61668-696-3
Editor: D. G. Macri and L. D. Procaccini, pp. 155-167

Chapter VI

POLYMORPHISM A1/A2 IN CELL SURFACE INTEGRIN ALPHAIIB/BETA3 AND THE DEVELOPMENT OF INCREASED RISK FOR VENOUS THROMBEMBOLISM AND RECURRENT PREGNANCY LOSS

Ivanov Petar, Komsa-Penkova Regina and Tsvetomira Tsvyatkovska
Medical University, Pleven, Bulgaria.

ABSTRACT

The investigation of the risk factors, development and treatment of venous thrombembolism (VTE) is probably one of the fields in medicine that possesses one of the most evidence-based labors of knowledge. The complexity of finding and understanding the main causes and pathological mechanism of thrombosis process extended the time of the study. Therefore, there are still several controversial issues in the understanding of thrombosis development. Many factors have played a role in venous thrombosis development. The acquired risk factors such as trauma, surgery, prolonged immobilization, etc. affect many persons, but frequently a combination of some risk factors in one person, is necessary for thrombus formation. Indeed, multiple risk factors are a prerequisite for thrombosis development. In our days, the importance of inherited risk factors in the development of venous thromboembolism, has been increasingly recognized. The knowledge for relatively rare conditions take part in VTE development, such as protein C, protein S and antitrombin III deficiency [1], have been expanded with the discovery of the impact of mutation in coagulation factors. Recently, the most frequent prothrombotic genetic defects in patients with VTE have been considered to be Factor V Leiden mutation [2] (FVL) and Factor II 20210 G>A mutation (FII 20210 G>A) [3]. Along with mutation in natural anticoagulants and factors from cascade of coagulation, an inherited changes in platelet membrane receptors was discussed as a possible cause for abnormal thrombosis development. The surface glycoproteins (integrins), such as the GP Ib/IX/V complex, GP IIb/III, GP Ia/IIa and GPVI , play major roles in platelet activity, and so inherited changes in glycoproteins' structure could be associated with pathologic disorders without change in platelet count. Some of the heritable differences in glycoproteins' structure influence the expression and avidity of these receptors, which lead to enhanced platelet activity and increase risk for thrombus development.

This review discusses the role of inherited changes in cell surface glycoproteins, in increased risk for development of deep venous thrombosis (DVT), venous thrombembolism, as well as thrombotic events in intervillous space of placenta of the pregnant women, which could leaded to pregnancy loss. The establishment of clinically significant inherited changes in cell integrins could help to identify high-risk patients with a genetic predisposition, who have had a permanently risk for venous thrombosis development. An important impact of the genetic profile is into those individuals, who have risk of recurrent venous thrombotic events, as the identification of the polymorphisms in cell surface integrins could have influence in further antithrombotic therapy. This chapter manly focused on carrier status for polymorphism A1/A2 (PL A1/A2) in beta3 subunits of integrins alphaIIb/beta3 (GP IIb/IIIa), because of a common spread of this polymorphism in Caucasian and the important role of GP IIb/IIIa in platelet aggregation, and the risk of thrombus development. The significance of PL A1/A2 in integrin alphaV/beta3 is not connected precisely with thrombosis development, but it could be referred as possible factor in implantation failure of the concepsus in the early part of gestation. The contribution of platelet glycoprotein polymorphisms as genetic risk factors for the disease is a relatively new area of human genomics, that is still evolving. The role of PL A1/A2 in the development of venous thrombosis, as well as the impact in early and late pregnancy loss, needs conformation in more and larger studies.

STRUCTURE AND FUNCTION OF PLATELED GLYCOPROTEIN IIB/IIIA. MOLECULAR CHARACTERISTICS OF POLIMORPHYSM A1/A2

Structure and Function of Platelet Glycoprotein IIb/IIIa

The most important role of platelet is to maintain vascular integrity and to stop bleeding. In case of vessel injury, the platelet surface plays a crucial role of cell contacts, first ensuring adhesion to the exposed subendothelium components and then aggregation of platelets to build the platelet plug.

The platelet activity has been mediated by many types of receptors, situated on the cell membrane: GP Ib/IX/V comlex (constitutively active receptor for VWF related with platelet adhesion), GP Ia/IIa and GP VI (receptors for collagen [4]), receptors for Adenosine Diphosphate (ADP), Tromboxan A_2 and serotonin (5-HT-2 subtype) [5] etc. Although this large number of platelet membrane receptors, GP IIb/IIIa have a crucial role in platelet functions. The main function of GP IIb/IIIa is connected with platelet aggregation. GP IIb/IIIa is a member of the integrin family of membrane receptors, named so because the integrins integrate extracellular ligands with the intracellular cytoskeleton [6]. Platelets are the first cells with which have been made the discovery and the initial description of the structure of the integrin family receptors, and their role in diseases [7].

GP IIb/IIIa forms from two separated polypeptide chains: subunits IIb and IIIa. In the integrin nomenclature, GP IIb is the alphaIIb subunit, and GP IIIa is the beta3 subunit. The two protein subunits must associate stoichiometrically into a 1:1 noncovalent complex for efficient cell-surface expression [8,9].

The genes for the synthesis of both subunits of GP IIb/IIIa are situated in chromosome 17. GP IIb synthesis is restricted to megakaryocytes and platelets, whereas GP IIIa synthesis also occurs in endothelial cells and in many other cells (including endometrial cells, cells of preimplantated embryo), as the beta3 subunit of integrin alphaV/beta3.

GP IIb/IIIa is the most abundant GP on the cell surface membrane. After activation of the platelets, the surface density of functional GP IIb/IIIa receptors can increase by 30% to 50% (from approximately 40,000 available molecules per platelet to approximately 80,000) [10]. After the activation of the platelet GP IIb/IIIa, along with the increasing number of molecules on cells surface, GP IIb/IIIa undergo a transformation from a resting low-affinity state to an activated high-affinity state. Platelet activation caused a conformational change in GP IIb/IIIa that markedly enhances ligand binding affinity of the receptor [11]. GP IIb/IIIa had many ligands: fibrin [12], VWF, fibronectin, vitronectin, thrombospondin [13,14], but principally it is the receptor for fibrinogen, who is the main mediator of platelet aggregation [15].

Molecular Characteristics of Polymorphism A1/A2 in GP IIb/IIIa.

Inherited changes in the structure of GP IIb/IIIa lead to variation of number and function of the receptor. One common spread polymorphism in beta3 subunit of GP IIb/IIIa is Leucin-Prolin substitution at place 33 in the amino-terminal loop of the peptide chain (replacement of Timine with Cytocine at 1565 place in nucleotide sequence of the gene [16]). This substitution defined two haplotypes of the polymorphism: alloantigen PL A1 and alloantigens PL A2.

The influence of PL A1/A2 on platelet function has been vigorously debated. Several reports have provided data that confers either an enhanced function of GP IIb/IIIa or an increased resistance to platelet aggregation inhibitors.

Epidemiology of Polymorphism A1/A2

In 1989, Newman et al., [16] established 15% carriers of PL A1/A2 in health subjects (Americans, Caucasian). In a few other studies, a wide variation of allele A2 in health individuals was specified (from 14.3% [29] to 28.5% [62]). Investigation in the populations of Asia established a very low prevalence of allele A2, in comparison with those in the White race. In Indians, Malaysians, Chinese was found 0.01% to 0.1% carriers of PL A1/A2 in health subjects [17].

Clinical Manifestations in Presence of Polymorphism A1/A2

A number of reports have found an association between the expression of allele A2 of PL A1/A2 and the risk for arterial thrombosis. Particularly, some studies [18,19] have found association of PL A1/A2 and increased risk for myocardial infarction among young individuals. Other studies [20] on large patient cohorts have failed to find a relation to the risk for myocardial infarction or stroke. Interestingly, one meta-analysis concluded that there is no association between PL A1/A2 and increased thrombotic risk [21], whereas a second recent meta-analysis [22] concluded that there is a weak but significant correlation.

Laboratory Diagnosis. Detection of Carrier Status for Polymorphism A1/A2

To detect the 1565 T>C substitution in exon 2 of the glycoprotein IIIa gene, that is responsible for the PL A1/A2 polymorphism, a modified PCR-based restriction fragment length polymorphism (RFLP) analysis have been used [16]. A T>C substitution creates a Msp I enzyme restriction site that is present in the allele A2 allele, but not in the allele A1. After Msp I digestion, the restricted PCR fragments were loaded onto 3.5% agarose gel and then were visualized by UV transillumination.

Contribution of Polymorphism A1/A2 in GP IIb/IIIa for the Development of Increased Risk of Venous Thrombembolism

Recent family-based studies indicate that venous thromboembolism is highly heritable and follows a complex mode involving interaction between environmental and inherited risk factors [23,24]. Inherited predisposition to thrombus formation (called thrombophilia) was referred mainly for the elevated risk of venous thrombosis [25]. Thrombophilia is not a disease per se, but may be associated with a disease as an underlying predisposition for thrombus formation [26]. Prospective cohort studies indicate that the elevated risk for VTE is connected with increased basal fibrin formation [27,28]. Therefore, patients with inherited predisposition for thrombosis, caused by either variation of coagulation factors' activity, or increased function of platelets, have had multiplicity of risk for venous thrombosis. So, the assessment and demonstration of increased platelet activity had substantial role in the evaluation of risk for VTE development. Indeed, little data is available about the impact of polymorphism A2 in GP IIb/IIIa in patients with VTE and especially about its role in combined presence with other inherited thrombophilic factors (FVL, FII 20210 G>A).

Our study [29] have shown a 35.3% carriers of PL A1/A2 in patients with pulmonary embolism versus 14.3% in healthy control subjects (OR 3.3, 95%CI 1.3–7.9, p=0.003). Patients with recurrent VTE incidence showed a higher prevalence of the polymorphism (OR 3.5, 95% CI 1.2–10.3, p=0.017). In a large prospective cohort of men, Ridker et al. [20] have not found association between PL A1/A2 and increased risk of deep venous thrombosis

(DVT). These authors investigated 121 patients with DVT and found 14.5% carriers of PL A1/A2 (similar to control subjects). They [20] calculated a relative risk of 1.07 (0.7-1.6) for DVT development in presence of A2 allele. Renner et al. [30] found a slightly higher prevalence of PL A1/A2 (31.6%) in 310 patients with DVT, unlike the results of Ridker et al. [20] The result of Renner et al. does not reach significant difference in comparison with controls (OR 1.21, 95%CI 0.85-1.71) and remains insignificant after the adjustment of factor V Leiden and FII 20210 G>A. These two studies concern only the presence of PL A1/A2 in patients with DVT, but do not include investigation of carrier status in patients with pulmonary embolism. In our study [29], we found also a slight higher prevalence of PL A1/A2 in patients with isolated pulmonary embolism, comparing with the prevalence in the patients with PE and DVT (respectively 41.7% and 33.3%). Also the results of Ridker et al. [20] should be revised in further prospective study, due to a relatively short followed up period (8.6 years).

Podciechowski et al. [31] investigated the relationship between PL A1/A2 and the increased risk for DVT development in the group of women in labour. They have not found any significant difference in the carrier status for PL A1/A2 in 72 women with DVT during pregnancy or labor and 173 women in childbirth.

Hooper et al. [32] investigated 71 African Americans with VTE and 185 health subjects for carrier status for PL A1/A2. They do not found relationship between the polymorphism and VTE development. Surprisingly the authors established a relatively high prevalence of PL A1/A2 in controls (21%), in comparison to the previously reported [33] very low population frequency of allele A2 among Black race. As the authors noted, this discrepancy could be related to regional differences in gene frequencies among African Americans.

Whether PL A1/A2 is an independent risk factor for DVT and pulmonary edembolism development, or it increases the risk only in associatiation with other risk factors, is a subject of future investigation. In conclusion, recent clinical and epidemiologic studies have established that VTE is not a consequence of a single gene or any one environmental factor, but rather represent a complex pathology that is caused by multiple interactions between genetic and environmental factors.

Possibility to Influence the Increased Risk of Venous Thrombosis in Presence of PL A1/A2. Resistance to Antithrombotic Drugs due to PL A1/A2

The initial management of DVT or pulmonary embolism in patients with heritable thrombophilia does not differ from the management of venous thrombosis in any other patient, according to the British Society of Haematology [34]. In general, patients who have had recurrent spontaneous VTE or those with established inherited thrombophilia, need to be considered for indefinite anticoagulant thromboprophylaxis. According to American College of Chest Physicians (Antithrombotic therapy for venous thromboembolic disease, 2008) [35], the duration of thromboprophylaxis in patients with genetic thrombophilic variations should be individualized. A common practice is to use low-molecular-weight heparin in patients with VTE, carriers of FVL or FII 20210 G>A, to cover periods of increased thrombotic risk (for example, surgery, trauma, or immobilization) [35]. Affected asymptomatic relatives of patients with inherited thrombophilia merit consideration for short-term thromboprophylaxis to cover similar periods of increased thrombotic risk.

The thrombembolic prophylaxis in subjects, carriers of platelet genetic defects, is not yet exactly defined. The most used antiplatelet drug – acetyl-salicylic acid (ASA), is a relatively ineffective drug for prophylaxis of DVT recurrence, and the somewhat sparse data suggest that it will be used only infrequently for this indication [36,37]. The most impressive result with aspirin in this regard was a 36% reduction in DVT or pulmonary embolism in 13,000 patients with hip fracture [38]. Overall, aspirin is much less effective than anticoagulants in DVT/pulmonary embolism prevention [36]. So, using of ASA to avoid recurrent venous thrombotic events should be discussed only in context of combination therapy of antiplatelet agents with low-molecular-weight heparins (LMWHs) or antiplatelet drugs with indirect anticoagulants [39].

Resistance to Antithrombotic Drugs due to PL A1/A2

The pattern for genetic resistance to antiplatelet drugs is aspirin resistance (ASAR). It was defined, that exactly about 75 to 150 mg ASA daily, is an effective antiplatelet regimen for long-term use among patients with increased risk for occlusive vascular events [36]. Those genetic differences that influence the rate and efficiency of platelet responses might also influence the ability of an inhibitor, such as ASA, attenuate or enhance platelet function.

Several studies emphasized an increased sensitivity of the PL A1/A2 (allele A2) to a variety of platelet agonists. In one of the first studies [40] of this nature, bleeding times before and after ASA ingestion were shown to be influenced by the presence or absence of allele A2 of the polymorphism: in 80 healthy men, aged 20 to 25 years, the bleeding time prior and after ASA ingestion was shorter in carriers of PL A1/A2 than in those homozygous for the allele A1. These authors concluded that carriers of the haplotype A2 appear to be more resistant to the antithrombotic action of ASA. The phenomenon of "resistance" to ASA is generally detected by nonspecific means, such as the bleeding time in the previously mentioned study, or as the occurrence of a thrombotic event in an aspirin-treated patient [41]. These findings forced to identify the patients with a reduced response to aspirin and investigate whether or not such individuals should receive an alternate antiplatelet agent, such as clopidogrel [42].

The assessment of the antiplatelet effect of clopidogrel or ASA with the recently developed method of multiple electrode platelet aggregometry (MEA) [43,44,45] have had a predictive value for thrombosis risk estimation. This method could identify the overall platelet activation and might better estimate the risk of thrombosis development. The evaluation of low response to ASA or clopidogrel reached significance because of the recently raised data [40,46] for ASA resistance, as well as the reduced inhibition of platelet activity by GP IIb/IIIa receptor specific antagonists (abciximab) [47] in presence of PL

A1/A2. Further studies are warranted to evaluate the ability of MEA to optimize the antiplatelet therapy according to genetic resistance, due to the PL A1/A2 presence.

Polymorphism A1/A2 in GP IIb/IIIa and Poor Fetal Outcome

The pathology of pregnancy loss is complex and still poorly understood. About 30 to 40% of the miscarriages cannot be explained on the basis of serological, endocrine or chromosomal investigations [48]. Therefore the association between thrombophilia and poor fetal outcome is now widely discussed [49]. Both congenital and acquired types of thrombophilia are found to be overrepresented in cases with recurrent first- and second-trimester miscarriages, intrauterine fetal death, intrauterine growth retardation (IUGR), placental abruption, or preeclampsia. As these disorders are associated with thrombotic complications of the placental vasculature, it is biologically plausible that thrombophilia is a potential mechanism contributing to the pathophysiology of these conditions [49,50,51].

On the basis of available data from case–control and retrospective cohort studies, women who have a deficiency of antithrombin, protein C, or protein S have a twofold to fivefold risk of spontaneous pregnancy loss compared to women without these defects [52,53]. Although there are inconsistencies between the studies, available data also suggests that FVL is associated with a twofold to fourfold risk of fetal loss, particularly in the second or third trimester [54]. Also, our and other recent studies showed the impact of FVL [55] and FII 20210 G>A [56] in very early fetal loss (developed before 10th week of gestation). There are conflicting data on whether other mutations (for example the methylenetetrahydrofolate reductase 677 C>T mutation is also associated with a higher risk of fetal wastage) [57,58,59].

To the best of recently knowledge, a few observations have been published on the possible association between the platelet integrin polymorphisms and recurrent pregnancy loss development. The hypothesis for the connection between PL A1/A2 of GP IIb/IIIa and increased risk of pregnancy loss has been based on the supposition that impairment of platelet function is related with disturbance in uteroplacental vascular system. Increased platelet aggregation, as a result of the presence of allele A2, could establish prothrombotic conditions and increase thrombus formation in intervillous space, leading to poor fetal outcome.

In a recent study, Ruzzi et al. [60] have showed significant difference in carrier status for PL A1/A2 when comparing 98 women with spontaneous fetal loss in first and second trimester of pregnancy, and 38 healthy volunteers (heterozygous carriers for PL A1/A2 42.9% and 18.4% respectively in patients and controls). These authors [60] heard as undivided group women with recurrent pregnancy loss (RPL) in first and second trimester. Because of that, it is hard to evaluate the significance of the impact of PL A1/A2 in different stages of pregnancy.

Other authors [61] investigated 105 women with RPL in first and second trimester of pregnancy and found a slight difference in the carrier status for PL A1/A2 between the groups of patients and controls (28.4 % and 24.2% respectively in women with RPL and health subjects). The found high prevalence of PL A1/A2 in health subjects in this paper [61] could have been due to the relatively smaller group of controls (85 individuals), and also could have been connected with the ethnicity of the investigated population (Uruguayan).

Gerhardt et al. [62] investigated the prevalence of PL A1/A2 in 104 women with RPL and in 277 controls. They have not found a possible impact of the polymorphism on the development of RPL (prevalence in patients and controls respectively 21.2% and 28.5%). The authors divided the women with RPL in two groups: women with RPL before and after 12 week of gestation. They did not include embryonic pregnancy loss (before 10 week of gestation) in the group of women with RPL in first trimester of pregnancy. Approximately 50-60% of the women in both groups had at least one successful pregnancy (condition termed as secondary infertility). The found prevalence of PL A1/A2 in the two groups is 20.6% and 21.4%, respectively in women with early and late pregnancy loss (both results not significantly differ from those of the controls).

In our pilot study [63] of 67 women with primary sterility and 96 healthy control subjects, we found a significantly higher prevalence of PL A1/A2 in women with implantation failure after assisted reproduction technology (ART) in comparison with controls (OR: 2.6, 95% CI: 1.1-6.3, p=0.033). These data suggest that the carriers of PL A1/A2 are at higher risk of implantation failure and do not have successful ART outcome.

To study the role of PL A1/A2 in the development of recurrent spontaneous abortion we investigated [64] 56 women with recurrent miscarriages before 10 week of gestation, 38 women with RPL between 10 to 20 week of gestation and 98 healthy women with at least one uncomplicated full-term pregnancy. The prevalence of PL A1/A2 in women with recurrent miscarriages in the first 10 week of gestation, adjusted for combined carriage of other thrombophilic factors (FVL or FII 20210 G>A), was not significant in comparison with controls The carriage status of PL A1/A2 in women with recurrent pregnancy loss in the period from 10 to 20 week of gestation was significantly higher as compared to controls (OR = 8.8; 95% CI: 3.5-22.6, p <0.0001).

Considering the sample size, design and limitations of presented investigations, the importance of PL A1/A2 for the increased risk of recurrent pregnancy loss, needs confirmation in further large studies, but agreement, that platelet-dependent pathomechanism is involved in recurrent pregnancy failure, could be laid down. In future, establishment of carrier status for PL A1/A2 in women undergoing IVF or/and those who have recurrent pregnancy loss, could be grounded for antiplatelet prophylaxis to prevent further pregnancy complications.

Trend for Influence the poor fetal Outcome in Presence of PL A1/A2

The benefit of aspirin in patients with thrombophilia and gestational vascular complications now remains uncertain. Although the role of thrombosis in placental insufficiency and preeclampsia is somewhat unclear, aspirin has been studied in detail in this regard and found to be moderately effective [65,66]. A broad overview of data shows that aspirin reduces preeclampsia by 15% and fetal or near-term infant deaths by 14% [67]. Another study compared the benefit of treatment with dalteparin and/or low-dose aspirin in 43 women (110 pregnancies) with severe early-onset preeclampsia or fetal growth restriction and found equivalent effects of these two drugs in gain of good fetal outcome.

Recent randomized trial [68] found a few advantages of ASA only treatment (43 patients) compared to LMWH/ASA combined prophylaxis (45 patients), in women with recurrent pregnancy loss and inherited thrombophilia or antiphospholipid autoantibodies. But the efficacy and safety of aspirin alone or in combination with low-molecular-weight heparin needs further large randomized investigations.

CONCLUSION

Recently, exponential rised genetic information established that not only the assessment of risk for individual patients, but also the design of tailored therapeutic strategies and the pharmacogenetic approach to therapy should be included in venous thrombembolism management. There is substantial data that PL A1/A2 in GP IIb/IIIa can contribute to the risk and morbidity of venous thrombotic disease and poor fetal outcome. Likewise, there is growing body of literature that A2 haplotype seems to impede the antithrombotic efficacy of ASA prophylaxis. These findings reinforce the concept that in future genetic studies, the cumulative effects of platelet glycoprotein gene polymorphism and other inherited thrombophilic factors must be evaluated concurrently.

REFERENCES

[1] Sanson B-J, Simioni P, Tormene D, et al. The incidence of venous thromboembolism in asymptomatic carriers of a deficiency of antithrombin, protein C, or protein S: a prospective cohort study. *Blood* 1999;94:3702–3706

[2] Dahlbäck B, Carlsson M, Svensson PJ. Familial thrombophilia due to a previously unrecognized mechanism characterized by poor anticoagulant response to activated protein C: prediction of a cofactor to activated protein C. *Proc Natl Acad Sci U S A*. 1993 Feb 1;90(3):1004-8

[3] Poort SR, Rosendaal FR, Reitsma PH, Bertina RM. A common genetic variation in the three untranslated regions of the prothrombin gene is associated with elevated plasma prothrombin levels and an increase in venous thrombosis. *Blood* 1996;88:3698

[4] Nieswandt B, Watson SP. Platelet-collagen interaction: is GP VI the central receptor? *Blood* 2003;102:449–461.

[5] Julius D, Huang KN, Livelli TJ, et al. The 5HT2 receptor defines a family of structurally distinct but functionally conserved serotonin receptors. *Proc Natl Acad Sci U S A* 1990;87:928–932

[6] Hynes RO. Integrins: bidirectional, allosteric signaling machines. *Cell* 2002; 110:673–687

[7] Kunicki TJ, Pidard D, Rosa JP, et al. The formation of calcium-dependent complexes of platelet membrane glycoproteins IIb and IIIa in solution as determined by crossed immunoelectrophoresis. *Blood* 1981;58:268–276

[8] Duperray A, Troesch A, Berthier R, et al. Biosynthesis and assembly of platelet GPIIb-IIIa in human megakaryocytes: evidence that assembly between pro-GPIIb and GPIIIa is

a prerequisite for expression of the complex on the cell surface. *Blood* 1989;74:1603–1611

[9] Phillips DR, Charo IF, Parise LV, et al. The platelet membrane glycoprotein IIb-IIIa complex. *Blood* 1988;71:831–843

[10]Wagner CL, Mascelli MA, Neblock DS, et al. Analysis of GP IIb/IIIa receptor number by quantification of 7E3 binding to human platelets. *Blood* 1996;88:907–914

[11]Shattil SJ, Kashiwagi H, Pampori N. Integrin signaling: the platelet paradigm. *Blood* 1998;91:2645–2657

[12]Hantgan RR. Fibrin protofibril and fibrinogen binding to ADP-stimulated platelets: evidence for a common mechanism. *Biochim Biophys Acta* 1988; 968:24–35

[13]Ruggeri ZM, Bader R, de Marco L. Glanzmann thrombasthenia: deficient binding of von Willebrand factor to thrombin-stimulated platelets. *Proc Natl Acad Sci U S A* 1982;79:6038–6041

[14]Ginsberg MH, Forsyth J, Lightsey A, et al. Reduced surface expression and binding of fibronectin by thrombin-stimulated thrombasthenic platelets. *J Clin Invest* 1983;71:619–624

[15]Bennett JS, Vilaire G. Exposure of platelet fibrinogen receptors by ADP and epinephrine. *J Clin Invest* 1979;64:1393–1401

[16]Newman PJ, Derbes RS, Aster RH. The human platelet alloantigens, Pl(A1) and Pl(A2), are associated with a leucine(33)/proline(33) amino acid polymorphism in membrane glycoprotein IIIa, and are distinguishable by DNA typing. *J. Clin. Invest.* 1989;83: 1778-1781

[17]Lim J, Lal S, Ng KC, Ng KS, Saha N, Heng CK. Variation of the platelet glycoprotein IIIa PI(A1/A2) allele frequencies in the three ethnic groups of Singapore. *Int J Cardiol.* 2003;90(2-3):269-73

[18]Carter AM, Ossei-Gerning N, Grant PJ. Platelet glycoprotein IIIa PIA polymorphism in young men with myocardial infarction. *Lancet* 1996; 348:485–486

[19]Ardissino D, Mannucci PM, Merlini PA, et al. Prothrombotic genetic risk factors in young survivors of myocardial infarction. *Blood* 1999;94:46–51

[20]Ridker PM, Hennekens CH, Schmitz C, et al. Polymorphism of platelet glycoprotein IIIa and risks of myocardial infarction,stroke, and venous thrombosis. *Lancet* 1997;349:385–388

[21]Zhu MM, Weedon J, Clark LT. Meta-analysis of the association of platelet glycoprotein IIIa PlA1/A2 polymorphism with myocardial infarction. *Am J Cardiol* 2000;86:1000–1005

[22]Di Castelnuovo A, De Gaetano G, Donati MB, et al. Platelet glycoprotein receptor IIIa polymorphism PLA1/PLA2 and coronary risk: a meta-analysis. *Thromb Haemost* 2001;85:626–633

[23]Souto J, Almasy L, Borrel 1 M, et al. Genetic susceptibility to thrombosis and its relationship to physiological risk factors: the GAIT study. Genetic analysis of idiopathic thrombophilia. *Am J Hum Genet* 2000;67(6): 1452–1459

[24]Heit JA, Phelps MA, Ward SA, et al. Familial segregation of venous thromboembolism. *J Thromb Haemost* 2004;2:731–736

[25]Kupferminc MJ. Thrombophilia and pregnancy. *Curr Pharm Des.* 2005;11(6):735-48

[26]Heit JA. Thrombophilia: Common Questions on Laboratory Assessment and Management. *Hematology Am Soc Hematol Educ Program*. 2007;2007:127-35
[27]Folsom AR, Cushman M, Heckbert SR, et al. Prospective study of fibrinolytic markers and venous thromboembolism. *J Clin Epidemiol* 2003; 56:598–603
[28]Cushman M, Folsom AR, Wang L, et al. Fragmin fragment D-dimer and the risk of future venous thrombosis. *Blood* 2003;101:1243–1248
[29]Ivanov P, Komsa-Penkova R, Kovacheva K, Ivanov Y, Stoyanova A, Ivanov I, Pavlov P, Glogovska P, Nojarov V. Impact of genetic factors on pulmonary embolism - early onset and recurrent incidences. *Lung*. 2008 Jan-Feb;186(1):27-36
[30]Renner W, Winkler M, Hoffmann C, Koppel H, Seinost G, Brodmann M, Pilger E. The PlA1/A2 polymorphism of platelet glycoprotein IIIa is not associated with deep venous thrombosis. *Int Angiol*. 2001 Jun;20(2):148-51
[31]Podciechowski L, Dabrowska K, Nowakowska D, Bielak A, Wilczynski J.Polymorphism of the glycoprotein Ia and IIIa in the group of women in childbirth does not correlate with an increased risk of developing thrombosis. *Neuro Endocrinol Lett*. 2005 Dec;26(6):789-94
[32]Hooper WC, Lally C, Austin H, Benson J, Dilley A, Wenger NK, Whitsett C, Rawlins P, Evatt BL. The relationship between polymorphisms in the endothelial cell nitric oxide synthase gene and the platelet GPIIIa gene with myocardial infarction and venous thromboembolism in African Americans. *Chest*. 1999 Oct;116(4):880-6
[33]Weiss EJ, Bray PF, Tayback M, et al. A polymorphism of a platelet glycoprotein receptor as an inherited risk factor for coronary thrombosis. *N Engl J Med* 1996; 334:1090–1094
[34]British Society for Haematology Investigation and Management of Heritable Thrombophilia. *Br J Haematol* 2001; 114(3):512–528
[35]Kearon C, Ginsberg JS, Kovacs MJ, et al. for the Extended Low-Intensity Anticoagulation for Thrombo-Embolism Investigators. Comparison of low-intensity warfarin therapy with conventional-intensity warfarin therapy for long-term prevention of recurrent venous thromboembolism. *N Engl J Med*. 2003;349:631– 639
[36]Antiplatelet Trialists' Collaboration. Collaborative overview of randomized trials of antiplatelet therapy: III Reduction in venous thrombosis and pulmonary embolism by antiplatelet prophylaxis among surgical and medial patients. *Br Med* J 1994;308:235–243
[37]Sors H, Meyer G. Place of aspirin in prophylaxis of venous thromboembolism. Lancet 2000;355:1288–1289
[38]Pulmonary Embolism Prevention (PEP) Trial Collaborative Group. Prevention of pulmonary embolism and deep vein thrombosis with low dose aspirin. Pulmonary Embolism Prevention (PEP) trial. *Lancet* 2000;355: 1295–1302
[39]Sherman DG. Prevention of venous thromboembolism, recurrent stroke, and other vascular events after acute ischemic stroke: the role of low-molecular-weight heparin and antiplatelet therapy. *J Stroke Cerebrovasc Dis*. 2006 Nov-Dec;15(6):250-9
[40]Szczeklik A, Undas A, Sanak M, et al. Relationship between bleeding time, aspirin and the PlA1/A2 polymorphism of platelet glycoprotein IIIa. *Br J Haematol* 2000;110:965–967

[41]McKee SA, Sane DC, Deliargyris EN. Aspirin resistance in cardiovascular disease: a review of prevalence, mechanisms, and clinical signif icance. *Thromb Haemost* 2002;88:711–715

[42]Patrono C. Aspirin resistance: definition, mechanisms and clinical read-outs. *J Thromb Haemost* 2003;1:1710–1713

[43]Sibbing D, Morath T, Braun S, Stegherr J, Mehilli J, Vogt W, Schömig A, Kastrati A, von Beckerath N. Clopidogrel response status assessed with Multiplate point-of-careanalysis and the incidence and timing of stent thrombosis *Thromb Haemost* 2009; 102 (article in press)

[44]Sibbing D, Braun S, Morath T, Mehilli J, Vogt W, Schömig A, Kastrati A, von Beckerath N.Platelet reactivity after clopidogrel treatment assessed with point-of-care analysis and early drug-eluting stent thrombosis. *J Am Coll Cardiol.* 2009 Mar 10;53(10):849-56

[45]Velik-Salchner C, Maier S, Innerhofer P, et al. Point-ofcare whole blood impedance aggregometry versus classicallight transmission aggregometry for detecting aspirin and clopidogrel: the results of a pilot study. *Anesth Analg.* 2008;107:1798-1806

[46]Pamukcu B, Oflaz H, Nisanci Y. The role of platelet glycoprotein IIIa polymorphism in the high prevalence of in vitro aspirin resistance in patients with intracoronary stent restenosis. *Am Heart J.* 2005 Apr;149(4):675-80

[47]Wheeler GL, Braden GA, Bray PF, Marciniak SJ, Mascelli MA, Sane DC. Reduced inhibition by abciximab in platelets with the PlA2 polymorphism. *Am Heart J.* 2002 Jan;143(1):76-82

[48]Kutteh WH, Triplett DA. Thrombophilias and recurrent pregnancy loss. *Semin Reprod Med* 2006; 24:54–66

[49]Brenner B. Thrombophi l ia and fetal loss. *Semin Thromb H*emost 2003; 29(2):165–170.

[50]Mousa HA, Alfirevicl Z. Do placental lesions reflect thrombophilia state in women with adverse pregnancy outcome? *Hum Reprod* 2000;15(8): 1830–1833

[51]Gris JC, Quere I, Monpeyroux F, et al. Case-control study of the frequency of thrombophi lic disorders in couples with late fetal loss and no thrombotic antecedent—the Nimes Obstetricians and Haematologists Study5 (NOHA5). *Thromb Haemost* 1999;81(6):891–899

[52]Alfirevic Z, Roberts D, Martlew V. How strong is the association between maternal thrombophilia and adverse pregnancy outcome? A systematic review. *Eur J Obstet Gynecol Reprod Biol* 2002;101(1):6–14

[53]Lockwood CJ. Inherited thrombophilias in pregnant patients: detection and treatment paradigm. *Obstet Gynecol* 2002; 99:333–341

[54]Preston FE, Rosendaal FR, Walker ID, et al. Increased fetal loss in women with heritable thrombophilia. *Lancet* 1996;348(9032):913–916

[55]Langhoff-Roos J, Paidas MJ, Ku DH, et al. Inherited thrombophilias and early pregnancy loss. In: Mor G, editor. *Immunology of pregnancy*. Eurekah.com 2005 and Springer Science & Business Media; 2006. pp. 229–243

[56]Ivanov PD, Komsa-Penkova RS, Konova EI, Kovacheva KS, Simeonova MN, Popov JD. Association of inherited thrombophilia with embryonic and postembryonic recurrent pregnancy loss, Blood Coagulation & Fibrinolysis. 2009 March; Vol. 20(2): 134-140

[57]Brenner B, Sarig G, Weiner Z, et al. Thrombophilic polymorphisms are common in women with fetal loss without apparent cause. *Thromb Haemost* 1999;82(1):6–9

[58]Sarig G, Younis JS, Hoffman R, et al. Thrombophilia is common in women with idiopathic pregnancy loss and is associated with late pregnancy wastage. *Fertil Steril* 2002;77(2):342–347

[59]Martinelli I, Taioli E, Cetin I, et al. Mutations in coagulation factors in women with unexplained late fetal loss. *N Engl J Med* 2000;343(14): 1015–1018

[60]Ruzzi L, Ciarafoni I, Silvestri L, Semeraro ML, Abeni D. Association of PLA2 polymorphism of the ITGB3 gene with early fetal loss. *Fertil Steril* 2005 Feb;83(2):511-2

[61]Lens D, Brugnini A, Trías N, Piquinela M, Pierri S, Diaz A, Juri M, De Lisa E, Otero A. M. Association between recurrent pregnancy loss and prothrombotic gene polymorphisms. *J Thromb and Haemostasis* 2003; 1 Suppl 1 July: abstract number P0951

[62]Gerhardt A, Scharf RE, Mikat-Drozdzynski B, Krüssel JS, Bender HG, Zotz RB. The polymorphism of platelet membrane integrin alpha2beta1 (alpha2807TT) is associated with premature onset of fetal loss. *Thromb Haemost.* 2005 Jan;93(1):124-9

[63]Ivanov P, Komsa-Penkova R, Kovacheva K, Konova E, Todorova K, Simeonova M, Ivanov I, Stoĭkov S, Popov I, Tanchev S, Bozhinova S. Risk of thrombophilia in carriers of thrombophilic genetic factors in unsuccessful assisted reproduction. *Akush Ginekol* (Sofiia). 2007;46(6):3-8 [Article in Bulgarian]

[64]Ivanov P, Komsa-Penkova R, Ivanov I, Konova E, Kovacheva K, Stoĭkov S, Popov I. High risk of recurrent spontaneous abortion during second trimester in women carriers of polymorphism A2 in platelet glycoprotein IIb/IIIa *Akush Ginekol (Sofiia)*. 2008;47(4):3-9 [Article in Bulgarian]

[65]Caritis S, Sibai B, Hauth J, et al. Low-dose aspirin to prevent pre-eclampsia in women at high risk. *N Engl J Med* 1998;338:701–705

[66]Duley L, Henderson-Smart D, Knight M, et al. Antiplatelet drugs for prevention of pre-eclampsia and its consequences:systematic review. *Br Med J* 2001;322:329–333

[67]Duley L, Henderson-Smart D, Knight M, et al. Antiplatelet drugs for prevention of pre-eclampsia and its consequences:systematic review. *Br Med J* 2001;322:329–333

[68]Laskin CA, Spitzer KA, Clark CA, Crowther MR, Ginsberg JS, Hawker GA, Kingdom JC, Barrett J, Gent M. Low molecular weight heparin and aspirin for recurrent pregnancy loss: results from the randomized, controlled HepASA Trial. *J Rheumatol.* 2009 Feb;36(2):279-87

In: Thrombosis: Causes, Treatment and Prevention ISBN 978-1-61668-696-3
Editor: D. G. Macri and L. D. Procaccini, pp. 169-178

Chapter VII

SIMULTANEOUS DETERMINATION OF FOUR ACTIVE COMPONENTS IN CHINESE MEDICINE 'TONGMAI' ORAL LIQUID BY HPLC-DAD

Xue-jia Zhai*

Huazhong University of Science and Technology, Wuhan, People's Republic of China.

ABSTRACT

An effective, accurate and reliable method for the simultaneous separation and determination of four active components (3,4-dihydroxyphenyllactic acid, protocatechuic aldehyde, puerarin and ferulaic acid) in Chinese medicine 'TONGMAI' oral liquid was developed using reverse phase high-performance liquid chromatography (RP-HPLC) coupled with diode array detection. The chromatographic separation was performed on a Lichrospher C_{18} column (250 mm × 4.6 mm i.d. with 5.0 μm particle size) with a simple linear gradient elution programme. Due to the different UV characteristic of these components, three detection wavelengths were utilized for the quantitative analysis (UV wavelength 250 nm for puerarin, 281 nm for 3,4-dihydroxyphenyllactic acid and protocatechuic aldehyde, and 323 nm for ferulaic acid, respectively). Excellent linear behaviors over the investigated concentration ranges were observed with the value of R^2 higher than 0.99 for all the analytes. The recoveries, measured at three concentration levels, varied from 98.6% to 102.0%. The validated method was successfully applied to the simultaneously determination of these active components in 'TONGMAI' oral liquid from different production batches.

Keywords: High-performance liquid chromatography; Quantitative analysis; Active components; Chinese medicine; 'TONGMAI' oral liquid; Quanlity control.

---

* Correspondence concerning this article should be addressed to: Xue-jia Zhai, Department of Pharmacy, Union Hospital, Huazhong University of Science and Technology, Wuhan, 430022, People's Republic of China. E-Mail: zhaixuejia@gmail.com.

1. Introduction

Traditional Chinese medicine (TCM) has a robust history in China and some Asian countries for thousands of years [1,2]. 'TONGMAI' oral liquid, derived from the well known TCM formal named 'TONGMAI FANG' and composed of three commonly used herbs *Radix Salviae Miltiorrhizae*, *Pueraria Radix* and *Rhizoma Chuanxiong*, has been officially listed in the Drug Standard of Ministry of Public Health of the Peoples Republic of China for a long time [3]. 'TONGMAI FANG' has therapeutic effects on coronary heart disease, hepatitis, menstrual disorders, bone loss, chronic renal failure, blood circulation diseases and other cardiovascular diseases. Accordingly, the derived botanical drug 'TONGMAI' oral liquid id used for the treatment of arteriosclerosis, cerebral thrombosis, coronary artery disease, angina pectoris and also effective for the treatment of ischemia cardiovascular diseases [4,5].

By now, some analytical methods have been developed for the quantitative analysis of the target components in the final products derived from 'TONGMAI FANG' [6-9]. However, most of the current studies concentrate on the determination of the target components from only one medicinal plant, and are lack of the quantitative information about the other two medicinal compositions. Generally, all the medicinal plants composing 'TONGMAI FANG' play the important roles for the therapeutic effects, according to the theory of TCM and thousands of years of medicinal practice. The modern pharmacology studies have also revealed that the phenolic acids from *Radix Salviae Miltiorrhizae*, isoflavones from *Pueraria Radix*, and phenolic acids from *Rhizoma Chuanxiong* are the active components contained in these herbs [10-14]. Although the methods for the determination of the target components in the medicinal plants, such as puerarin, 3,4-dihydroxyphenyllactic acid and other chemical matrices have been well reported using different analytical techniques [15-20], the method about the simultaneous separation and determination of multiple active components (including the phenolic acids in *Radix Salviae Miltiorrhizae*, isoflavones in *Pueraria Radix*, and phenolic acids in *Rhizoma Chuanxiong*) in a single running are not available in the literatures. It is in common thought that taking into account as many as possible components will provide much valuable qualitative and quantitative information for the quality control of the TCM made by multiple medicinal plants. Therefore, the development of an analytical method for the simultaneous determination of phenolic acids and isoflavones compounds is in urgent need to improve the quality control of 'TONGMAI' oral liquid and the other related botanical drugs.

In this study, a simple , accurate and reliable analytical method for the simultaneous determination of four active components including 3,4-dihydroxyphenyllactic acid, protocatechuic aldehyde, puerarin and ferulaic acid (their chemical structures were shown in Figure 1) contained in 'TONGMAI' oral liquid was developed using reverse phase high-performance liquid chromatography coupled with diode array detection. The baseline separation of the target components was achieved within 30 min using a simple gradient elution programme. To improve the sensitivity and selectivity of the separation, the detections at three different wavelengths were employed for the quantitative analysis because of the different UV characteristic of the investigated compounds. The validated method was successfully applied to the quantitative analysis of these four active components contained in 'TONGMAI' oral liquid from different production batches. As a result, the developed HPLC method is particularly suitable for the routine analysis of 'TONGMAI' oral liquid and the other related botanical drugs.

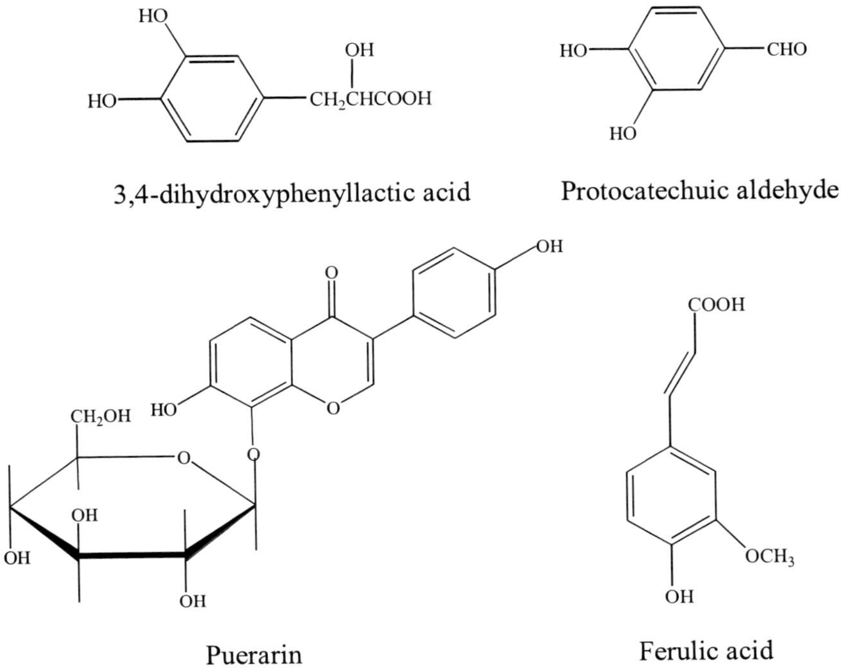

Figure 1. The chemical structures of the investigated four active components.

2. EXPERIMENTAL

2.1. Chemicals and Reagents

Botanical drug 'TONGMAI' oral liquid was supplied by a Chinese pharmaceutical manufacturer (Jinshi, Shantou, China). Standard substances including 3,4-dihydroxyphenyllactic acid, protocatechuic aldehyde, puerarin and ferulaic acid were all purchased from National Institute for the Control of Pharmaceutical and Biological Products (Beijing, China). HPLC-grade acetonitrile was obtained from Merck (Darmstadt, Germany), HPLC-grade formic acid (96%) and glacial acetic acid were purchased from Tedia (USA). All other reagents were of analytical-grade purity, at least, and used without further purified. The water used for HPLC was purified by use of a Milli-Q system (Millipore, Milford, MA, USA).

2.2. Instrumentation and Analytical Conditions

The HPLC system HP 1100 series (Agilent Technologies, Waldbronn, Germany), equipped with the ChemStation software (Agilent Technologies) and comprised a quaternary pump, an online vacuum degasser, an autosampler, a thermostated column compartment and a diode array detector, was used for the chromatographic analysis. All separations were carried out on a Lichrospher C_{18} column (250 mm × 4.6 mm i.d., 5.0 μm particle size) from Hangbang Science & Technology (Jiangsu, China). A linear gradient elution of eluents A (0.05% aqueous formic acid) and B (acetonitrile) was used to run the separation. The elution programme was well optimized and conducted as follows: an isocratic elution of 10% B with the first 10 min, a linear gradient of 10-27% B with the range of 10-20 min, and then 27-35% B with the range of 20-30 min. The solvent flow rate was 1.0 ml/min, the injection volume was 20 μl, and the column temperature was maintained at 30°C.

2.3. Standard Solution Preparation

The standard stock solutions of 3,4-dihydroxyphenyllactic acid (1.49 mg/ml), protocatechuic aldehyde (3.57 mg/ml), puerarin (3.15 mg/ml) and ferulaic acid (1.55 mg/ml) were prepared in methanol containing 1% acetic acid and stored away from light at 4°C. Working solutions of the lower concentration were prepared by appropriate dilution of the stock solutions.

2.4. Sample Solution Preparation

An accurately measured amount (1.0 ml) of the 'TONGMAI' oral liquid was diluted to 50 ml with methanol and well mixed. After the centrifugation at 10,000 rpm for 10 min, the supernatant was injected into HPLC system after filtering through a 0.45 μm syringe filter.

3. Result and Discussion

3.1. Chromatographic Separation

Due to the complex composition of the sample solution, different mobile phases (such as H_2O-CH_3OH, H_2O-CH_3CN, 0.5% (*v/v*) $HCOOH$-H_2O-CH_3CN, 1% (*v/v*) CH_3COOH-H_2O-CH_3CN, 0.2% (*v/v*) H_3PO_4-H_2O-CH_3CN) were attempted to eluted the investigated four components. At first, H_2O-CH_3CN system resulted in better separation than H_2O-CH_3OH system. Then, the acid in the mobile phase was used to reduce peak tailing of phenolic compounds. The results showed that peak shape was improved by use of 0.5% (*v/v*) HCOOH. When the effect of formic acid concentration was investigated 0.1% formic acid resulted in the best separation.

Column temperatures of 20, 25, 30, 35, and 40°C were examined. Considering the total resolution of the chromatograohic separation, the running time and solvent/reagent consumption, 30°C was chosen as the column temperature for the separation.

The typical chromatographic profiles of the negative samples and the real sample solutions were shown in Figure 2. The negative samples used here were all prepared according to the preparation technology of 'TONGMAI' oral liquid. Almost no interference was presented in the chromatographic separation, and each target peak had a good resolution. Because of the different UV characteristic of these three categories compounds investigated, the detections at three wavelengths (250 nm for puerarin, 281 nm for 3,4-dihydroxyphenyllactic acid and protocatechuic aldehyde, and 323 nm for ferulaic acid, respectively) were carried out to improve the sensitivity and selectivity for the quantitative analysis. The chromatograms of the standard solution at three different detection wavelengths were shown in Figure 3. The target components in the chromatographic profile of the real sample solution were identified by comparing the retention times and the characteristic of the UV spectra of these peaks with those presented in the chromatogram of the mixture standard solution.

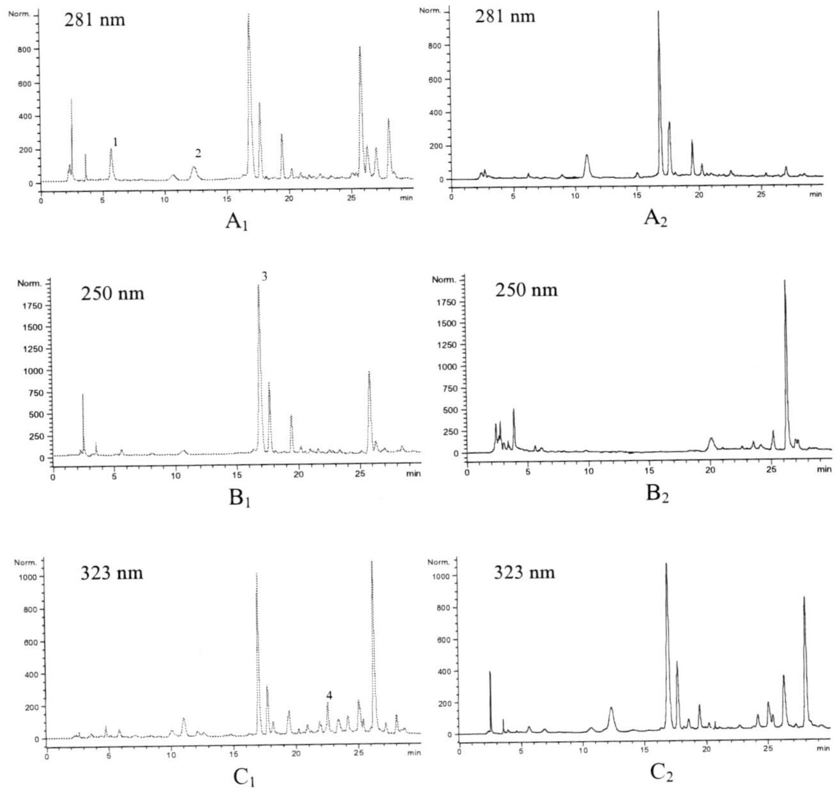

Figure 2. The typical chromatographic profiles of the real sample solutions (A_1, B_1, C_1) and the negative samples (A_2. negative sample without Radix Salviae Miltiorrhizae, B_2. negative sample without Radix Puerariae, C_2. negative sample without Rhizoma Chuanxiong). The peaks marked with 1-4 are 3,4-dihydroxyphenyllactic acid, protocatechuic aldehyde, puerarin and ferulaic acid, respectivity. The separation condition was described in Section 2.2.

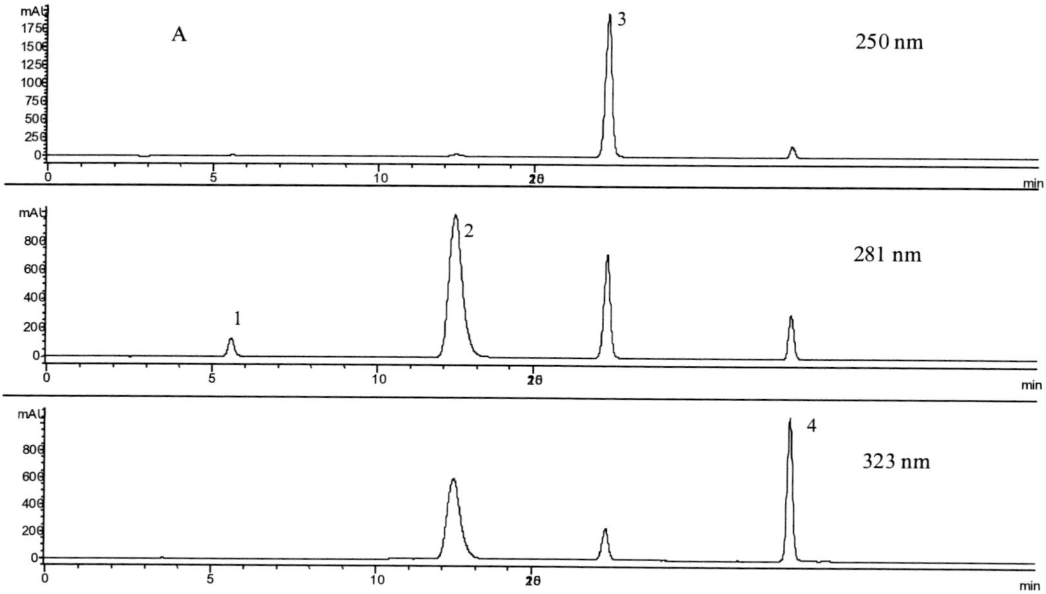

Figure 3. Representative chromatograms of the mixture standard solution at three different detection wavelengths. The peaks marked with 1-4 are 3,4-dihydroxyphenyllactic acid, protocatechuic aldehyde, puerarin and ferulaic acid, respectivity. The separation condition was described in Section 2.2.

Table 1. Results of regression analysis on calibration curves and detection limits

Components	Regression equation ($y=ax+b$)[a]	R^2	Linear range (mg/l)	LOD (mg/l)	LOQ (mg/l)
3,4-dihydroxyphenyllactic acid	$y = (12.4 \pm 0.2)\,x + (1.67 \pm 2.10)$	0.9992	0.745-149	0.745	0.373
protocatechuic aldehyde	$y = (80.6 \pm 0.3)\,x + (24.9 \pm 4.6)$	0.9998	1.79-357	1.79	0.893
puerarin	$y = (94.0 \pm 0.5)\,x + (59.8 \pm 13.1)$	0.9991	1.58-315	1.58	0.788
ferulaic acid	$y = (81.8 \pm 0.3)\,x + (17.3 \pm 3.40)$	0.9998	0.775-155	0.775	0.388

[a] y is the peak area, x the corresponding injection concentration, a is the slope and b is the intercept of the regression line, respectively. Both values of a and b are given as the form of mean ± S.D.

3.2. Linearity, Work Range and Limits of Detection

Integrated chromatographic peak areas were plotted against the corresponding concentration of the injected standard solutions to obtain the calibration curves. The injection concentration, which could be detected at the signal-to-noise ratio of 3, was considered to be the limit of detection (LOD). Limit of quantification (LOQ) was the injection concentration corresponding to the peak height with signal-to-noise ratio of 10. The regression equations were established using seven concentration levels on the consecutive 6 days. The detailed descriptions of the regression curves were presented in Table 1. The good linearity (Coefficient of determination R^2>0.99) was achieved in the investigated ranges for all the analytes. Moreover, the developed calibration curves were considerable stable because the relative standard derivation (R.S.D.) values of the slope were all less than 1.6%. Although the

R.S.D. values of intercept were a little higher, the quantification results were still stable, due to the fact that the values of intercept were not in the same order of magnitude of the corresponding values of peak area.

3.3. Intra-assay and Inter-assay Precision and Stability

The instrument precision was examined by performing the intra-day and inter-day assays by six replicate injections of the real sample solution. The intra-assay precision was performed with the interval of 4 h in 1 day, while the inter-assay precision was performed over 6 days. The precision result of the solution was presented in Table 2, and it was shown that the R.S.D. values were lower than 2.5% both for the intra-assay and inter-assay precision. For the stability test, the same real sample was analyzed within 48 h at the room temperature, and the solution was found to be rather stable (R.S.D. values of the retention time and peak area were both lower than 2.0%).

Table 2. Intra-assay and inter-assay precision of the developed method (n=6)

Components	Intra-assay[a]		Inter-assay[b]	
	Contents (± SD, mg/l)	R.S.D.(%)	Contents (± SD, mg/l)	R.S.D.(%)
3,4-dihydroxyphenyllactic acid	47.00 ± 0.70	1.49	47.69 ± 1.18	2.48
protocatechuic aldehyde	7.16 ± 0.10	1.33	7.19 ± 0.07	0.93
puerarin	77.95 ± 0.50	0.64	78.20 ± 0.49	0.62
ferulaic acid	2.55 ± 0.02	0.96	2.58 ± 0.05	2.03

[a] The sample was analyzed 6 times during one day.
[b] The sample was analyzed once a day over six consecutive days.

Table 3. Recovery test of the develop method (n=6)

Components	Content (mg/l)	Amount added (mg/l)	Amount found (mg/l)	Recovery (%)	R.S.D. (%)
	23.55	19.11	42.40	98.6	0.97
3,4-dihydroxyphenyllactic acid	23.55	23.52	46.93	99.4	0.67
	23.55	27.93	52.07	102.0	0.76
	3.55	2.86	6.39	99.6	1.47
protocatechuic aldehyde	3.55	3.57	7.09	99.4	0.82
	3.55	4.28	7.84	100.1	1.24
	39.42	31.5	71.41	101.6	1.02
puerarin	39.42	39.38	78.47	99.2	1.57
	39.42	47.25	86.78	100.3	0.55
	1.29	1.01	2.30	99.8	1.83
ferulaic acid	1.29	1.27	2.58	101.3	0.46
	1.29	1.71	2.98	98.9	0.74

3.4. Recovery Test

Because of the complexity of Chinese medicines, there has neither a standard method for the determination of these active components nor a standard reference. Therefore, recovery of the standard from samples is generally used to evaluate the accuracy of the newly developed analytical method. There different quantities (low, medium and high) of the authentic standards were added into the known real sample. The mixtures were extracted as described in Section 2.4, and was analyzed using the developed HPLC method mentioned above. Then, the quantity of each component was subsequently achieved from the corresponding calibration curves. As was shown in Table 3, the recovery of the investigated components ranged from 98.6% to 102.0%, and their R.S.D. values were all less than 1.83%. It was known from the recovery tests that the developed method manifested the reliability and accuracy for the measurement of these components.

3.5. Application

The developed HPLC method was applied to the simultaneous determination of 3,4-dihydroxyphenyllactic acid, protocatechuic aldehyde, puerarin and ferulaic acid in Chinese medicine 'TONGMAI' oral liquid from different production batches, and the results were presented in Table 4. It was shown that the content of puerarin was quite stable, because it was the target component for the quality control of 'TONGMAI' oral liquid by the current method accepted by the Drug Standard of Ministry of Public Health of the Peoples Republic of China [3]. Meanwhile, the content of some important components such as 3,4-dihydroxyphenyllactic acid, protocatechuic aldehyde and ferulaic acid were relative stable. Therefore, our work can offer a general analytical method for the quality control of 'TONGMAI' oral liquid.

Table 4. Determination of the acive components in 'TONGMAI' oral liquid by the developed HPLC method

No. of batches	Content (n=3, man ± S.D., mg/l)			
	3,4-dihydroxyphenyllactic acid	protocatechuic aldehyde	puerarin	ferulaic acid
060701	47.28 ± 0.60	7.19 ± 0.06	78.11 ± 0.43	2.54 ± 0.05
060702	47.61 ± 0.22	7.12 ± 0.04	78.12 ± 0.48	2.58 ± 0.04
060704	47.36 ± 0.15	7.18 ± 0.11	77.93 ± 0.40	2.59 ± 0.01
060706	48.02 ± 0.07	7.1 ± 0.03	78.06 ± 0.33	2.56 ± 0.06
060709	47.54 ± 0.20	7.18 ± 0.12	78.18 ± 0.42	2.54 ± 0.05
060711	47.49 ± 0.17	7.11 ± 0.04	78.07 ± 0.47	2.57 ± 0.02
060903	48.22 ± 0.43	7.21 ± 0.08	77.62 ± 0.75	2.61 ± 0.05
060907	48.57 ± 0.49	7.18 ± 0.07	77.83 ± 0.46	2.63 ± 0.04
Average	47.76	7.16	77.99	2.58
R.S.D. (%)	0.96	0.59	0.24	1.24

4. Conclusion

In the present study, an accurate and reliable analytical method for the simultaneous determination of four active components (3,4-dihydroxyphenyllactic acid, protocatechuic aldehyde, puerarin and ferulaic acid) in Chinese medicine 'TONGMAI' oral liquid was developed using reversing phasing high-performance liquid chromatograohy coupled with diode array detection, accuracy and reliability were presented in the method validation procedure. The proposed method is promising to improve the quality control of 'TONGMAI' oral liquid and other related botanical drugs.

Acknowledgments

This study was financially supported by the National Basic Research Program of China (no. 2005CB523402).

References

[1] WHO/EDM/TRM (2002) WHO traditional medicine strategy 2002-2005, Geneva.
[2] WHO/Policy perspectives on medicine (2002) Traditional medicine-growing needs and potential, Geneva.
[3] The Drug Standard of Ministry of Public Health of the Peoples Republic of China (1998) People's Health Press, Beijing, pp. 302.
[4] Wang Y, Niu F, Zhao M, Zhong B, Hao J, Yan W, Lu X, Wang W, Li Q, Lin Q, Dai Y, Zhao Y, Xiao M, Tang L, He L, Jiang X, Guo W, Wang S, Lu W (2002) *J Tradit Chin Med 22*: 87-92.
[5] Zhang J, Sun M, Zhou HY (2007) *Zhong Nan Da Xue Xue Bao Yi Xue Ban 32*: 895-898.
[6] Huang C, Fang S (2005) *Zhong Yao Cai 28*: 229-231.
[7] Yang YL (2007) *Central South Pharmacy 5*: 31-33.
[8] Tong LQ, Zhu CF, Wang GZ, Zheng YG (2004) Chin. *Tradit Herb Drugs 35*: 1248-1249.
[9] Liang YK, Xiong LH (2004) *J Jiangxi Coll Tradit Chin Med 16*: 40-41.
[10] Zhou LM, Zuo Z, Chou MSS (2005) *J Clin Pharmacol 45*: 1345-1351.
[11] Chan K, Chui SH, Wong DYL, Ha WY, Chan CL, Wong RNS (2004) *Life Sci 75*: 3157-3163.
[12] Ma ZZ, Wu QL, Lee DYW, Tracy M, Lukas SE (2005) *J Chromatogr B 823*: 108-114.
[13] Yan B, Xing DM, Ding Y, Tao JL, Du LJ (2005) *J Pharm Biomed Anal 37*: 297-301.
[14] Li YJ, Bi KS (2006) *Chem Pharm Bull 54*: 847-851.
[15] Liu AH, Li L, Xu M, Lin YH, Guo HZ, Guo DA (2006) *J Pharm Biomed Anal 41*: 48-56.
[16] Hu P, Luo GA, Zhao ZZ, Jiang ZH (2005) *Chem Pharm Bull 53*: 481-486.
[17] Zhou LM, Chow M, Zuo Z (2006) *J Pharm Biomed Anal 41*: 744-750.
[18] Wang CY, Huang HY, Kuo KL, Hsieh YZ (1998) *J Chromatogr A 802*: 225-231.

[19]Yu BS, Yan XP, Zhen GB, Rao YP (2002) *J Pharm Biomed Anal 30*: 843-849.
[20]Shi Z, Zhao M, Chang W (2005) *J Pharm Biomed Anal 37*: 469-473.

In: Thrombosis: Causes, Treatment and Prevention ISBN 978-1-61668-696-3
Editor: D. G. Macri and L. D. Procaccini, pp. 179-190

Chapter VIII

A Comprehensive Analysis of the Risk of Thrombosis after Drug Eluting Stent Implantation

Alexandre S. Quadros*[*] and Cristiano Cardoso
Universitary Foundation of Cardiology, Porto Alegre, Brazil.

Abstract

Drug eluting stents are associated with significantly lower restenosis rates than bare metal stents. However, recent reports of an increased risk of thrombosis with these devices have cast some doubt on the clinical effectiveness of this new technology. In this review, the most recent studies in this field are evaluated, showing that drug eluting stents are a safe and effective technology when adequately used in its approved indications.

Keywords: Interventional Cardiology – Drug eluting Stents – Thrombosis.

Introduction

According to Prof. Patrick Serruys, co-idealizer of bare-metal and drug-eluting coronary stents and also one of the principal researchers in the field of interventional cardiology, "stent thrombosis is an old foe, which we have pursued and fought repeatedly throughout the history of interventional cardiology"[1]. The analysis of the evolution of this technique, since

[*] Correspondence concerning this article should be addressed to: Prof. Alexandre Quadros, Unidade de Pesquisa do IC/FUC, Av. Princesa Isabel, 395 Santana 90.620-001 Porto Alegre – RS. E-mail address: editoracao-pc@cardiologia.org.br / alesq@terra.com.br. Telephone: 51-3230.3600 R.3757 / 3777 Fax: 51-3217.2035.

its appearance 20 years ago, confirms the words of Prof. Serruys and is an interesting example of how medical technology and scientific knowledge, in general, develop.

Sigwart and cols [2] initially described the procedure for the implantation of coronary stents in 1987 with the aim of treating acute occlusion after conventional angioplasty, and, at this time, it was associated to a rate of thrombosis above 20% [3]. The appearance of new models of stents and the introduction of vigorous anticoagulation schemes decreased the rate of thrombosis to between 3% and 4% in 1994 when the BENESTENT and STRESS studies were published [4,5]. The following year, Colombo and coworkers [6] proved that the risk of thrombosis could be lowered to less than 1% with proper stent apposition to the arterial wall, using high pressure, and double anti-platelet therapy (aspirin and thienopyridines). By the end of the 90s, reestenosis was the great limitation to the bare metal stents (BMS) implantation and intracoronary brachitherapy was introduced for its treatment [7]. In spite of being very effective in reducing neointimal hyperplasia and new revascularization, this therapy was unappealably condemned and progressively abandoned, since it brought back the "old enemy": thrombosis in more than 5% in treated patients [8,9].

Drug-eluting stents (DES) entered the scene in 2001 with the pioneering work of Souza and Serruys [10,11]. DES use promoted a reduction in restenosis rates not seen until then, with a reduction of relative risk up to 70% [12,13]. However, the history repeated itself and after an initial spurt of enthusiasm, that benefit seemed not free of problems. Recent studies suggest a small increase in the rates of thrombosis in the long run [14-18]. The "old enemy" was rehearsing a comeback, one more time.

Therefore, the aim of this revision is to analyze the scientific evidence that sustain the use of DES in daily clinical practice, proving that the risk of thrombosis is small and does not supersede the benefit of this technology in its indications.

Studies Suggesting Increased Risk with Drug - Eluting Stents

The eluted stents with sirolimus (SES - Cypher) and paclitaxel (PES - Taxus) were approved by the FDA in 2003 [19] and 2004 [20], respectively. The SIRIUS and TAXUS studies, clinical randomized trials with more than 1000 patients, were used as a basis for the approval of those devices. A significant reduction of angiographic restenosis, when compared to BMS, was achieved in approximately 70% with no increased risk of thrombosis [12,13].

The first study which suggested an association between drug-eluting stents and an increase in the rate of thrombosis was a case report of 4 patients published by McFadden and coworkers [21] in 2004. In that study, DES thrombosis was observed over a year after stent implantation, and all patients shared thienopyridine discontinuation a few days before. A year later, the same group of researchers published an analysis of 2000 patients followed up to 26 months, and the incidence of late thrombosis was 0.35%. Surprisingly, DES thrombosis happened also in patients under dual anti-platelet therapy (aspirin and clopidogrel) [22]. At that time, experimental studies with animals demonstrated the lack of endothelization and adverse vascular reactions in those treated with drug-eluting stents, providing a physiopatologic basics for late thrombosis [23].

The BASKET study [24,25] was designed to assess the cost-effectiveness of DES, including a pre-specified subgroup analysis for the assessment of clinical events after thienopyridine discontinuation. Considering mortality and myocardial infarction (MI), there was no difference between DES and BMS during the clinical follow up (18 months). Additionally, the significant benefit in reduction of revascularization was maintained in the follow up. Meanwhile, in the period after discontinuation of clopidrogel (between the 7th and 18th month), MACE occurred in 4.9% of the patients in the DES group versus 1.3% in BMS. The rates of late thrombosis were more frequent in DES than in BMS (2.6% vs. 1.3%).

The criticism in relation to the safety of DES was increased after the presentation of two meta-analysis in the European Society of Cardiology (ESC) / World Congress of Cardiology (WCC), in September 2006 in Barcelona. In the meta-analysis reported by Camenzind and coworkers [26], increased rates of death or MI, presumably due to thrombosis of the stents, were reported in the late follow up with SES (relative risk 1.60; IC 95% 1.06-2.43) but not with PES (relative risk 1.15; IC 95%, 0.79 to 1.69). In Nordmann's meta-analysis [27], with 4 randomized clinical trials, the use of SES was not associated with significant difference in cardiac mortality in 3 years, but non-cardiac mortality was significantly increased when compared to BMS (rate of chance 2.04; IC 95% 1.00 to 4.15). Although these findings still do not have a clear explanation, it has been suggested that either systemic effects of the drug applied to the stents or methodological problems of the studies could have played a role [28].

Recently, a large register with approximately 20.000 patients and clinical follow up of 3 years, sponsored by the Swedish government, also revealed an increased mortality with DES [29]. In that study, DES were associated with 0.5% more risk of death after 6 months of follow up, and the increase in the composite outcome of death/MI was 0.5-1.0% per year. These authors suggest that the safety of these devices must be assessed in long term clinical trials with a large number of patients.

Studies Demonstrating the Safety of Drug Eluting Stents

The great concern generated by the results of the aforementioned studies, made the American FDA, maximum body for the regulation of the use of drugs and medical devices in the United States, to summon a panel of the experts and scientists in this field to analyze all the data [30,31]. In that document, the safety analysis of DES was performed taking into account if the clinical and angiographic indication of the device were in accordance either the specifications of the label (*on-label* indications) (Table 1) or other indications different to those (*off-label* indications) [19,20]. The main conclusions of that meeting, which have marked out the use of these devices in many centers worldwide, are the following:

On - Label Indications

Both DES approved for use in the United States are associated with a small increase of thrombosis when compared to BMS, which becomes apparent 1 year after the procedure.

However, based upon the available data, this increased risk of thrombosis was not associated with an increase in death or MI, when compared to BMS. These findings might be due to an insufficient number of patients in the available studies, or to the fact that the increase of deaths and MI was compensated by the reduction of in-stent restenosis and additional revascularization procedures.

When compared to BMS, DES are not associated with increased general mortality.

The concern regarding thrombosis do not overcome the benefits of the DES when implanted within the approved limits for their use.

Larger and longer follow up studies are necessary, with uniform definitions of the stent thrombosis and with more attention to the adherence to the dual anti-platelet therapy.

Table 1. On label Indications of Drug – eluting stents

CYPHER Sirolimus-eluting Coronary Stent De-novo lesions Length < 30 mm Native coronary arteries Diameter of the vessel > 2.5 mm and <3.5mm
TAXUS Express Paclitaxel – eluting Coronary Stent De-novo lesions Length < 28 mm Native coronary arteries Diameter of the vessel > 2.5 mm and <3.75mm

Off-Label Indications

In complex patients, it is expected an increased risk of adverse events with any device. The Panel agreed that the *off-label* use of DES is associated with higher risk of thrombosis, death or MI than the *on-label* use.

The available data is insufficient to determine if the higher event risk is equal or not between the two current approved platforms.

Data about the *off-label* use are limited and additional studies are necessary to determine which is the optimal treatment for complex patients. Until more data are available, it must be clear that, when DES is used *off-label*, the clinical outcomes may not be the same as those verified in clinical trials conducted to obtain their approval.

Many of the FDA Panel conclusions were obtained originated from four important studies that were published in a recent issue of the *New England Journal of Medicine*.

Kastrati performed a meta-analysis of the individual data of 4958 patients included in 14 randomized clinical trials which compare SES with BMS [32]. The global death risk (hazard ratio, 1.03; IC 95%, 0.80 – 1.30) and the combined death and heart attack risk (hazard ratio, 0.97; IC 95%, 0.81 – 1.16) were not significantly different between the groups. A significant reduction was observed in the combined end-point of death, MI or re-intervention (hazard ratio, 0.43; IC 95%, 0.34 – 0.54) associated to SES. There was no difference in the global risk of thrombosis with SES versus BMS (hazard ratio, 1.09; IC 95%, 0.64 to 1.86), although a discreet increase in thrombosis risk was observed after the first year.

Spaulding and coworkers [33] performed a joint analysis of 1748 patients in 4 clinical trials, comparing SES with BMS, the data being analyzed, patient by patient, by independent statisticians in two independent academic institutions. This analysis concluded that there was not a significant statistical difference in MI, death or thrombosis rates.

Stone and cols [34] performed a joint analysis of the data of 4 clinical trials with 1748 patients who received SES or BMS, and of 5 clinical trials that included 3513 patients who received PES or BMS. The thrombosis rate in 4 years was 1.2% in the patients who received SES versus 0.6% in those patients treated with BMS ($P = 0.20$), and 1.3% in the patients treated with PES 0.9% in BMS ($P = 0.30$). Yet, after 1 year, 5 thrombosis episodes were observed in patients treated with SES versus none in the BMS group ($P = 0.025$), and nine episodes in PES versus 2 patients with BMS ($P = 0.028$). The 4-year target vessel revascularization (TVR) rates were markedly reduced in the patients who received DES, and death and MI rates were not different in both groups. The main conclusion of this study was that that the incidence of stent thrombosis after one year was higher in DES, and these devices were associated to a marked reduction in the necessity of new revascularization and similar death and MI rates.

Mauri and cols [35] assessed the definitions of thrombosis used in the principal clinical trials, due to restrictive or non uniform criteria which were used in these studies. A hierarchical classification of thrombosis developed by the *Academic Research Consortium* [36] *(ARC)* was applied in studies with 878 patients treated with SES and 1400 patients treated with PES and 2267 treated with BMS, combining 4 year outcomes and awarded by independent clinical event committees. The definitions of stent thrombosis are described in Table 2. The conclusions of this analysis did not show statistically different incidence between DES and BMS, although the power to detect such differences had been small.

Table 2. Stent thrombosis definitions*

Period of time Acute: 0 – 24 hours Subacute: > 24 hours – 30 days Late: > 30 days – 1 year Very late: > 1 year
Evidence of thrombosis Definitive: confirmation through angiography or necropsy Probable: Any death during the first months after the implantation or IAM in the territory related to the target vessel Possible: Any unexplained death after 30 days after the implantation

* Defined by American Research Consortium [36].

These studies were also commented on by an editorial and two clinical perspectives in the same edition of a journal, and their analysis, as a whole, reinforce the notion that, when used according to their indications, DES are safe and are associated to significant clinical benefit [37-39].

Recently, two important registries were published, with a large number of patients, which also showed the safety of DES in daily clinical practice. Jensen and cols relate the experience of the Danish register, a study with a design and importance very similar to the Swedish register mentioned in the previous section [40]. The data of all the percutaneous procedures performed in the West of Denmark from January 2002 until June 2005, were prospectively collected in the Western Denmark Heart Registry. Twelve thousand, three hundred and ninety five consecutive patients were admitted, 3,548 with DES and 8,847 with BMS, with a 15 month follow up period. Defined, probable or possible thrombosis was found in 2.15% of patients treated with BMS and 1.80% in those treated with DES. The risk of a defined thrombosis, according to the definition of the ARC, was similar in both groups (0.65% vs 0.61%), but the incidence of thrombosis within 12 and 15 months after implantation was slightly higher in those patients with DES. The conclusion of the study is that the small risk of late thrombosis should not supersede the benefits of DES.

Marzochi and cols [41] reported data regarding 10,629 patients, 3064 treated with DES and 7565 treated with BMS, in a prospective registry of 13 hospitals in Italy with a 2 year follow up. The rate of major cardiovascular events was significantly lower in the DES group (17.8% vs 21%; $p<0.003$), and stent thrombosis confirmed through angiography was 1.0% in DES and 0.6% in BMS ($p=0.09$). There were no differences regarding death or MI rates in both groups, and the patients treated with DES presented a significant reduction in TVR ($p<0.00001$). The authors' conclusion was that, in this large representative population of patients of the "real world", the beneficial effects of DES in reducing the need of a new revascularization extended itself for 2 years –with no evidence of an adverse risk profile.

A collaborative network meta-analysis recently brought new evidences regarding the safety of DES. In this study, a network group led by Stettler performed an important analysis including 38 randomized trials (18,023 patients) comparing either BMS versus DES or SES and PES in a head-head comparison. With a follow up of up to 4 years, there was no difference in mortality among the three groups. Also, definite stent thrombosis by ARC definition was similar and all groups. These authors concluded that stent thrombosis were not different between BMS and DES, although SES was associated with lower rates of TVR.

RAVEL [42] trial was the first of several randomized trials comparison DES and BMS for prevention of restenosis and neointimal hyperplasia. In that study, 238 patients, with de novo coronary stenosis which could be treated with a single 18mm stent length in vessels between 2.5 to 3.5mm of diameter, were enrolled and randomized to receive SES or BMS. Currently this is the study with the longest follow up, and those results have already been published43. About 92.5% of patients in SES and 89.1% in BMS group were followed up for five years. Patients treated with SES presented improved 5-year survival free of TVR (89.7% in SES vs 74% in BMS, $p<0.001$) and lower MACE rates (25.8% in SES vs 35.2% in BMS, $p=0.03$) than those treated with BMS. Stent thrombosis rates were similar in both groups (3.3% in SES vs 6.8% BMS, p=NS). The authors conclude that, although not powered to address specific questions about late thrombosis, RAVEL is the trial with the longest follow up and it shows safe results using SES.

Possible Mechanisms and Clinical Predictors for Late Thrombosis

According to the ARC definition, late thrombosis and very late thrombosis are defined as stent thrombosis later than 30 days and 1 year, respectively. Since its first report, we still try to understand the mechanisms to prevent this process. It is likely that stent thrombosis is a multifactorial entity, and not only one but also many components can be involved. Pre clinical studies have clearly demonstrated that there is a lack of endothelization in the struts of DES after stent implantation when compared to BMS [44-46]. Similar finds were also described regarding the pathology of DES in humans [23,47], and the concept that improper stent endothelialization plays an important role in late stent thrombosis is generally accepted. Uncovered stent struts may be vulnerable to platelet activation and thrombus formation, and this is potentially aggravated by thienopyridine discontinuation. Additional factors, such as premature withdrawal of dual anti-platelet therapy, stent malapposition or incomplete apposition and *off label* indications possibly contribute to this phenomenon.

Clinical and angiographic predictors of stent thrombosis have been identified. Premature discontinuation of thienopyridine seems to be the most important predictor [48], as cited in a shared science advisory from the several societies [49]. Other identified predictors are stent length, brachytherapy, final pressure at stent implantation, reference vessel diameter, excentric [48] lesion and low left ventricle ejection fraction. In the EVASTENT matched-cohort registry [50], risk factors for stent thrombosis after implantation of SES were analyzed in diabetic and nondiabetic patients. In this analysis, diabetic population presented significant higher incidence of stent thrombosis (3.2% versus 1.7, $p=0.03$). In multivariated analysis, in addition to the interruption of antithrombotic treatment, independent stent thrombosis predictors were previous stroke, renal failure, lower ejection fraction, calcified lesion, length stented, and insulin-requiring diabetes. Okabe and coworker [51] led a coronary intravascular ultrasound analysis in 13 patients who experienced DES thrombosis and compared to controls. At the time of stent thrombosis, 38% of patients were not taking dual anti-platelet therapy. Additionally, a small post-procedural stent area was also identified as a predictor of thrombosis.

Open Questions Regarding the Safety of Drug Eluting Stents

The questions which remain open are related to aspects of the *on-label* and *off-label* indications and the duration of the thienopyridines.

Regarding the *on-label* indications, it is still unclear why the slight increase in stent thrombosis rates in late follow up does not translate into an increase in MI or mortality rates. The most acceptable explanation is that the reduction in restenosis, provided by DES, compensated for the small increase of thrombosis [52-54].

It is known that *off-label* indications are rather frequent and associated with an increased risk of thrombosis either in DES or with BMS [55,56]. However, *off-label* indications are quite a heterogeneous group of clinical and angiographic conditions, and recent evidence suggests that the risk of DES is not the same in all those situations. For instance, Vermeesch and cols recently reported an increase in death rate with DES in a small randomized clinical trial in patients treated with vein grafts, one of the *off-label* indications [57]. On the other hand, Valgimigli et al [58] demonstrated the safety of DES in those who had suffered a ST elevation MI (another off-label indication), with no increase of thrombosis rates even after stopping the thienopyridine. Therefore, we must evolve towards a more accurate characterization of what is an *off-label* indication, because it seems to be a very heterogenous group of patients with quite different safety profiles.

The FDA panel and most specialists recommend the use of clopidogrel for at least one year after the implant of a DES, taking into account that continuous use must always be considered among those without side effects [30,31,59]. The question of adherence to clopidogrel has been much valorized [49]. A recent study with 500 ST elevation MI patients submitted to implantation of DES showed that 13% of the subjects discontinued the drug during the first month, and this group had a significant increase of the mortality rate within one year. Patients with a planned non-cardiac surgery in the short term represent an additional problem. The current recommendation is to postpone the surgery for at least one year or to maintain the anti-platelet during the surgical period in those at high risk [60]. The resistance to clopidogrel is also another open question and, in spite of its frequency and treatment are not well established, it is one more predictor of stent thrombosis [61].

Conclusions

Drug-eluting stents have become the most successful strategy for the prevention of restenosis after percutaneous coronary interventions, which is an important clinical problem due to its association with recurrent events and worsening of quality of life [52-54,62]. The initial optimism led to the idea that restenosis would be completely abolished, a fact which has not been corroborated by recent evidences.

However, DES are still a relatively young technology, but gifted with a great potential for improvement. Recent skepticism about the long-term safety of these devices is not justified by the available evidence, which have demonstrated that the rates of thrombosis are small and that death and MI rates are very similar in several clinical and angiographic substrata.

Exaggerated optimism and skepticism are equally deleterious for good medical practice, which must rest on good sense and judicious assessment, aiming at what is best for the patient. As physicians, we must resist the temptation, so common in the lay press, in prematurely proclaiming both success and failure of any given medical treatment. Only in this way we will be able to win the battle over our old common enemy, stent thrombosis, having our patients as winners.

REFERENCES

[1] Serruys PW, Daemen J. Are drug-eluting stents associated with a higher rate of late thrombosis than bare metal stents? Late stent thrombosis: a nuisance in both bare metal and drug-eluting stents. *Circulation.* Mar 20 2007; 115(11):1433-1439; discussion 1439.

[2] Sigwart U, Puel J, Mirkovitch V, et al. Intravascular stents to prevent occlusion and restenosis after transluminal angioplasty. *N Engl J Med.* Mar 19 1987;316(12):701-706.

[3] Serruys PW, Strauss BH, Beatt KJ, et al. Angiographic follow-up after placement of a self-expanding coronary-artery stent. *N Engl J Med.* Jan 3 1991; 324(1):13-17.

[4] Serruys PW, de Jaegere P, Kiemeneij F, et al. A comparison of balloon-expandable-stent implantation with balloon angioplasty in patients with coronary artery disease. Benestent Study Group. *N Engl J Med.* Aug 25 1994; 331(8):489-495.

[5] Fischman DL, Leon MB, Baim DS, et al. A randomized comparison of coronary-stent placement and balloon angioplasty in the treatment of coronary artery disease. Stent Restenosis Study Investigators. *N Engl J Med.* Aug 25 1994;331(8):496-501.

[6] Colombo A, Hall P, Nakamura S, et al. Intracoronary stenting without anticoagulation accomplished with intravascular ultrasound guidance. *Circulation.* Mar 15 1995;91(6):1676-1688.

[7] Teirstein PS, Massullo V, Jani S, et al. Catheter-based radiotherapy to inhibit restenosis after coronary stenting. *N Engl J Med.* Jun 12 1997;336(24):1697-1703.

[8] Waksman R. Late thrombosis after radiation. Sitting on a time bomb. *Circulation.* Aug 24 1999;100(8):780-782.

[9] Costa MA, Sabate M, van der Giessen WJ, et al. Late coronary occlusion after intracoronary brachytherapy. *Circulation.* Aug 24 1999;100(8):789-792.

[10] Sousa JE, Costa MA, Abizaid A, et al. Lack of neointimal proliferation after implantation of sirolimus-coated stents in human coronary arteries: a quantitative coronary angiography and three-dimensional intravascular ultrasound study. *Circulation.* Jan 16 2001;103(2):192-195.

[11] Sousa JE, Costa MA, Abizaid AC, et al. Sustained suppression of neointimal proliferation by sirolimus-eluting stents: one-year angiographic and intravascular ultrasound follow-up. *Circulation.* Oct 23 2001;104(17):2007-2011.

[12] Stone GW, Ellis SG, Cox DA, et al. A polymer-based, paclitaxel-eluting stent in patients with coronary artery disease. *N Engl J Med.* Jan 15 2004;350(3):221-231.

[13] Moses JW, Leon MB, Popma JJ, et al. Sirolimus-eluting stents versus standard stents in patients with stenosis in a native coronary artery. *N Engl J Med.* Oct 2 2003;349(14):1315-1323.

[14] Luscher TF, Steffel J, Eberli FR, et al. Drug-eluting stent and coronary thrombosis: biological mechanisms and clinical implications. *Circulation.* Feb 27 2007;115(8): 1051-1058.

[15] Kuchulakanti PK, Chu WW, Torguson R, et al. Correlates and long-term outcomes of angiographically proven stent thrombosis with sirolimus- and paclitaxel-eluting stents. *Circulation.* Feb 28 2006;113(8):1108-1113.

[16]Spertus JA, Kettelkamp R, Vance C, et al. Prevalence, predictors, and outcomes of premature discontinuation of thienopyridine therapy after drug-eluting stent placement: results from the PREMIER registry. *Circulation.* Jun 20 2006;113(24):2803-2809.

[17]Iakovou I, Schmidt T, Bonizzoni E, et al. Incidence, predictors, and outcome of thrombosis after successful implantation of drug-eluting stents. *Jama.* May 4 2005;293(17):2126-2130.

[18]Daemen J, Wenaweser P, Tsuchida K, et al. Early and late coronary stent thrombosis of sirolimus-eluting and paclitaxel-eluting stents in routine clinical practice: data from a large two-institutional cohort study. *Lancet.* Feb 24 2007;369(9562):667-678.

[19]Cypher™ Sirolimus-eluting coronary stent on RAPTOR™ over-the-wire delivery system and Cypher™ sirolimus-eluting coronary stent RAPTORAIL rapid exchange delivery system. Available at: http://www.fda.gov/cdrh/pdf2/p020026c.pdf. Accessed 16 september 2007.

[20]TAXUS™ EXPRESS 2™ paclitaxel-eluting coronary stent system. Available at: http://www.fda.gov/cdrh/pdf3/P030025c.pdf. Accessed 16 september, 2007.

[21]McFadden EP, Stabile E, Regar E, et al. Late thrombosis in drug-eluting coronary stents after discontinuation of antiplatelet therapy. *Lancet.* Oct 23-29 2004;364(9444):1519-1521.

[22]Ong AT, McFadden EP, Regar E, et al. Late angiographic stent thrombosis (LAST) events with drug-eluting stents. *J Am Coll Cardiol.* Jun 21 2005;45(12):2088-2092.

[23]Joner M, Finn AV, Farb A, et al. Pathology of drug-eluting stents in humans: delayed healing and late thrombotic risk. *J Am Coll Cardiol.* Jul 4 2006;48(1):193-202.

[24]Kaiser C, Brunner-La Rocca HP, Buser PT, et al. Incremental cost-effectiveness of drug-eluting stents compared with a third-generation bare-metal stent in a real-world setting: randomised Basel Stent Kosten Effektivitats Trial (BASKET). *Lancet.* Sep 10-16 2005;366(9489):921-929.

[25]Pfisterer M, Brunner-La Rocca HP, Buser PT, et al. Late clinical events after clopidogrel discontinuation may limit the benefit of drug-eluting stents: an observational study of drug-eluting versus bare-metal stents. *J Am Coll Cardiol.* Dec 19 2006;48(12):2584-2591.

[26]Camenzind E, Steg PG, Wijns W. Stent thrombosis late after implantation of first-generation drug-eluting stents: a cause for concern. *Circulation.* Mar 20 2007;115(11):1440-1455; discussion 1455.

[27]Nordmann AJ, Briel M, Bucher HC. Mortality in randomized controlled trials comparing drug-eluting vs. bare metal stents in coronary artery disease: a meta-analysis. *Eur Heart J.* Dec 2006;27(23):2784-2814.

[28]Kaul S, Shah PK, Diamond GA. As time goes by: current status and future directions in the controversy over stenting. *J Am Coll Cardiol.* Jul 10 2007;50(2):128-137.

[29]Lagerqvist B, James SK, Stenestrand U, et al. Long-term outcomes with drug-eluting stents versus bare-metal stents in Sweden. *N Engl J Med.* Mar 8 2007;356(10):1009-1019.

[30]Laskey WK, Yancy CW, Maisel WH. Thrombosis in coronary drug-eluting stents: report from the meeting of the Circulatory System Medical Devices Advisory Panel of the Food

and Drug Administration Center for Devices and Radiologic Health, December 7-8, 2006. *Circulation.* May 1 2007;115(17):2352-2357.

[31]Update to FDA statement on coronary drug-eluting stents. Accessed 16 september, 2007.

[32]Kastrati A, Mehilli J, Pache J, et al. Analysis of 14 trials comparing sirolimus-eluting stents with bare-metal stents. *N Engl J Med.* Mar 8 2007;356(10):1030-1039.

[33]Spaulding C, Daemen J, Boersma E, et al. A pooled analysis of data comparing sirolimus-eluting stents with bare-metal stents. *N Engl J Med.* Mar 8 2007;356(10): 989-997.

[34]Stone GW, Moses JW, Ellis SG, et al. Safety and efficacy of sirolimus- and paclitaxel-eluting coronary stents. *N Engl J Med.* Mar 8 2007;356(10):998-1008.

[35]Mauri L, Hsieh WH, Massaro JM, et al. Stent thrombosis in randomized clinical trials of drug-eluting stents. *N Engl J Med.* Mar 8 2007;356(10):1020-1029.

[36]Cutlip DE, Windecker S, Mehran R, et al. Clinical end points in coronary stent trials: a case for standardized definitions. *Circulation.* May 1 2007;115(17):2344-2351.

[37]Maisel WH. Unanswered questions--drug-eluting stents and the risk of late thrombosis. *N Engl J Med.* Mar 8 2007;356(10):981-984.

[38]Farb A, Boam AB. Stent thrombosis redux--the FDA perspective. *N Engl J Med.* Mar 8 2007;356(10):984-987.

[39]Shuchman M. Debating the risks of drug-eluting stents. *N Engl J Med.* Jan 25 2007;356(4):325-328.

[40]Jensen LO, Maeng M, Kaltoft A, et al. Stent thrombosis, myocardial infarction, and death after drug-eluting and bare-metal stent coronary interventions. *J Am Coll Cardiol.* Jul 31 2007;50(5):463-470.

[41]Marzocchi A, Saia F, Piovaccari G, et al. Long-term safety and efficacy of drug-eluting stents: two-year results of the REAL (REgistro AngiopLastiche dell'Emilia Romagna) multicenter registry. *Circulation.* Jun 26 2007;115(25):3181-3188.

[42]Morice MC, Serruys PW, Sousa JE, et al. A randomized comparison of a sirolimus-eluting stent with a standard stent for coronary revascularization. *N Engl J Med.* Jun 6 2002;346(23):1773-1780.

[43]Morice MC, Serruys PW, Barragan P, et al. Long-term Clinical Outcomes with Sirolimus-Eluting Coronary Stents. *J Am Coll Cardiol.* 2007;50:1299-12304.

[44]Farb A, Heller PF, Shroff S, et al. Pathological analysis of local delivery of paclitaxel via a polymer-coated stent. *Circulation.* Jul 24 2001;104(4):473-479.

[45]Finn AV, Kolodgie FD, Harnek J, et al. Differential response of delayed healing and persistent inflammation at sites of overlapping sirolimus- or paclitaxel-eluting stents. *Circulation.* Jul 12 2005;112(2):270-278.

[46]Suzuki T, Kopia G, Hayashi S, et al. Stent-based delivery of sirolimus reduces neointimal formation in a porcine coronary model. *Circulation.* Sep 4 2001;104(10):1188-1193.

[47]van Beusekom HM, Saia F, Zindler JD, et al. Drug-eluting stents show delayed healing: paclitaxel more pronounced than sirolimus. *Eur Heart J.* Apr 2007;28(8):974-979.

[48]Airoldi F, Colombo A, Morici N, et al. Incidence and predictors of drug-eluting stent thrombosis during and after discontinuation of thienopyridine treatment. *Circulation.* Aug 14 2007;116(7):745-754.

[49]Grines CL, Bonow RO, Casey DE, Jr., et al. Prevention of premature discontinuation of dual antiplatelet therapy in patients with coronary artery stents: a science advisory from the American Heart Association, American College of Cardiology, Society for Cardiovascular Angiography and Interventions, American College of Surgeons, and American Dental Association, with representation from the American College of Physicians. *Circulation.* Feb 13 2007;115(6):813-818.

[50]Machecourt J, Danchin N, Lablanche JM, et al. Risk factors for stent thrombosis after implantation of sirolimus-eluting stents in diabetic and nondiabetic patients: the EVASTENT Matched-Cohort Registry. *J Am Coll Cardiol.* Aug 7 2007;50(6):501-508.

[51]Okabe T, Mintz GS, Buch AN, et al. Intravascular ultrasound parameters associated with stent thrombosis after drug-eluting stent deployment. *Am J Cardiol.* Aug 15 2007;100(4):615-620.

[52]Nayak AK, Kawamura A, Nesto RW, et al. Myocardial infarction as a presentation of clinical in-stent restenosis. *Circ J.* Aug 2006;70(8):1026-1029.

[53]Chen MS, John JM, Chew DP, et al. Bare metal stent restenosis is not a benign clinical entity. *Am Heart J.* Jun 2006;151(6):1260-1264.

[54]Al Suwaidi J, Holmes DR, Jr., Salam AM, et al. Impact of coronary artery stents on mortality and nonfatal myocardial infarction: meta-analysis of randomized trials comparing a strategy of routine stenting with that of balloon angioplasty. *Am Heart J.* May 2004;147(5):815-822.

[55]Beohar N, Davidson CJ, Kip KE, et al. Outcomes and complications associated with off-label and untested use of drug-eluting stents. *Jama.* May 9 2007;297(18):1992-2000.

[56]Win HK, Caldera AE, Maresh K, et al. Clinical outcomes and stent thrombosis following off-label use of drug-eluting stents. *Jama.* May 9 2007;297(18):2001-2009.

[57]Vermeersch P, Agostoni P, Verheye S, et al. Increased late mortality after sirolimus-eluting stents versus bare-metal stents in diseased saphenous vein grafts: results from the randomized DELAYED RRISC Trial. *J Am Coll Cardiol.* Jul 17 2007;50(3):261-267.

[58]Valgimigli M, Campo G, Arcozzi C, et al. Two-year clinical follow-up after sirolimus-eluting versus bare-metal stent implantation assisted by systematic glycoprotein IIb/IIIa Inhibitor Infusion in patients with myocardial infarction: results from the STRATEGY study. *J Am Coll Cardiol.* Jul 10 2007;50(2):138-145.

[59]Holmes DR, Jr., Kereiakes DJ, Laskey WK, et al. Thrombosis and drug-eluting stents: an objective appraisal. *J Am Coll Cardiol.* Jul 10 2007;50(2):109-118.

[60]Schouten O, van Domburg RT, Bax JJ, et al. Noncardiac surgery after coronary stenting: early surgery and interruption of antiplatelet therapy are associated with an increase in major adverse cardiac events. *J Am Coll Cardiol.* Jan 2 2007;49(1):122-124.

[61]Buonamici P, Marcucci R, Migliorini A, et al. Impact of platelet reactivity after clopidogrel administration on drug-eluting stent thrombosis. *J Am Coll Cardiol.* Jun 19 2007;49(24):2312-2317.

[62]Rinfret S, Grines CL, Cosgrove RS, et al. Quality of life after balloon angioplasty or stenting for acute myocardial infarction. One-year results from the Stent-PAMI trial. *J Am Coll Cardiol.* Nov 15 2001;38(6):1614-1621.

In: Thrombosis: Causes, Treatment and Prevention ISBN 978-1-61668-696-3
Editor: D. G. Macri and L. D. Procaccini, pp. 191-206

Chapter IX

ADVANCES IN ANTIPLATELET THERAPY TO PREVENT STENT THROMBOSIS

A. Schäfer[1,*]*, J. Bauersachs*[1] *and M. Eigenthaler*[2]
[1]Medizinische Klinik und Poliklinik I, Würzburg, Germany;
[2]Julius-Maximilians-Universität Würzburg, Germany.

ABSTRACT

The integral role of pathologic platelet activation for progression of atherosclerosis and acute clinical events such as myocardial infarction and stroke has been recognized in the last decades. Consequently, treatment with oral antiplatelet agents — particularly acetylsalicylic acid (ASA) and the thienopyridines clopidogrel and ticlopidine— constitutes a cornerstone in the therapy of vascular diseases. Coronary angioplasty and stent implantation furthermore dramatically improved the therapy of coronary artery disease and especially the treatment of acute myocardial infarction. Sustained success with regard to prevention of reocclusion was achieved when dual antiplatelet therapy had been introduced. This combination of ASA and clopidogrel reduced the risk of stent thrombosis to ~1% following elective stenting in stable coronary artery disease. However, targeting more complex lesions or performing the intervention in states of increased platelet reactivity such as in acute coronary syndromes or in diabetic patients is still associated with an increased risk of stent thrombosis. Additionally, incomplete ADP-receptor inhibition by thienopyridine treatment is associated with increased cardiovascular events and mortality after coronary intervention.

This review displays the underlying pathophysiology of stent thrombosis and its pharmacological prevention by dual antiplatelet therapy. Furthermore, it discusses the assessment of antiplatelet therapy by different analytical methods and the phenomenon of clopidogrel non-responsiveness. The last part highlights current strategies in improving the efficacy of clopidogrel treatment as well as the next generation anti-platelet

* Correspondence concerning this article should be addressed to: Andreas Schäfer, MD, Medizinische Klinik und Poliklinik I, Universitätsklinikum Würzburg, Josef-Schneider-Str. 2, 97080 Würzburg, Germany. E-mail address: a.schaefer@medizin.uni-wuerzburg.de. Tel. +49-931-201-1. Tel. +49-931-201-36131.

substances such as novel thienopyridines and non-thienopyridine $P2Y_{12}$-receptor blocking agents.

Keywords: ADP, Platelet activation, diabetes, P2Y12 receptor, clopidogrel.

INTRODUCTION

Platelet activation is a major component in the pathogenesis of coronary thrombosis, myocardial infarction and cerebral ischemia. Therefore, anti-platelet therapy has become a cornerstone in the therapy of cardiovascular diseases including ischemic heart disease and stroke. At the site of vascular lesions, adhesion and aggregation of platelets is the initial step in the pathogenesis of atherosclerosis [1,2]. Although adhesion molecules like von Willebrand factor and selectins initiate the first contact of the platelet to the vessel wall, the generation and release of agonists stored in platelet granules is – together with the activation of the coagulation cascade - the main mechanism of further platelet recruitment and occlusion of the blood vessel. Among all the platelet agonists present at the site of the vessel lesion, adenosine-5'-diphosphate (ADP) plays a pivotal role. Various pharmacological possibilities to prevent platelet aggregation are currently available, however, two approaches have been established in the last decade for long-term therapeutical platelet inhibition. While actetylsalicylic acid (ASA) irreversibly inhibits platelet cyclooxygenase (COX)-1 and thereby prevents platelet granula secretion and platelet activation by various agonists, thienopyridines selectively inhibit the ADP-induced platelet activation via direct interaction with platelet ADP receptor signaling. Both treatments are very effective in anti-platelet regimens, however, the temporary combination of both strategies has proven even more effective in cardiovascular patients at high risk.

PLATELET ADP-RECEPTORS

As described above, ADP plays a crucial role in hemostasis and is probably the most important in vivo mediator of platelet activation and thrombosis. As depicted in figure 1, ADP acts mainly through two G-protein-coupled P2 receptors, $P2Y_1$ and $P2Y_{12}$ [3]. The $G_{\alpha q}$-coupled $P2Y_1$ receptor initiates ADP-induced aggregation via phospholipase C (PLCβ) and mobilization of calcium. The $G_{\alpha i}$-coupled $P2Y_{12}$ receptor is involved in amplification of the aggregation response mainly via activation of IP_3-kinase and calcium regulation [4]. $P2Y_{12}$ receptor signalling completes activation of the GPIIb/IIIa receptor (fibrinogen receptor, integrin $\alpha_{IIb}b_3$) and stabilizes the platelet thrombus. In addition to these signalling pathways, $P2Y_{12}$ receptor activation inhibits cyclic adenosine monophosphate (cAMP) production by inhibition of adenylyl cyclase (AC). AC can be stimulated by platelet inhibitory prostaglandins, and this effect is used in some laboratory testing (Platelet-Reactivity-Index (PRI)-test) as described below in detail [5]. Due to its key role in thrombus formation, the $P2Y_{12}$ receptor has become an established antithrombotic target in cardiovascular diseases.

$P2Y_{12}$ receptor signaling has further been shown to be involved in the formation of platelet microaggregates in diabetic patients [6].

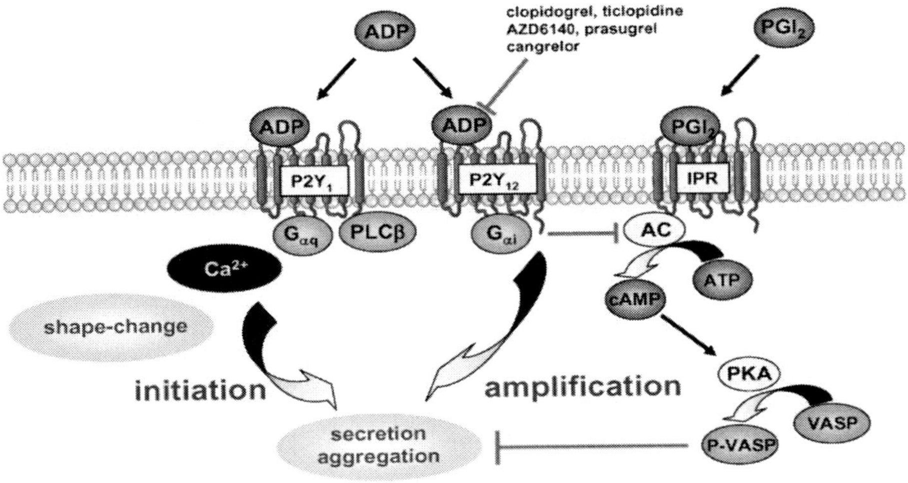

Figure 1. Adenosine-5'-diphosphate (ADP) activates platelets through two G protein-coupled P2 receptors, $P2Y_1$ and $P2Y_{12}$. The $G_{\alpha q}$-coupled $P2Y_1$ receptor initiates ADP-induced aggregation via phospholipase C (PLCβ) and mobilization of calcium (Ca^{2+}), while the $G_{\alpha i}$-coupled $P2Y_{12}$ receptor mediates amplification and completion of the aggregation response. In addition, $P2Y_{12}$ is linked to the inhibition of cyclic adenosine monophosphate (cAMP) production by adenylyl cyclase (AC), which can be stimulated by prostaglandins (e.g. PGE_1 or PGI_2). cAMP-dependent protein kinase (PKA) phosphorylates the vasodilator-stimulated phosphoprotein (VASP) and inhibits platelet aggregation and secretion. The extent of ADP-induced attenuation of prostaglandin-mediated VASP phosphorylation is used in the platelet reactivity index to determine $P2Y_{12}$-specific ADP-activity. Thienopyridines and new ADP-antagonists inhibit multiple pro-aggregatory actions of ADP, mostly by preventing the $P2Y_{12}$-mediated secondary ADP-response contributing to amplification of platelet activation.

ADP Receptor Antagonism

Thienopyridines (ticlopidine, clopidogrel) inhibit multiple pro-aggregatory actions of the platelet agonist ADP by selectively and irreversibly blocking the $P2Y_{12}$ platelet ADP receptor and preventing the secondary ADP-triggered amplification of platelet activation (Figure 1). Compared to ticlopidine, clopidogrel has an increased pharmacological activity and less side effects. Clopidogrel requires hepatic metabolization by an cytochrome P450 isoenzyme, however, approximately 85% of the inactive prodrug clopidogrel are already hydrolyzed by circulating blood esterases to an inactive metabolite before the remaining 15% undergo hepatic metabolization to generate the active metabolite [7]. This active metabolite forms disulfide bridges with the extracellular part of the $P2Y_{12}$ receptor and inactivates the receptor in this way. Large clinical trials demonstrated the superiority of clopidogrel to aspirin for preventing ischemic events in selected patients with atherosclerotic disease [8,9]. Current guidelines from the American College of Cardiology (ACC)/ American Heart Association (AHA)/ Society for Cardiovascular Angiography and Interventions (SCAI) as well as from the European Society of Cardiology (ESC) recommend (class IB) that clopidogrel 75 mg daily should be given for at least 4 weeks after stent implantation [10,11]. Both guidelines recommend a 300 mg loading dose of clopidogrel at least 6 hours prior to PCI [10,11]. The ESC guidelines further recommend to initiate the loading dose even a day before the procedure if possible [10]. The daily dose of 75 mg clopidogrel had been chosen based on initial data in healthy volunteers demonstrating approximately 50% inhibition of platelet aggregation by this dosing regimen [12]. However, some patients experience thromboembolic events despite daily dual anti-platelet therapy, and so-called aspirin and clopidogrel "non-responsiveness" has been observed [13-17].

LABORATORY ASSESSMENT OF $P2Y_{12}$ INHIBITION

The method most commonly used to assess treatment efficacy of clopidogrel is conventional ADP-induced light transmission platelet aggregation, which measures the change in light absorbance through platelet-rich plasma in response to the agonist ADP. However, this 'gold standard' procedure needs rapid in vitro preparation, is labour-intensive, not well standardized and not specific for $P2Y_{12}$ receptors [18,19]. The method itself has a high interindividual variability and only adequately assesses the platelet inhibitory effect of the therapy when pre- and post treatment samples are obtained [20].

Another routine laboratory method is electrical impedance aggregometry which can be performed in diluted whole blood in the presence of ADP. While the use of whole blood makes this assay technically less challenging, the responses are still variable and this technique has only rarely been used to investigate clopidogrel responsiveness [21]. Multiplate electrode whole blood aggregometry is a novel method for assessment of platelet inhibition by various inhibitors. Using ADP stimulation in the absence and presence of prostaglandin E1, this technique gives rapid results from a whole blood assay, however, its specificity for $P2Y_{12}$ inhibition is not optimal compared to more specific assays [22].

Point-of-care assays such as the platelet function analyzer PFA-100 are widely used to test platelet activation under high shear stress conditions using test cartridges containing a membrane coated with type I collagen and ADP [23]. It represents an easy to use system, is automated, rapidly produces results, and only requires a small sample volume. Technically, anticoagulated blood is aspirated through a capillary and an aperture, which are used to mimick shear conditions of small arteries and the injured part of a vessel, respectively. The time from the beginning of the test until formation of an occlusive platelet plug over the aperture is measured in seconds as closure time, which is considered an *in vitro* bleeding time. While it is sensitive to detect von Willebrand disease and severe platelet function disorders such as Glanzmann thrombasthenia and Bernard-Soulier syndrome, its sensitivity to drug-induced defects of platelet function is low [24]. The PFA-100 device has failed to reliably detect thienopyridine-induced inhibition of ADP-mediated platelet activation and does not correlate with platelet aggregation [25,26] or $P2Y_{12}$ specific assays [27]. Therfore, it is commonly accepted that the PFA-100 is not an adequate method for monitoring thienopyridines effectiveness [28].

A more recent development to monitor responses to clopidogrel treatment is the Ultegra Rapid Platelet function Assay (RPFA)-Verify Now P2Y12. It is a modification of a point-of-care bedside test, which was initially developed to assess the anti-platelet effects of glycoprotein IIb/IIIa antagonists and is based on the measurement of agglutination of fibrinogen-coated beads by stimulated platelets in citrated whole blood. The VerifyNow-P2Y12 is a rapid assay that tests platelet activity over three minutes and by using a combination of ADP and prostaglandin E_1 to measure the effects of clopidogrel on the $P2Y_{12}$ receptor [29].

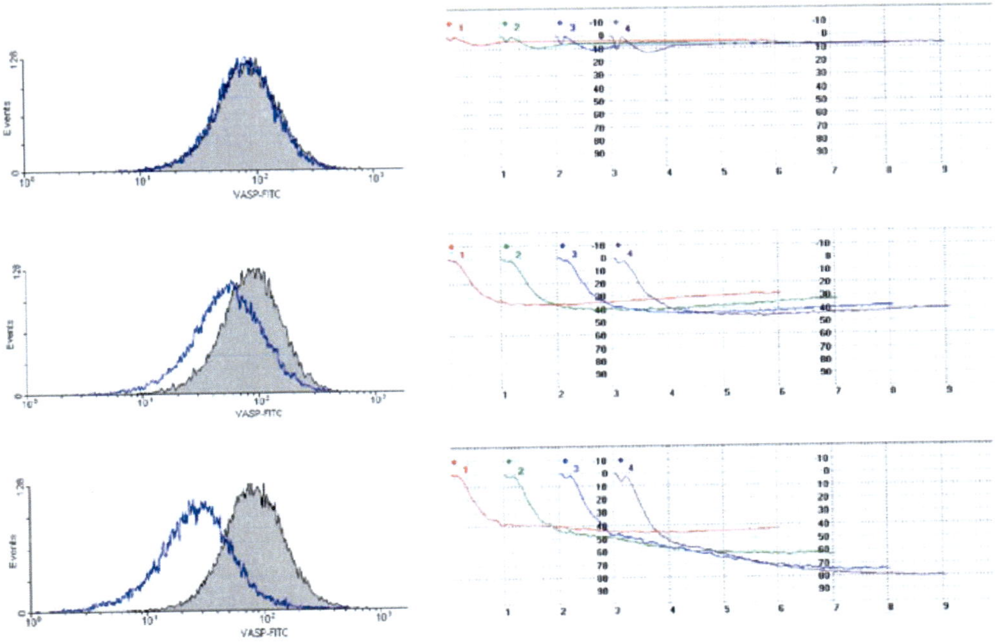

Figure 2. Typical flow-cytometry histograms for determination of the platelet reactivity index (PRI, left) and ADP-induced platelet aggregation (right) depicting a good response (top), a borderline response (middle), and a non-response to clopidogrel (bottom). The PRI is calculated after measurement of Phospho-VASP levels following stimulation with PGE_1 (0.5 µmol/L, filled grey) by mean fluorescence intensity (MFI PGE_1) as well as stimulation with PGE_1 in the presence of ADP (20 µmol/L, MFI PGE_1 + ADP, blue curve). The P2Y12 platelet reactivity index is defined as: ([MFI PGE_1] - [MFI PGE_1 + ADP]) / [MFI PGE_1] * 100% following subtraction of the background value. The lower the detected $P2Y_{12}$ PRI, the better is the clopidogrel inhibition of $P2Y_{12}$ activity. Platelet aggregation is registered over 6 minutes following stimulation with ADP (5 µM = curve 1, red; 10 µM = curve 2, green; 15 µM = curve 3, blue; 20 µM = curve 4, black).

The probably most specific assay to determine clopidogrel non-response is the measurement of cAMP-dependent phosphorylation of the vasodilator-stimulated phosphoprotein (VASP) [30]. As described above, $P2Y_{12}$ receptor activation also inhibits cAMP production by inhibition of AC. AC is an essential enzyme in platelet inhibition by endogenous vasodilators from the group of prostaglandins. By costimulation of platelets in vitro with ADP and prostaglandins, this inhibitory clopidogrel effect on AC activation by prostaglandin can effectively be used to determine and quantitate the activation of $P2Y_{12}$ via ADP [5]. This test system is based on flow cytometry and assesses the difference in PGE_1-induced, cAMP-mediated phosphorylation of VASP in the absence and presence of ADP [31]. The remaining platelet reactivity is calculated and expressed as $P2Y_{12}$ platelet reactivity index (PRI) and is currently the only standardized $P2Y_{12}$-specific assay broadly available. Typical analysis of a good, a borderline and a non-responder are depicted in figure 2. If the $P2Y_{12}$ receptor is completely inhibited, the PRI is 0% because of the inability of ADP to inhibit adenylyl cyclase via $P2Y_{12}$, and a PRI of 100% indicates complete ineffectiveness of clopidogrel [32]. Since pre-treatment variability of this assay is very low, PRI is currently the only test selectively assessing $P2Y_{12}$-mediated signalling without requiring a pre-treatment blood sample to be diagnostic [18,33].

Monitoring of Platelet Function in Cardiovascular Patients

Currently used clopidogrel dosage was chosen based on a 50% inhibition of platelet activation under therapy. However, platelet aggregability – as detected with standard in vitro laboratory aggregation assays – reveals a high intra- and inter-individual variability even in the absence of any anti-platelet therapy. Since pre-treatment maximum platelet aggregation can be significantly lower than 100%, a definition of 50% maximum aggregation to describe sufficient platelet inhibition could substantially overestimate the actual degree of platelet inhibition and thereby underestimate the incidence of an impaired clopidogrel response. $P2Y_{12}$ blockade inhibits a common signaling pathway responsible for amplification of platelet aggregation and thrombus growth. Therefore, for assessment of functional responses following clopidogrel treatment it is mandatory to investigate selectively $P2Y_{12}$-mediated platelet activation, which can not be achieved by measuring platelet aggregation that comprises both $P2Y_1$ and $P2Y_{12}$-mediated effects. Currently, the evaluation of PRI is the only commercially available assay, which assesses specific the $P2Y_{12}$ ADP-activity, the drug target of thienopyridines. Furthermore, this assay is not affected by variable ADP-mediated signalling through the $P2Y_1$ receptor and correlates with clinical events such as subacute stent thrombosis [32,33]. Therefore, it might be proposed as a new reference standard for the assessment of functional $P2Y_{12}$ receptor inhibition and response to thienopyridines in the future [34].

Impaired Responsiveness

The currently recommended daily dose of 75 mg clopidogrel is based on a phase II trial in healthy volunteers. In this study, daily doses of 100 mg or 150 mg clopidogrel resulted in marked prolongation of bleeding time compared to 75 mg, while there was no relevant additional inhibition of platelet aggregation [12]. The term clopidogrel "non-response", or initially "resistance", was introduced after clopidogrel 75 mg/day had been initiated as a standard therapy following PCI. Initially, variability of clopidogrel response was reported, when strong platelet reactivity to ADP following a 300 mg loading dose and a 75 mg maintenance dose of clopidogrel had been found [35]. Several larger observational trials could later confirm this phenomenon: there was marked interindividual variability in clopidogrel response measured by platelet aggregation, activation of glycoprotein IIb/IIIa determined by PAC-1 antibody, and the expression of P-selectin in response to ADP. Furthermore, the patients with the highest pre-treatment response to ADP remained the most reactive after one day [15]. Similarly, variability in response to clopidogrel has been found in patients with intermittent claudication: while a small proportion of these patients responded excessively to clopidogrel, another small group showed no response at all [36]. This phenomenon has now been widely described and its hypothetical implications have been discussed [18-20,37,38].

The high variability ranging from nearly complete inhibition of ADP-induced platelet activation to almost complete failure of detectable platelet inhibition raised the question, whether patients with less pronounced inhibition would be at risk for thrombotic complications, e.g. subacute stent thrombosis following percutaneous coronary intervention (PCI). Over time, several studies demonstrated that maximum aggregation of >50% as well as a PRI >50% were associated with increased stent thrombosis and major adverse cardiovascular events [33,39-41]. A first, retrospective analysis using $P2Y_{12}$-specific PRI among 1,684 consecutive patients undergoing PCI compared patients who had suffered a subacute stent thrombosis with stented patients free of subacute stent thrombosis. Patients with stent thrombosis had a significantly higher PRI (63%) compared to patients without stent thrombosis (39%) [33]. Another study with 100 patients who suffered subacute stent thrombosis verified that high post-treatment platelet reactivity and incomplete $P2Y_{12}$ receptor inhibition are indeed risk factors for the development of subacute stent thrombosis [42]. Afterwards, ischemic event occurrence was prospectively examined over six months and high platelet reactivity was discovered as a novel risk factor for ischemic events after PCI [41].

Depending on the criteria used to define "non-responsiveness", up to 30% of patients undergoing coronary stenting are clopidogrel "non-responders" [14-16,32,41] that might therefore have an increased risk for recurrent or subacute stent thrombosis [39,42,43]. Clopidogrel "non-responsiveness" is also associated with increased risk of adverse cardiovascular events in patients with acute myocardial infarction [16,44]. A residual platelet reactivity of >50% was associated with an increased risk for stent thrombosis and adverse events [33,40,41].

The pathophysiologic origin of clopidogrel non-response is still not fully elucidated and several mechanisms have been discussed (reviewed by Siller-Matula et al. [30]): Non-compliance and underdosing occur probably more often than expected, especially if the patient ignores the loading dose that is essential for rapid onset of the platelet inhibitory effect. However, variable absorption of clopidogrel as well as variable metabolism and clearance of the active metabolite might be involved in inadequate clinical effects. Furthermore, $P2Y_{12}$ receptor polymorphisms as well as variations of the hepatic cytochrome

P450 enzyme have been discussed in the context of reduced clopidogrel effects [45,46], however, this alone does not explain the high incidence of clopidogrel non-responders.

Complications in Non-responders

The standard loading dose of clopidogrel (300 mg) is preferably given 12-24 hours before PCI to achieve platelet inhibition [38]. Interindividual variability in the platelet inhibitory response from clopidogrel determined by platelet aggregation, activation of glycoprotein IIb/IIIa and platelet degranulation occurs in patients undergoing elective coronary stenting [15]. Several authors have therefore suggested a higher loading dose of clopidogrel (600 mg) to achieve sufficient platelet activation more rapidly, which is reached at 2-4 hours [47,48]. However, patients with high pre-treatment reactivity at more than 2 hours after receiving the higher loading dose had an increased risk for development of major adverse cardiac events within 30 days after elective PCI [49]. Considering that patients with the highest pre-treatment platelet reactivity remained the most reactive over the first 24 hours [15], the CREST-study investigated whether patients, who suffered a subacute stent thrombosis, had higher post-treatment reactivity than those who do not encounter stent thrombosis. In this study, patients with subacute stent thrombosis showed higher platelet reactivity determined by ADP-induced platelet aggregation, PRI, and glycoprotein IIb/IIIa activation [42]. Retrospectively, several studies have shown that patients with stent thrombosis display impaired response to antiplatelet therapy and, therefore, incomplete $P2Y_{12}$-receptor inhibition might confer a risk factors for stent thrombosis [33,39,50]. Different study groups have recently reported that the level of platelet aggregation before coronary stenting in patients pre-treated with clopidogrel is correlated with short-, mid-, and long-term outcome after the procedure [41,49,51]. In patients with acute ST segment elevation myocardial infarction, who showed inadequate response to clopidogrel as determined by baseline and repetitive ADP-induced aggregation after 6 days, 40% sustained a recurrent cardiovascular event during a 6-month follow-up [16]. The high rate of impaired clopidogrel responsiveness in combination with the huge number of electively performed PCIs is a reason for distinct concern: performing PCI in patients with impaired clopidogrel responsiveness yields an increased risk of stent thrombosis resulting in complete occlusion, which might clinically appear as acute myocardial infarction with all its risks for arrhythmias, chronic heart failure, and sudden cardiac death. Paradoxically, while preventive PCI does not reduce the risk of myocardial infarction by itself [52,53], performing the procedure in a clopidogrel non-responder might actually increase the risk of myocardial infarction in a patient with otherwise stable coronary artery disease.

Treatment Modification in Non-responders

The high variability in clopidogrel responsiveness appears to be predominantly related to inefficient metabolisation of the prodrug clopidogrel to its active metabolite [17]. *In vitro* addition of the specific, directly active $P2Y_{12}$ antagonist AR-C69931MX has previously been shown to overcome the observed clopidogrel non-responsiveness resulting in transient aggregation only, which is highly suggestive for complete $P2Y_{12}$ inhibition. Furthermore, a PRI of <5% was achieved in blood from patients who had an initial PRI of ~60% under chronic treatment with clopidogrel [34].

The significant inter-individual variability in pharmacological response to clopidogrel suggests a potential benefit by increasing the maintenance dose of clopidogrel, which however is a strategy currently not yet recommended by guidelines [18,20]. Increasing the maintenance dose of clopidogrel has been shown to improve $P2Y_{12}$ inhibition demonstrated by enhanced reduction of PRI [54]. The occurrence of major adverse cardiac events following PCI is increased in patients with a PRI >50% [33,55], while a PRI <50% has a negative predictive value of 100% [55]. In non-ST segment elevation myocardial infarction patients undergoing coronary stenting, a 600-mg loading dose of clopidogrel showed a benefit on platelet reactivity and clinical prognosis [44]. Furthermore, trials using higher loading or maintenance doses suggest that a suboptimal bioavailability of the active metabolite might contribute to clopidogrel non-responsiveness [14,44,48,54]. However, this approach might bear some risk for additional bleeding, since daily doses of more than 75 mg clopidogrel resulted in prolonged bleeding time during the initial dose-finding studies [12]. Recently, the use of ticlopidine as an alternative therapy in the case of clopidogrel non-response has been suggested [56]. However, this approach is based on three cases observed and requires further investigation in clinical trials if more potent novel antiplatelet agents might no become available.

FUTURE PERSPECTIVES / NOVEL ANTIPLATELET SUBSTANCES

Further need for sufficient $P2Y_{12}$ inhibition has arisen, when late stent thrombosis following implantation of drug-eluting stents (DES) had been reported after premature antiplatelet therapy discontinuation [57] as well as under stable antiplatelet monotherapy (e.g. acetylsalicylic acid) [58]. Recent data demonstrate a high rate of thrombus-occluded DES at autopsies [59]. These reports as well as case reports about asymptomatic complete occlusions [50] or stent thrombosis in DES up to 41 months after implantation [60] suggest that it might be feasible for the future to demand routine measurements of platelet function before implantation of DES [18] to provide optimal $P2Y_{12}$ inhibition. Recent analyses have shown that the risk of DES thrombosis is increased both in diabetics as well as in patients with ACS [61]. In parallel, a very high incidence of clopidogrel "non-responsiveness" (62.5%) was reported in type II-diabetic patients with coronary artery disease [54].

Since metabolic differences might contribute to the variability in response to clopidogrel [62,63], novel substances which are metabolized more consistently and achieve more reliable platelet inhibition are needed. One such novel orally active thienopyridine prodrug with potent and long-lasting antiplatelet effects is prasugrel. Previous studies have shown that the antiplatelet potency of prasugrel is at least 10 times higher than that of clopidogrel and first promising results have been shown in patients undergoing elective PCI [64,65]. *In vivo* treatment with the newer $P2Y_{12}$ receptor antagonist prasugrel reduced platelet aggregation more rapidly and effectively than clopidogrel [62]. In healthy subjects, prasugrel (60 mg loading dose) inhibited platelet aggregation more effectively and more rapidly than clopidogrel (300 mg loading dose). Its effects start already 15 minutes after oral application. Furthermore, the response to prasugrel was more consistent compared to clopidogrel and the lower inhibition of platelet aggregation by clopidogrel was associated with lower plasma concentrations of its active metabolite [62]. In stable aspirin-treated patients with coronary artery disease no non-responders (defined as inhibition of platelet aggregation by less than 20%) to prasugrel were detetcted, while the rate for clopidogrel-treated patients was 45%. Furthermore, prasugrel given with a 40-60 mg loading dose and maintained at 10-15 mg daily achieved greater inhibition of platelet aggregation in this population [64]. Recently, the TRITON-TIMI 38-study compared prasugrel to clopidogrel in moderate to high risk patients with acute coronary syndrome and PCI. Treatment with prasugrel significantly reduced ischaemic events including stent thrombosis, however, it was also associated with significantly increased bleeding risk including fatal bleedings and major bleeding during coronary artery bypass grafting [66].

Cangrelor is an intravenously administered, reversible agent, which has a rapid onset of activity and inhibits $P2Y_{12}$ reversibly. It inhibits platelet aggregation with rapid onset and offset and does not require metabolism for therapeutic activity [38,67]. Given as an adjunct to reduced thrombolytic therapy it has a similar safety profile than full-dose thrombolysis in patients with acute myocardial infarction and achieves similar coronary patency [68].

A new class of $P2Y_{12}$ receptor antagonist are the cyclopentyltriazolopyrimidines. The reversible $P2Y_{12}$ receptor antagonist AZD6140 is the first of these new compounds of antiplatelet agents. It is given orally and does not require metabolic activation [67]. Similar to thienopyridines, AZD6140 blocks the platelet $P2Y_{12}$ receptor to inhibit the prothrombotic effects of ADP. Unlike thienopyridines, which are irreversible antagonists, AZD6140 binds reversibly to the $P2Y_{12}$ receptor at a distinct, noncompetitive site [69]. For AZD6140, maximum inhibition of platelet aggregation is observed already after 2-4 hours, whereas clopidogrel only minimally inhibits platelet aggregation at this time. AZD6140 produces approximately 90-95% inhibition of platelet aggregation 4 hours after dosing during chronic treatment, while clopidogrel reaches only approximately 60% inhibition [69]. AZD6140 showed no difference in major bleeding in an initial investigation in patients with non ST elevation ACS [70]. It has been shown to reduce platelet aggregation more rapidly and effectively in patients with ACS compared with clopidogrel exhibiting greater inhibition of platelet aggregation than a standard regimen of clopidogrel and further suppressing platelet aggregation in clopidogrel pretreated patients [71]. The efficacy and safety of AZD6140 is currently assessed in the phase 3 trial PLATO in patients with acute coronary syndromes.

Conclusion

Thienopyridines, especially clopidogrel, have a highly significant effect in clinical trials with regard to reduction of stent thrombosis and functional inhibition of ADP-induced platelet activation in cardiovascular patients. Nevertheless, there is a high incidence of impaired clopidogrel responsiveness in patients associated with adverse cardiovascular events following PCI. Individual testing and adjusted anti-platelet therapy might be recommendable under certain circumstances, e.g. high-risk interventions such as last patent vessel, dominant vessel, or planned DES implantation. Further prospective studies are needed to determine the risk reduction by individually adjusted anti-platelet therapy. Newly developed $P2Y_{12}$ antagonists in combination with inhibitors of other platelet receptors that are currently under development or in clinical trials will provide safe and efficient anti-platelet therapy in cardiovascular medicine in the near future.

REFERENCES

[1] Huo Y, Schober A, Forlow SB, Smith DF, Hyman MC, Jung S, Littman DR, Weber C, Ley K. Circulating activated platelets exacerbate atherosclerosis in mice deficient in apolipoprotein *E. Nat Med* 2003; 9(1):61-67.

[2] Massberg S, Brand K, Gruner S, Page S, Muller E, Muller I, Bergmeier W, Richter T, Lorenz M, Konrad I, Nieswandt B, Gawaz M. A critical role of platelet adhesion in the initiation of atherosclerotic lesion formation. *J Exp Med* 2002; 196(7):887-896.

[3] Gachet C, Hechler B. The platelet P2 receptors in thrombosis. *Semin Thromb Hemost* 2005; 31(2):162-167.

[4] Gachet C. Regulation of platelet functions by P2 receptors. *Annu Rev Pharmacol Toxicol* 2006; 46:277-300.

[5] Geiger J, Brich J, Honig-Liedl P, Eigenthaler M, Schanzenbacher P, Herbert JM, Walter U. Specific impairment of human platelet P2Y(AC) ADP receptor-mediated signaling by the antiplatelet drug clopidogrel. *Arterioscler Thromb Vasc Biol* 1999; 19(8):2007-2011.

[6] Matsuno H, Tokuda H, Ishisaki A, Zhou Y, Kitajima Y, Kozawa O. P2Y12 receptors play a significant role in the development of platelet microaggregation in patients with diabetes. *J Clin Endocrinol Metab* 2005; 90(2):920-927.

[7] Savi P, Pereillo JM, Uzabiaga MF, Combalbert J, Picard C, Maffrand JP, Pascal M, Herbert JM. Identification and biological activity of the active metabolite of clopidogrel. *Thromb Haemost* 2000; 84(5):891-896.

[8] The Clopidogrel in Unstable Angina to Prevent Recurrent Events Trial Investigators. Effects of clopidogrel in addition to aspirin in patients with acute coronary syndromes without ST-segment elevation. *N Engl J Med* 2001; 345(7):494-502.

[9] A randomised, blinded, trial of clopidogrel versus aspirin in patients at risk of ischaemic events (CAPRIE). CAPRIE Steering Committee. *Lancet* 1996; 348(9038):1329-1339.

[10] Silber S, Albertsson P, Aviles FF, Camici PG, Colombo A, Hamm C, Jorgensen E, Marco J, Nordrehaug JE, Ruzyllo W, Urban P, Stone GW, Wijns W. Guidelines for percutaneous coronary interventions. The Task Force for Percutaneous Coronary Interventions of the European Society of Cardiology. *Eur Heart J* 2005; 26(8):804-847.

[11] Smith SC, Jr., Feldman TE, Hirshfeld JW, Jr., Jacobs AK, Kern MJ, King SB, III, Morrison DA, O'Neill WW, Schaff HV, Whitlow PL, Williams DO, Antman EM, Smith SC, Jr., Adams CD, Anderson JL, Faxon DP, Fuster V, Halperin JL, Hiratzka LF, Hunt SA, Jacobs AK, Nishimura R, Ornato JP, Page RL, Riegel B. ACC/AHA/SCAI 2005 guideline update for percutaneous coronary intervention--summary article: a report of the American College of Cardiology/American Heart Association Task Force on Practice

Guidelines (ACC/AHA/SCAI Writing Committee to Update the 2001 Guidelines for Percutaneous Coronary Intervention). *Circulation* 2006; 113(1):156-175.

[12]Thebault JJ, Kieffer G, Lowe GD, Nimmo WS, Cariou R. Repeated-dose pharmacodynamics of clopidogrel in healthy subjects. *Semin Thromb Hemost* 1999; 25 Suppl 2:9-14.

[13]Wiviott SD, Antman EM. Clopidogrel resistance: a new chapter in a fast-moving story. *Circulation* 2004; 109(25):3064-3067.

[14]Muller I, Besta F, Schulz C, Massberg S, Schonig A, Gawaz M. Prevalence of clopidogrel non-responders among patients with stable angina pectoris scheduled for elective coronary stent placement. *Thromb Haemost* 2003; 89(5):783-787.

[15]Gurbel PA, Bliden KP, Hiatt BL, O'Connor CM. Clopidogrel for coronary stenting: response variability, drug resistance, and the effect of pretreatment platelet reactivity. *Circulation* 2003; 107(23):2908-2913.

[16]Matetzky S, Shenkman B, Guetta V, Shechter M, Bienart R, Goldenberg I, Novikov I, Pres H, Savion N, Varon D, Hod H. Clopidogrel resistance is associated with increased risk of recurrent atherothrombotic events in patients with acute myocardial infarction. *Circulation* 2004; 109(25):3171-3175.

[17]Cattaneo M. Aspirin and clopidogrel: efficacy, safety, and the issue of drug resistance. *Arterioscler Thromb Vasc Biol* 2004; 24(11):1980-1987.

[18]Gurbel PA, Tantry US. Aspirin and clopidogrel resistance: consideration and management. *J Interv Cardiol* 2006; 19:439-448.

[19]Angiolillo DJ, Fernandez-Ortiz A, Bernardo E, Alfonso F, Macaya C, Bass TA, Costa MA. Variability in individual responsiveness to clopidogrel: clinical implications, management, and future perspectives. *J Am Coll Cardiol* 2007; 49:1505-1516.

[20]O'Donoghue M, Wiviott SD. Clopidogrel response variability and future therapies: clopidogrel: does one size fit all? *Circulation* 2006; 114(22):e600-e606.

[21]Ivandic BT, Schlick P, Staritz P, Kurz K, Katus HA, Giannitsis E. Determination of clopidogrel resistance by whole blood platelet aggregometry and inhibitors of the P2Y12 receptor. *Clin Chem* 2006; 52(3):383-388.

[22]Mueller T, Dieplinger B, Poelz W, Calatzis A, Haltmayer M. Utility of whole blood impedance aggregometry for the assessment of clopidogrel action using the novel Multiplate(R) analyzer-comparison with two flow cytometric methods. *Thromb Res* 2007.

[23]Kundu SK, Heilmann EJ, Sio R, Garcia C, Davidson RM, Ostgaard RA. Description of an in vitro platelet function analyzer--PFA-100. *Semin Thromb Hemost* 1995; 21 Suppl 2:106-112.

[24]Hayward CP, Harrison P, Cattaneo M, Ortel TL, Rao AK. Platelet function analyzer (PFA)-100 closure time in the evaluation of platelet disorders and platelet function. *J Thromb Haemost* 2006; 4(2):312-319.

[25]Agarwal S, Coakley M, Reddy K, Riddell A, Mallett S. Quantifying the effect of antiplatelet therapy: a comparison of the platelet function analyzer (PFA-100) and modified thromboelastography (mTEG) with light transmission platelet aggregometry. *Anesthesiology* 2006; 105:676-683.

[26]Mani H, Linnemann B, Luxembourg B, Kirchmayr K, Lindhoff-Last E. Response to aspirin and clopidogrel monitored with different platelet function methods. *Platelets* 2006; 17:303-310.

[27]Geiger J, Teichmann L, Grossmann R, Aktas B, Steigerwald U, Walter U, Schinzel R. Monitoring of clopidogrel action: comparison of methods. *Clin Chem* 2005; 51(6): 957-965.

[28]Cattaneo M. Resistance to antiplatelet drugs: molecular mechanisms and laboratory detection. *J Thromb Haemost* 2007; 5 suppl1:230-237.

[29]Malinin A, Pokov A, Swaim L, Kotob M, Serebruany V. Validation of a VerifyNow-P2Y12 cartridge for monitoring platelet inhibition with clopidogrel. *Methods Find Exp Clin Pharmacol* 2006; 28(5):315-322.

[30]Siller-Matula J, Schrör K, Wojta J, Huber K. Thienopyridines in cardiovascular disease: focus on clopidogrel resistance. *Thromb Haemost* 2007; 97:385-393.

[31]Schwarz UR, Geiger J, Walter U, Eigenthaler M. Flow cytometry analysis of intracellular VASP phosphorylation for the assessment of activating and inhibitory signal transduction pathways in human platelets. *Thromb Haemost* 1999; 82:1145-1152.

[32]Grossmann R, Sokolova O, Schnurr A, Bonz A, Porsche C, Obergfell A, Lengenfelder B, Walter U, Eigenthaler M. Variable extent of clopidogrel responsiveness in patients after coronary stenting. *Thromb Haemost* 2004; 92:1201-1206.

[33]Barragan P, Bouvier J-L, Roquebert P-O, Macaluso G, Commeau P, Comet B, Lafont A, Camoin L, Walter U, Eigenthaler M. Resistance to thienopyridines: clinical detection of coronary stent thrombosis by monitoring of vasodilator-stimulated phosphoprotein phoshorylation. *Catheter Cardiovasc Interv* 2003; 59:295-302.

[34]Aleil B, Ravanat C, Cazenave JP, Rochoux G, Heitz A, Gachet C. Flow cytometric analysis of intraplatelet VASP phosphorylation for the detection of clopidogrel resistance in patients with ischemic cardiovascular diseases. *J Thromb Haemost* 2005; 3(1):85-92.

[35]Jaremo P, Lindahl TL, Fransson SG, Richter A. Individual variations of platelet inhibition after loading doses of clopidogrel. *J Intern Med* 2002; 252(3):233-238.

[36]Cassar K, Bachoo P, Ford I, Greaves M, Brittenden J. Variability in responsiveness to clopidogrel in patients with intermittent claudication. *Eur J Vasc Endovasc Surg* 2006; 32(1):71-75.

[37]Bhatt DL, Topol EJ. Scientific and therapeutic advances in antiplatelet therapy. *Nature Reviews Drug Discovery* 2003; 2:15-28.

[38]Steinhubl S, Roe MT. Optimizing platelet P2Y12 inhibition for patients undergoing PCI. *Cardiovasc Drug Rev* 2007; 25(2):188-203.

[39]Wenaweser P, Dorffler-Melly J, Imboden K, Windecker S, Togni M, Meier B, Haeberli A, Hess OM. Stent thrombosis is associated with an impaired response to antiplatelet therapy. *J Am Coll Cardiol* 2005; 45(11):1748-1752.

[40]Bliden KP, DiChiara J, Tantry US, Bassi AK, Chaganti SK, Gurbel PA. Increased risk in patients with high platelet aggregation receiving chronic clopidogrel therapy undergoing percutaneous coronary intervention: is the current antiplatelet therapy adequate? *J Am Coll Cardiol* 2007; 49:657-666.

[41]Gurbel PA, Bliden KP, Guyer K, Cho PW, Zaman KA, Kreutz RP, Bassi AK, Tantry US. Platelet reactivity in patients and recurrent events post-stenting: results of the PREPARE POST-STENTING study. *J Am Coll Cardiol* 2005; 46(10):1820-1826.

[42]Gurbel PA, Bliden KP, Samara W, Yoho JA, Hayes K, Fissha MZ, Tantry US. Clopidogrel effect on platelet reactivity in patients with stent thrombosis: results of the CREST Study. *J Am Coll Cardiol* 2005; 46(10):1827-1832.

[43]Glowczynska R, Malek LA, Spiewak M, Filipiak KJ, Grabowski M, Kisiel B, Kochman J, Kostrzewa G, Ploski R, Opolski G. Clinical, biochemical and genetical resistance to clopidogrel in a patient with the recurrent coronary stent thrombosis--a case report and review of the literature. *Int J Cardiol* 2006; 111(2):326-328.

[44]Cuisset T, Frere C, Quilici J, Morange PE, Nait-Saidi L, Carvajal J, Lehmann A, Lambert M, Bonnet JL, Alessi MC. Benefit of a 600-mg loading dose of clopidogrel on platelet reactivity and clinical outcomes in patients with non-ST-segment elevation acute coronary syndrome undergoing coronary stenting. *J Am Coll Cardiol* 2006; 48(7):1339-1345.

[45]Angiolillo DJ, Fernandez-Ortiz A, Bernardo E, Ramirez C, Cavallari U, Trabetti E, Sabate M, Hernandez R, Moreno R, Escaned J, Alfonso F, Banuelos C, Costa MA, Bass TA, Pignatti PF, Macaya C. Contribution of gene sequence variations of the hepatic cytochrome P450 3A4 enzyme to variability in individual responsiveness to clopidogrel. *Arterioscler Thromb Vasc Biol* 2006; 26(8):1895-1900.

[46]Fontana P, Dupont A, Gandrille S, Bachelot-Loza C, Reny JL, Aiach M, Gaussem P. Adenosine diphosphate-induced platelet aggregation is associated with P2Y12 gene sequence variations in healthy subjects. *Circulation* 2003; 108(8):989-995.

[47]Hochholzer W, Trenk D, Frundi D, Blanke P, Fischer B, Andris K, Bestehorn HP, Buttner HJ, Neumann FJ. Time dependence of platelet inhibition after a 600-mg loading dose of clopidogrel in a large, unselected cohort of candidates for percutaneous coronary intervention. *Circulation* 2005; 111(20):2560-2564.

[48]Montalescot G, Sideris G, Meuleman C, Bal-dit-Sollier C, Lellouche N, Steg PG, Slama M, Milleron O, Collet JP, Henry P, Beygui F, Drouet L. A randomized comparison of high clopidogrel loading doses in patients with non-ST-segment elevation acute coronary syndromes: the ALBION (Assessment of the Best Loading Dose of Clopidogrel to Blunt Platelet Activation, Inflammation and Ongoing Necrosis) trial. *J Am Coll Cardiol* 2006; 48(5):931-938.

[49]Hochholzer W, Trenk D, Bestehorn HP, Fischer B, Valina CM, Ferenc M, Gick M, Caputo A, Buttner HJ, Neumann FJ. Impact of the degree of peri-interventional platelet inhibition after loading with clopidogrel on early clinical outcome of elective coronary stent placement. *J Am Coll Cardiol* 2006; 48(9):1742-1750.

[50]Schäfer A, Bonz A, Eigenthaler M, Bauersachs J. Late thrombosis of a drug eluting stent during combined anti-platelet therapy in a clopidogrel non-responsive diabetic patient: shall we routinely test platelet function ? *Thromb Haemost* 2007; 97:862-865.

[51]Campo G, Valgimigli M, Gemmati D, Percoco G, Tognazzo S, Cicchitelli G, Catozzi L, Malagutti P, Anselmi M, Vassanelli C, Scapoli G, Ferrari R. Value of platelet reactivity in predicting response to treatment and clinical outcome in patients undergoing primary

coronary intervention: insights into the STRATEGY Study. *J Am Coll Cardiol* 2006; 48(11):2178-2185.

[52]Boden WE, O'Rourke RA, Teo KK, Hartigan PM, Maron DJ, Kostuk WJ, Knudtson M, Dada M, Casperson P, Harris CL, Chaitman BR, Shaw L, Gosselin G, Nawaz S, Title LM, Gau G, Blaustein AS, Booth DC, Bates ER, Spertus JA, Berman DS, Mancini GBJ, Weintraub WS, the COURAGE Trial Research Group. Optimal Medical Therapy with or without PCI for Stable Coronary Disease. *N Engl J Med* 2007; 356:1503-1516.

[53]Hochman JS, Steg PG. Does Preventive PCI Work? *N Engl J Med* 2007; 356:1572-1574.

[54]Angiolillo DJ, Shoemaker SB, Desai B, Yuan H, Charlton RK, Bernardo E, Zenni MM, Guzman LA, Bass TA, Costa MA. Randomized Comparison of a High Clopidogrel Maintenance Dose in Patients With Diabetes Mellitus and Coronary Artery Disease. Results of the Optimizing Antiplatelet Therapy in Diabetes Mellitus (OPTIMUS) Study. *Circulation* 2007; 115:708-716.

[55]Bonello L, Paganelli F, Arpin-Bornet M, Auquier P, Sampol J, Dignat-George F, Barragan P, Camoin-Jau L. Vasodilator-stimulated phosphoprotein phosphorylation analysis prior to percutaneous coronary intervention for exclusion of postprocedural major adverse cardiovascular events. *J Thromb Haemost* 2007; 5(8):1630-1636.

[56]Aleil B, Rochoux G, Monassier JP, Cazenave JP, Gachet C. Ticlopidine could be an alternative therapy in the case of pharmacological resistance to clopidogrel: a report of three cases. *J Thromb Haemost* 2007; 5(4):879-881.

[57]Iakovou I, Schmidt T, Bonizzoni E, Ge L, Sangiorgi GM, Stankovic G, Airoldi F, Chieffo A, Montorfano M, Carlino M, Michev I, Corvaja N, Briguori C, Gerckens U, Grube E, Colombo A. Incidence, predictors, and outcome of thrombosis after successful implantation of drug-eluting stents. *JAMA* 2005; 293(17):2126-2130.

[58]Ong AT, McFadden EP, Regar E, de Jaegere PP, van Domburg RT, Serruys PW. Late angiographic stent thrombosis (LAST) events with drug-eluting stents. *J Am Coll Cardiol* 2005; 45(12):2088-2092.

[59]Joner M, Finn AV, Farb A, Mont EK, Kolodgie FD, Ladich E, Kutys R, Skorija K, Gold HK, Virmani R. Pathology of drug-eluting stents in humans: delayed healing and late thrombotic risk. *J Am Coll Cardiol* 2006; 48(1):193-202.

[60]Henderson D, Gunalingam B. Very late stent thrombosis of a sirolimus-eluting stent. *Catheter Cardiovasc Interv* 2006; 68:406-408.

[61]Hodgson J, Stone GW, Lincoff AM, Klein L, Walpole H, Bottner R, Weiner BH, Leon MB, Feldman T, Babb J, Dehmer GJ. Late stent thrombosis: considerations and practical advice for the use of drug-eluting stents: a report from the Society for Cardiovascular Angiography and Interventions drug-eluting stent task force. *Cath Cardiovasc Interv* 2007; 69:327-333.

[62]Brandt JT, Payne CD, Wiviott SD, Weerakkody G, Farid NA, Small DS, Jakubowski JA, Naganuma H, Winters KJ. A comparison of prasugrel and clopidogrel loading doses on platelet function: magnitude of platelet inhibition is related to active metabolite formation. *Am Heart J* 2007; 153(1):66-16.

[63]Brandt JT, Close SL, Iturria SJ, Payne CD, Farid NA, Ernest CS, Lachno DR, Salazar D, Winters KJ. Common polymorphisms of CYP2C19 and CYP2C9 affect the

pharmacokinetic and pharmacodynamic response to clopidogrel but not prasugrel. *J Thromb Haemost* 2007.

[64] Jernberg T, Payne CD, Winters KJ, Darstein C, Brandt JT, Jakubowski JA, Naganuma H, Siegbahn A, Wallentin L. Prasugrel achieves greater inhibition of platelet aggregation and a lower rate of non-responders compared with clopidogrel in aspirin-treated patients with stable coronary artery disease. *Eur Heart J* 2006; 27(10):1166-1173.

[65] Wiviott SD, Antman EM, Gibson CM, Montalescot G, Riesmeyer J, Weerakkody G, Winters KJ, Warmke JW, McCabe CH, Braunwald E. Evaluation of prasugrel compared with clopidogrel in patients with acute coronary syndromes: design and rationale for the TRial to assess Improvement in Therapeutic Outcomes by optimizing platelet InhibitioN with prasugrel Thrombolysis In Myocardial Infarction 38 (TRITON-TIMI 38*). Am Heart J* 2006; 152(4):627-635.

[66] Wiviott SD, Braunwald E, McCabe CH, Montalescot G, Ruzyllo W, Gottlieb S, Neumann FJ, Ardissino D, De Servi S, Murphy SA, Riesmeyer J, Weerakkody G, Gibson CM, Antman EM. Prasugrel versus Clopidogrel in Patients with Acute Coronary Syndromes. *N Engl J Med* 2007; 357(20):2001-2015.

[67] Van Giezen JJ, Humphries RG. Preclinical and clinical studies with selective reversible direct P2Y12 antagonists. *Semin Thromb Hemost* 2005; 31(2):195-204.

[68] Greenbaum AB, Ohman EM, Gibson CM, Borzak S, Stebbins AL, Lu M, Le May MR, Stankowski JE, Emanuelsson H, Weaver WD. Preliminary experience with intravenous P2Y12 platelet receptor inhibition as an adjunct to reduced-dose alteplase during acute myocardial infarction: results of the Safety, Tolerability and Effect on Patency in Acute Myocardial Infarction (STEP-AMI) angiographic trial. *Am Heart J* 2007; 154(4): 702-709.

[69] Husted S, Emanuelsson H, Heptinstall S, Sandset PM, Wickens M, Peters G. Pharmacodynamics, pharmacokinetics, and safety of the oral reversible P2Y(12) antagonist AZD6140 with aspirin in patients with atherosclerosis: a double-blind comparison to clopidogrel with aspirin. *Eur Heart J* 2006; 27(9):1038-1047.

[70] Cannon CP, Husted S, Harrington RA, Scirica BM, Emanuelsson H, Peters G, Storey RF. Safety, tolerability, and initial efficacy of AZD6140, the first reversible oral adenosine diphosphate receptor antagonist, compared with clopidogrel, in patients with non-ST-segment elevation acute coronary syndrome: primary results of the DISPERSE-2 trial. *J Am Coll Cardiol* 2007; 50(19):1844-1851.

[71] Storey RF, Husted S, Harrington RA, Heptinstall S, Wilcox RG, Peters G, Wickens M, Emanuelsson H, Gurbel P, Grande P, Cannon CP. Inhibition of platelet aggregation by AZD6140, a reversible oral P2Y12 receptor antagonist, compared with clopidogrel in patients with acute coronary syndromes. *J Am Coll Cardiol* 2007; 50(19):1852-1856.

INDEX

A

B

C

D

E

F

G

H

I

K

L

M

N

O

P

Q

R

S

T

U

V

W

X

Y